Jefferson Heart Institute

HANDBOOK OF CARDIOLOGY

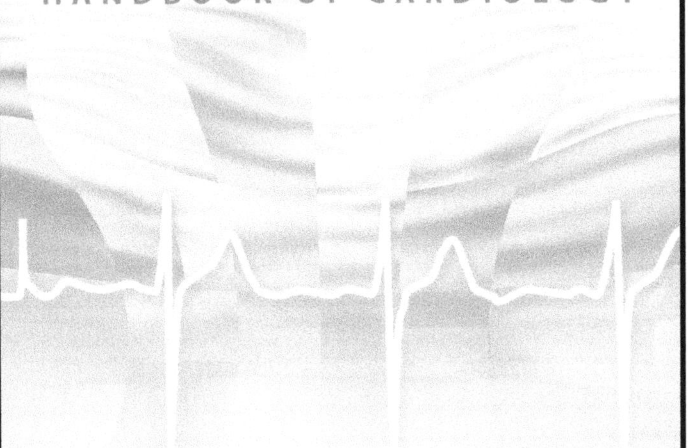

Edited by Paul J. Mather, MD
Professor of Medicine
Director, Advanced Heart Failure and
Cardiac Transplant Center at the Jefferson Heart Institute
Jefferson Medical College of Thomas Jefferson University
Philadelphia, PA

JONES & BARTLETT
LEARNING

World Headquarters
Jones & Bartlett Learning
40 Tall Pine Drive
Sudbury, MA 01776
978-443-5000
info@jblearning.com
www.jblearning.com

Jones & Bartlett Learning
Canada
6339 Ormindale Way
Mississauga, Ontario L5V 1J2
Canada

Jones & Bartlett Learning
International
Barb House, Barb Mews
London W6 7PA
United Kingdom

Jones & Bartlett Learning books and products are available through most bookstores and online booksellers. To contact Jones & Bartlett Learning directly, call 800-832-0034, fax 978-443-8000, or visit our website at www.jblearning.com.

Substantial discounts on bulk quantities of Jones & Bartlett Learning publications are available to corporations, professional associations, and other qualified organizations. For details and specific discount information, contact the special sales department at Jones & Bartlett Learning via the above contact information or send an email to specialsales@jblearning.com.

Production Credits
Executive Publisher: Christopher Davis
Editorial Assistant: Sara Cameron
Production Director: Amy Rose
Senior Production Editor: Daniel Stone
Associate Marketing Manager: Katie Hennessy
Manufacturing and Inventory
Control Supervisor: Amy Bacus
Printer: Malloy, Inc.
Composition: Auburn Associates, Inc.

Cover Credits
Cover Design: Kristin E. Parker
Cover Printing: Malloy, Inc.
Cover Images: © Bram Janssens/Dreamstime.com

Library of Congress Cataloging-in-Publication Data
Jefferson Heart Institute handbook of cardiology / [edited by] Paul J. Mather.
p. ; cm.
Other title: Handbook of cardiology
Includes bibliographical references and index.
ISBN 978-0-7637-6049-6
1. Heart—Diseases—Handbooks, manuals, etc. I. Mather, Paul J. II. Jefferson Heart Institute. III. Title: Handbook of cardiology.
[DNLM: 1. Heart Diseases. 2. Cardiology—methods. 3. Cardiovascular Surgical Procedures—methods. WG 210 J45 2011
RC669.15.J44 2011
616.1′2—dc22

2010018007

6048

Printed in the United States of America
14 13 12 11 10 10 9 8 7 6 5 4 3 2 1

Dedicated to
Pia
Nick and Chris
Grace and Stanley
Maria and Umberto

Table of Contents

Contributors

Editor

Paul J. Mather, MD
Jefferson Heart Institute
Thomas Jefferson University Hospital
Philadelphia, PA

Contributors

Suzanne Adams, RN, MPH
Jefferson Heart Institute
Thomas Jefferson University Hospital
Philadelphia, PA

Barbara Berko, MD
Jefferson Heart Institute
Thomas Jefferson University Hospital
Philadelphia, PA

Indranil Das Gupta, MD, MBA, MPH
Jefferson Heart Institute
Thomas Jefferson University Hospital
Philadelphia, PA

Matthew DeCaro, MD
Jefferson Heart Institute
Thomas Jefferson University Hospital
Philadelphia, PA

Danielle Duffy, MD
Jefferson Heart Institute
Thomas Jefferson University Hospital
Philadelphia, PA

David L. Fischman, MD
Jefferson Heart Institute
Thomas Jefferson University Hospital
Philadelphia, PA

Thomas Force, MD
Jefferson Heart Institute
Thomas Jefferson University Hospital
Philadelphia, PA

Daniel Frisch, MD
Jefferson Heart Institute
Thomas Jefferson University Hospital
Philadelphia, PA

Ethan J. Halpern, MD
Department of Radiology
Thomas Jefferson University
Philadelphia, PA

Christopher L. Hansen, MD
Jefferson Heart Institute
Thomas Jefferson University Hospital
Philadelphia, PA

Reginald T. Ho, MD
Jefferson Heart Institute
Thomas Jefferson University Hospital
Philadelphia, PA

Risto Kerkela
University of Oulu
Institute of Biomedicine
Department of Pharmacology and Toxicology
Oulu, Finland

Thomas J. Kiernan, MD
Massachusetts General Hospital
Department of Interventional Cardiology
Harvard Medical School
Boston, MA

Anish Koka, MD
Jefferson Heart Institute
Thomas Jefferson University Hospital
Philadelphia, PA

Li Shien Low, MD
Department of Medicine
Thomas Jefferson University Hospital
Philadelphia, PA

Gregary D. Marhefka, MD
Jefferson Heart Institute
Thomas Jefferson University Hospital
Philadelphia, PA

Geno J. Merli, MD, FACP, FHM
Thomas Jefferson University Hospital
Philadelphia, PA

Stephen Olex, MD
Cardiology Fellow
Albert Einstein Medical Center
Philadelphia, PA

Alyson Owen, MD
Jefferson Heart Institute
Thomas Jefferson University Hospital
Philadelphia, PA

Behzad B. Pavri, MD
Jefferson Heart Institute
Thomas Jefferson University Hospital
Philadelphia, PA

Christopher G. Roth, MD
Department of Radiology
Thomas Jefferson University Hospital
Methodist Hospital Division
Philadelphia, PA

Alexander Rubin, MD
Jefferson Heart Institute
Thomas Jefferson University Hospital
Philadelphia, PA

Nicholas J. Ruggiero, II, MD, FACC, FSCAI
Massachusetts General Hospital
Department of Interventional Cardiology
Harvard Medical School
Boston, MA

Sue Russell, MFA
Jefferson Heart Institute
Thomas Jefferson University Hospital
Philadelphia, PA

Michael P. Savage, MD
Jefferson Heart Institute
Thomas Jefferson University Hospital
Philadelphia, PA

Matthew Stopper, MD
Jefferson Heart Institute
Thomas Jefferson University Hospital
Philadelphia, PA

Marc Tecce, MD
Jefferson Heart Institute
Thomas Jefferson University Hospital
Philadelphia, PA

George Tzanis, MD
Jefferson Heart Institute
Thomas Jefferson University Hospital
Philadelphia, PA

Howard Weitz, MD
Jefferson Heart Institute
Thomas Jefferson University Hospital
Philadelphia, PA

David J. Whellan, MD, MHS, FACC
Jefferson Heart Institute
Thomas Jefferson University Hospital
Philadelphia, PA

James M. Yau, MD
Jefferson Heart Institute
Thomas Jefferson Hospital
Philadelphia, PA

Donna Zwas, MD
Hadassah-Hebrew University Medical Center
Adjunct Assistant Professor of Medicine
Jefferson Medical College of Thomas Jefferson University
Jerusalem, Israel

Foreword

Why do we need another cardiology textbook? There are plenty, but this work by the Jefferson Cardiology Faculty aims at providing a short, easy-to-use, and practical compendium of the important areas of cardiology. It is intended for use by residents and fellows, noncardiology providers, and cardiologists, but the essence of this work is the concise, quick-reference nature of the chapters.

The chapter on echocardiography provides a concise overview of the technology and a short review of the images relevant to common cardiac disorders. This will not turn a physician into an echocardiographer, but for the uninitiated, it provides in an easily understood and practical form a basic explanation of the echo principles and the features of many of the common cardiac disorders.

Similar approaches are found on the two chapters on arrhythmias. Practical approaches to ventricular arrhythmias and a discussion of managing serious ventricular arrhythmias are quite helpful in understanding cardiac arrhythmias, particularly in the patient with reduced left ventricular function. A short section on ablation therapy provides insight into its use and makes it clear that the decision process and the procedures are best left in the hands of an experienced electrophysiologist.

Atrial arrhythmias are also well reviewed, with concise information on their diagnosis and management. With the increasing incidence of atrial fibrillation, the information on diagnosis and medical and invasive management are essential to anyone who sees the high-risk older population in particular.

A separate chapter on device therapy for managing disorders of rhythm and conduction is quite helpful in understanding the issues involved in pacemakers and defibrillators.

The chapter on heart failure and heart transplant is written by a well-recognized expert in this area and provides important guidelines on management of all stages of heart failure. Dr. Mather's clinical insight into this disorder is welcomed. With the increasing incidence of heart failure to the aging population, this is another section that provides useful information when confronted with the inevitable patient with heart failure needing management. Although heart transplantation is a highly specialized field of cardiology, the principles used in selection of candidates, immunosuppression therapy, and the many and diverse complications are important to know.

The following chapter on hemodynamics supplements the heart failure information, as knowledge of hemodynamics in the normal and failing circulation is essential to understanding how to assess the cardiac patient at the bedside.

Several chapters are devoted to imaging. The chapter on nuclear imaging provides a compendium of indications, methods, and recommendations for appropriate use of nuclear imaging. This information is essential to efficient care in the future. Similar information is provided in the CT/MRI chapter, where the reader can also find details on the method for these two emerging imaging technologies and their application.

Clinical chapters on preoperative consultation, outpatient prevention, and management of peripheral arterial disease provide a quick reference for problems that arise frequently in cardiovascular practice; with the section on assessing clinical outcomes, all contribute to a comprehensive, easy-to-use compendium of cardiology.

The authors are to be commended for creating this easy-to-use practicum of clinical cardiology. It will ultimately reside in digital form in one of the many pocket media, where it can be used for quick reference at the bedside.

Alfred A. Bove, MD, PhD
Emeritus Professor of Medicine
Temple University School of Medicine

Introduction

Advances in medical technology appear to be outstripping the ability of the human mind to compile, assess, and understand these changes. Technological advances sometimes seem to bear down upon the human conscience like a runaway locomotive. As our scientific microscopes delve deeper into the human condition, their revelations challenge our capacity both to understand and to communicate these discoveries.

As scientific options become more numerous and complex, physicians and healthcare providers are faced with astounding, and seemingly overwhelming choices and data points, all competing for attention. The educational process has to also keep pace with the information being discovered and deciphered. This textbook attempts to translate state of the art information on cardiovascular diseases into a template which reinforces the necessary building blocks of knowledge while allowing easy access to the knowledge base. This format for learning hopefully increases the ability to absorb the content and tailor the data to one's own needs.

Technology, however, never substitutes for human interaction. At times it seems that the science of medicine is threatening to obliterate the art of medicine, and we must be careful not to let the medium obscure the message. Even as we struggle with the competing data streams assaulting our consciousness, we must not succumb to the urge to "do something" for the sake of using technology if it does not fit in with the needs and desires of our patients. At the crux of all our thought processes should be the patient. Our science should not overrule our reason. As healthcare providers we share privileged intimacies with patients that are unique and raw in their emotional intensity. Our white coats grant us entrance into the realms of their darkest fears and dreads—a privileged position we inherit from the countless physicians who have preceded us in our profession and whose care and dedication created this atmosphere of trust. In the end, it is the unspoken transactions in gentle human dignity—the occasions when we willingly meet our patient's eyes and conjoin inhuman touch—that play the greatest role in the well-being of a patient. No matter how far technology propels us, the common denominator in caring for the sick is human presence.

Along with the facts and opinions, we have also tried to convey the human face of this disease, reflecting its broad sweep and its ravages. We, and our patients, pursue each new promise of cure, because hope is forever at the heart of the human soul.

1 ■ Modifying Risk Factors in the Cardiac Patient: Part I

Marc Tecce, MD

Tremendous progress has taken place over the last century in understanding the pathophysiology and development of atherosclerotic vascular disease. Several environmental factors have been postulated to have had an impact on the development of this disease process, which was mostly unknown centuries ago. As populations began to migrate into early urban living environments, people began to change their behavioral patterns and adopted lifestyles that included less physical activity and diets that contained more saturated fats. The world became more industrialized, and tobacco usage became more prevalent in developing countries; it contributed to the advance of atherosclerotic disease.

More progress was made in understanding the formation of an atheroma, and several other risk factors for the development of vascular disease were established. We now know that cigarette smoking, diabetes, hypertension, hypercholesterolemia, sedentary lifestyles, obesity, and a pertinent family history are established risk factors that make patients more susceptible to the development of arteriosclerosis. Much research has been done over the past decades to determine how modification of these established risk factors can affect the development of atherosclerosis, and although much more needs to be done, we have developed methods of treatment for high-risk individuals who have proven to impact favorably on the development of vascular disease. These treatment options that are now available to clinicians form the cornerstone of modern-day preventive cardiology.

Cardiovascular disease has become a worldwide epidemic. It is estimated that by 2025 cardiovascular mortality will be the leading cause of death worldwide, surpassing cancer and infectious diseases. More people in the United States die from cardiovascular disease than the next two disease states (cancer and chronic obstructive pulmonary diseases) combined, and the cost to the U.S. healthcare system is hundreds of billions of dollars each year. The recognition and early treatment of high-risk individuals have become paramount in controlling this epidemic disease process and its economic strain not only on the U.S. healthcare system but on the worldwide healthcare budget as well.

Prevention of cardiovascular diseases is an area where tremendous progress has been made because of the identification of established risk factors and evidence that aggressive treatment of these pre-existing conditions can decrease mortality and morbidity. These risk factors include diabetes mellitus, hypercholesterolemia, smoking, hypertension, obesity, a strong family history of cardiovascular events, and a sedentary lifestyle. This chapter focuses on the recognition and treatment of these conditions that form the basis for a preventive strategy to deal with cardiovascular disease and its devastating impact on the livelihood of all people worldwide.

Hyperlipidemia

Pathologic data have shown that fatty streaks, which are the earliest evidence of the atherosclerotic process, are common in the aorta in patients in their late teens and early 20s. The formation of the atheromas in the endothelial lining of blood vessels is a complicated process that involves many factors and typically starts with accumulation of lipoprotein particles in the vessel intima. These particles then undergo modification because of release of local cytokines and enhanced leukocyte migration to adhesion molecules within the intima. Uptake of modified lipoproteins leads to oxidation of macrophages that then form foam cells. These foam cells are the source of additional cytokines that recruit smooth muscle cells into the developing atherosclerotic lesion. Plaque continues to grow with additional recruitment of smooth muscle cells and can change its makeup through cell apoptosis and fibrosis forming a fibrofatty lesion. The core can then become lipid rich and become surrounded by a fibrous capsule.

The role of low-density lipoprotein (LDL) cholesterol in this complex process led to the development of drugs that are capable of inhibiting 3-hydroxy-3-methyl-glutaryl-CoA reductase (controlling enzyme that works in the metabolic pathway (mevalonate) that produces cholesterol) and dramatically lowering the amount of LDL cholesterol available to partake in the development of the atherosclerotic plaque. The inhibition of HMG CoA reductase leads to an increased LDL cholesterol clearance from plasma and decreases hepatic production of LDL and very LDL. Statins also have anti-inflammatory properties that decrease the inflammatory component of plaque formation and can alter the collagen content of atherosclerotic plaque as well. The relationship between elevated serum cholesterol levels and the risk for coronary heart disease became clearer with the results of studies in the 1950s and the Framingham study, one of the earliest and most revealing trials. Many other trials subsequently followed and clearly established a clearcut relationship between elevated serum cholesterol levels and the risk for coronary heart disease.

Treatment of Elevated Levels of LDL Cholesterol

Treatment of elevated levels of LDL cholesterol remains a major goal in the treatment and prevention of coronary artery disease. Dietary intervention is typically used as an initial step, although the relationship between the reduction of LDL through dietary methods and subsequent coronary heart disease risk has not been clearly established. Diets rich in saturated and trans fatty acids and dietary cholesterol have been shown to raise LDL cholesterol; therefore, diets low in saturated fats and cholesterol are recommended and have been shown to decrease serum LDL levels by 5% to 10%. Table 1.1 contains the current National Cholesterol Education Program (NCEP) guidelines regarding the treatment of LDL cholesterol. Initial therapy should involve dietary measures aimed at reducing LDL cholesterol, as well as incorporating exercise and weight loss programs.

Several clinical trials have examined the effects of certain food groups on resultant serum lipids and cardiovascular disease with

Table 1.1 NCEP Guidelines for the Treatment of LDL Cholesterol

Risk Category	LDL Goal	Initiate Lifestyle Changes	Consider Drug Therapy
High Risk: CHD* or CHD Risk Equivalants	<100 mg/dL	≥100 mg/dL	≥100 mg/dL
Moderatly High Risk 2+ Risk Factors**	<130 mg/dL	≥130 mg/dL	≥130 mg/dL
Moderate Risk 1–2 Risk Factors	<130 mg/dL	≥130 mg/dL	≥160 mg/dL
Low Risk 0–1 Risk Factors	<160 mg/dL	≥160 mg/dL	≥190 mg/dL

*History of MI, unstable agents, prior PTCs or CASG, documented myocardial ischemia

**Risk factors include smoking, hypertension (BP≥140/90 mm/Hg or on anti-hypertensive medication), low HDL cholestrol (<40 mg/dL), family history of preventive CHD

some mixed results. Some early randomized trials examined the effects of cholesterol-lowering diets that were high in polyunsaturated fats, which led to a 25% to 50% reduction in cardiovascular end points, with patients having an average reduction in blood cholesterol levels of about 15%. These diets had about 30% to 40% of their calories come from fats. More recent trials have looked at diets with increased amounts of fruits, vegetables, fiber, and legumes with a lower amount of meats, butter, and cream but not cheese in patients with established coronary artery disease. The diet was also enriched with a fair amount of foods containing higher levels of omega-3 fatty acids. Both the controlled diet and the Mediterranean style diet had about a 30% calorie intake from fat. Despite no significant difference in serum lipid levels between the diet group and the controlled diet, there were significant reductions in all-cause mortality, cardiac mortality, and nonfatal myocardial infarction. Other studies have also since confirmed the current accepted concept that the amount of dietary fat consumed cannot in itself lower the risk of cardiovascular events. The American Heart Association guidelines recommend that saturated fats constitute no more than 7% to 10% of dietary calories and that trans saturated fats (trans fats), which are now well marked on food labels, are best kept to a minimum but not eliminated altogether. Serum LDL levels increase 2 to 3 mg/dl for every 100 mg/day of dietary cholesterol, and therefore, a goal of no more than 300 mg/day of dietary cholesterol is currently recommended.

Antilipid Drug Therapy

When patients are not able to lower their LDL cholesterol to their goal as per the NCEP guidelines by nonpharmacologic methods, then drug therapy is indicated to achieve this goal. No drug class has probably had a bigger impact on disease outcomes in the last 20 years than that seen with statin therapy with their associated reduction of risk of cardiovascular events and cardiovascular morbidity and mortality. Because of their safety and efficacy, statins are considered a first-line drug therapy to achieve the desired LDL cholesterol goal. Statins or HMG CoA reductase inhibitors work on the rate-limiting step of cholesterol synthesis and dramatically lower serum LDL cholesterol levels by having little overall effect on HDL and triglyceride levels. Currently available statin drugs in the United States include lovastatin, pravastatin, simvastatin, atorvastatin, fluvastatin, and rosuvastatin, and although they vary in potency, all are effective at lowering LDL cholesterol levels. The drugs are generally well tolerated, with the most common side effect being arthralgias, myalgias, serum transaminase elevation, and rarely myositis. Statins have been shown in numerous trials to provide primary prevention (patients without documented or proven disease but with risk factors) and secondary prevention (patients with established coronary heart disease) of cardiovascular events, including myocardial infarction, stroke, and reduced overall cardiovascular morbidity and mortality.

Bile acid-binding resins inhibit the reabsorption of bile acids in the intestine, leading to decreased cholesterol synthesis, and help to lower LDL cholesterol. Questran is available in 4-g unit doses and Colestid in 5-g unit doses; a typical daily dose is between 2- and 6-g unit doses. These drugs are usually used in conjunction with statins in patients with markedly elevated LDL cholesterol. The most common side effects include nausea, bloating, flatulence, and fullness, as they are not absorbed systemically and stay in the intestine. They may cause elevated triglyceride levels in some patients.

Ezetimibe is a relatively newer agent that limits selective uptake of cholesterol in the intestine by interfering with proteins involved in cholesterol absorption. The drug itself can lower serum LDL levels by approximately 15% but is most effective when combined with statins. The standard dose is 10 mg daily.

Fibrates are fibrinic acid derivatives and are indicated for the treatment of elevated triglyceride levels and for the secondary prevention of cardiovascular events in patients with low HDL levels. The two available agents in the United States are fenofibrate (48 to 245 mg daily) and gemfibrozil (600 mg twice daily). These agents are used for treatment of significantly elevated triglyceride levels in patients who have not responded to diet, exercise, and weight loss. They work via interaction with the nuclear transcription factor PPAR-2α, which affects transcription of the lipoprotein lipase (*LPL*), *apo CII*, and apoliprotein AI (*apo AI*) genes. Side effects include abdominal discomfort, bloating, elevated transaminases, erectile dysfunction, and an interaction with oral anticoagulants such as warfarin, and in some patients, there may be a slight rise in LDL cholesterol levels. Gemfibrozil can inhibit statin elimination and should be used cautiously with statins because of the increased risk of rhabdomyolysis and myotoxicity.

Niacin is the most effective agent available for treating low HDL cholesterol; it also causes a modest reduction in LDL cholesterol and triglycerides. It is very effective for LDL reduction, particularly when combined with a statin, although transaminase levels need to be followed closely on combination therapy. The dose is started usually around 500 mg daily of slow release niacin and titrated upward toward the goal of 2,000 mg daily. Flushing, the most common side effect, can be lessened by having the patients take aspirin 30 minutes before dosing. Other side effects include hyperglycemia, elevated uric acid levels, hepatotoxicity, and gastrointestinal upset. When combined with statins, niacin can slow the progression of coronary atherosclerosis and decrease cardiovascular event rates.

Additional Risk Factors

As discussed previously, it has been shown in multiple trials that a reduction of LDL cholesterol leads to a decrease in cardiovascular events and reduced cardiovascular morbidity and mortality. Although low levels of high-density lipoprotein (HDL) cholesterol are clearly an independent risk factor (regardless of LDL) for cardiovascular events, it remains unclear whether increasing HDL levels by nonpharmacologic methods clearly reduces risk. The VA HIT trial showed a reduction in myocardial infarction and coronary heart disease deaths in patients with established coronary artery disease with low HDL cholesterol (less than 40 mg/dl) with treatment with gemfibrozil.

Hypertriglyceridemia also predicts increased cardiac risk, although less strongly than cholesterol levels. When the levels are elevated, it typically identifies patients with other markers for dyslipidemia such as low HDL cholesterol, central obesity, type II diabetes, and metabolic syndrome.

Elevated plasma levels of homocysteine have also been shown in a recent meta-analysis to increase the risk for ischemic heart disease and stroke. Several trials have looked at the treatment of elevated homocysteine levels with vitamins B6 and B12 and folic acid, but the results were disappointing with no clearcut benefit established. Likewise, studies looking at the effects of antioxidant vitamins such as vitamin E, vitamin C, and beta carotene have also shown no clearcut reduction in CHD event rates or mortality.

Biomarkers

High-sensitivity C-reactive protein (CRP) is an acute-phase reactant that can be measured in the plasma and has been shown to identify patients who are at increased risk for cardiovascular events. C-reactive protein is a circulating protein that is a marker for inflammation. It is produced mostly in the liver, but cells within human coronary arteries are also able to release CRP. C-reactive protein has been shown to identify patients at increased cardiac risk across all levels of LDL cholesterol. C-reactive protein can be reduced by treatment with aspirin, statins, niacin, and fibrates. C-reactive protein is best used as an additional tool in assessing overall risk for patients but is probably most helpful in patients who are at intermediate risk when statins or other antilipid therapy is being considered. The recently released JUPITER trial showed that the treatment for low-risk patients who had an elevated CRP with rosuvastatin led to a markedly reduced rate of cardiovascular events.

Lp(a) is an LDL particle that when elevated also identifies patients at increased risk for cardiovascular events. Lp(a) levels can be reduced with high doses of niacin, but no studies have determined that this leads to a decreased cardiovascular event rate.

Homocysteine is an amino acid that is elevated in patients with an inherited defect with methionine metabolism, and when elevated in the plasma, it identifies patients who are at risk for early atherosclerosis and venous thrombosis. Studies on treatment with B-complex vitamins and folate have failed to demonstrate clearly the ability to lower cardiovascular risk in these patients.

Hypertension

Hypertension has clearly been identified as a risk factor for cardiovascular disease events and stroke. The Joint National Committee on Prevention, Detection, Evaluation, and Treatment of High Blood Pressure (JNC-7) report released in 2003 estimates that 65,000,000 Americans are hypertensive, with another 59,000,000 now being classified as prehypertension (systolic blood pressure 130 to 139 mm/Hg and diastolic blood pressure 80 to 89 mm/Hg). Hypertension is more common in blacks of both genders than in white patients, and blacks are felt to have lower renin hypertension, which may be less responsive to angiotensin-converting enzyme (ACE) inhibitors and angiotensin receptor blockers. Hypertension prevalence still increases with age, with 7% of patients between 18 and 39 years having high blood pressure and over 65% in patients over 60 years of age having hypertension as well.

The relationship between blood pressure and cardiovascular events is essentially linear throughout middle and older ages, and the risk begins to increase with blood pressures over 115/75 mm/Hg. Hypertension is also a risk factor for the development of renal failure (hypertensive nephrosclerosis), stroke, congestive heart failure, and hypertensive cardiomyopathy. The risk of cardiovascular disease doubles in patients with blood pressures between 115/75 to 185/115 with every 20 mm of mercury rise in the systolic blood pressure and 10 mm/Hg increase in diastolic blood pressure, with the systolic blood pressure being the more predictive value with respect to risk.

Many studies have shown that a reduction of blood pressure clearly reduces the risk of cardiovascular events across a wide range of patients, young and old, and across a wide variability in baseline blood pressure. In a large meta-analysis of blood pressure reduction trials, there was a consistent decrease in cardiovascular events with blood pressure reduction, no particular class of antihypertensive conferring more risk reduction, and there was more benefit observed with greater lowering of blood pressures. Treatment of hypertension therefore has clearly been proven to be beneficial, with a goal of less than 140/90 in low-risk patients and a goal of 130/80 in diabetics and higher risk patients with evidence of coronary heart disease.

Obesity and the Metabolic Syndrome

Obesity rates in the United States have steadily risen in the past few decades, with an estimated 64% of adults now classified as overweight (body mass index greater than 25), of which 30% are considered obese (body mass greater than 30). This compares to 31% and 13%, respectively, in the early 1960s; this is reflective of this growing epidemic. Comparable to the adult population, obesity has also been increasing among children and teenagers at an alarming rate, with 15% of 6 to 19 year olds being considered overweight and 10% of children age 2 to 5 years being considered overweight. The risk of coronary heart disease and stroke is clearly higher in patients considered to be overweight, but because these patients also have associated increases in the presence of hypertension, dyslipidemia, and type II diabetes, the risk caused by weight alone is hard to quantify accurately. With the advancement of technology, computers, and video games, children are not as active as they have been in previous generations; this may be contributing to this disturbing trend in obesity rates. We need to encourage our children to be more active, play outside, and limit time spent doing sedentary activities such as video games. Obesity increases patients' risk of developing type II diabetes mellitus, glucose intolerance, hypertension, and dyslipidemia and, as mentioned, is clearly linked to an increase in cardiovascular events. Few data are available that discuss the effect of solely decreasing weight and the risk of coronary heart disease; however, weight loss has multiple benefits in terms of improving serum lipids, lowering blood pressure, and improving glycemic control. Weight loss, exercise, and a heart healthy diet consisting of an abundance of fruits, vegetables, fish, and whole grains are part of a healthy lifestyle, the benefits of which need to be counseled aggressively to patients with high risk for coronary heart disease or with established disease.

Much has been written in the last few years about the metabolic syndrome. Although there have been some inconsistencies in its definition, the National Cholesterol Education Program Adult Treatment panel states that three of the following criteria must be present:

1. A waist circumference of more than 40 inches for men and 35 inches for women
2. Serum triglyceride levels over 150 mg/dl
3. Blood pressure over 130/85
4. HDL cholesterol less than 40 mg/dl and less than 50 mg/dl in women
5. Serum glucose greater than 110 mg/dl

This syndrome is used clinically as an additional tool to identify patients who are at increased risk for cardiovascular diseases and their associated morbidity and mortality. These patients should be treated aggressively with risk factor modification, lifestyle changes, exercise, and pharmacologic therapy when indicated.

Cardioprotection

Several drugs have been shown to be cardioprotective in patients with documented coronary heart disease and patients at high risk of developing coronary heart disease. Aspirin has been shown to reduce the risk of myocardial infarction and stroke in patients with established coronary heart disease (secondary prevention) and has shown primary prevention benefit in some groups, particularly those at high risk. Current guidelines in patients with established coronary heart disease recommend treatment with 75 to 162 mg of aspirin daily, as trials with higher doses did not reveal any additional benefit but did carry an increased risk of bleeding. In stable patients with coronary heart disease, clopidogrel did not offer any additional benefit over aspirin as antiplatelet therapy.

ACE inhibitors and angiotensin receptor blockers have been shown to reduce the risk of myocardial infarction and stroke in patients with established coronary heart disease with normal left ventricular function and are recommended for all patients with established coronary heart disease. β-Blockers have been shown to decrease the risk for a second myocardial infarction in patients with a previous infarction, but their use for prevention of a first event has come into question recently. In patients with established coronary artery disease and hypertension without prior infarction, ACE inhibitors and angiotensin receptor blockers may provide additional protective benefits in these patients and should be considered as a first-line antihypertensive therapy.

2 ■ Modifying Risk Factors in the Cardiac Patient: Part II

INDRANIL DAS GUPTA, MD, MBA, MPH

Diabetes

Cardiovascular disease is the major cause of morbidity and mortality in patients with type I and type II diabetes mellitus. Those with diabetes are three times more likely to develop cardiovascular disease than those without. This was established in the Multiple Risk Factor Intervention Trial. Coronary artery disease in type I diabetics occurs earlier in life and tends to be more aggressive. The disease is more diffuse, and this results in more heart failure and increased restenosis rates. The roles of hypoglycemia, endothelial dysfunction, and insulin resistance have been less established than hypertension, smoking, and high low-density lipoprotein (LDL) and low high-density lipoprotein (HDL).

The following sections provide a brief discussion relating to the pathophysiology of diabetes, trials that have provided insight to support evidence-based medicine, epidemiology, complications, medications, outcomes, and co-morbidities.

Pathophysiology

Multiple factors can contribute to atherosclerosis in diabetic patients. They include oxidated stress and glycoxidation, endothelia dysfunction, impaired endothelium-dependent vasodilation, inflammation, increased free fatty acids, and protein abnormalities.

Because diabetes—type II more than type I—is such a prevalent disease, the burden is substantially increased in macrovascular and microvascular circulation. Those with diabetes have increased rates of atherogenic complications in the setting of primary prevention and interventional procedures. Insulin resistance is instrumental in increasing the risk of congestive heart failure.

In the Nurses' Health Study of Women, the relative risk of myocardial infarction was statistically elevated before the diagnosis of diabetes itself was made.

Hyperglycemia causes deposition of glycation end products. These products result in vascular damage. A significant early step of atherogenesis is the increased leukocyte adhesion to vascular endothelium. Microalbuminuria accelerates this process.

Moreover, the relationship between the development of acute coronary syndromes and diabetics is multifactorial. There is an interaction with plaque disruption and the involvement of the local and systemic thrombogenic factors. By decreasing glycemic levels, one may decrease plaque rupture and improve outcome.

A clinical evaluation of risk factors that may lead to cardiovascular disease is as follows:

1. Access cigarette smoking pack years
2. Blood pressure
3. Serum lipids
4. Dietary habits
5. Alcohol intake
6. Amount of exercise
7. Family history
8. Lipid panel
9. Serum creatinine
10. Laboratory: hemoglobin A1C $> 126 \times 2$ fasting glucose 110 to 126×2

A fair number of studies have provided evidence-based medicine.

The Heart Outcome Prevention Evaluation study evaluated over 9,000 people and randomized subjects with Ramipril and placebo. Over a 5-year period, there was a 25% reduction in death, myocardial infarction, and stroke in patients taking the angiotensin-converting enzyme inhibitor Ramipril.

The Steno trial felt that a comprehensive approach would improve clinical outcome. This included lowering hemoglobin A1C less than 6.5% and blood pressure less than 130/80.

In the Hypertension Optimal Treatment Study, the risk for significant cardiovascular events in diabetics was drastically reduced if a diastolic pressure of less than or equal to 80 mm Hg was targeted.

The Captopril Prevention Project study showed the benefits of an angiotensin-converting enzyme inhibitor in reducing cardiovascular events. This effect was more affective than with β-blockers or diuretics.

The DIGAMI trial showed that aggressive and extensive therapy of insulin and glucose infusion in a setting of an acute myocardial infarction was beneficial over standard therapy.

In the EPISTENT (Evaluation of Platelet II B/III A Inhibition in Stenting) study, hope was provided to diabetics receiving stents, angioplasty, and abciximab over stents alone or angioplasty and abciximab alone.

Table 2.1 Alterations in Vascular Endothelium Associated with Diabetes

- Elevated plasma levels of von Willebrand factor endothelin-1
- Diminished prostacyclin release
- Decreased release of endothelium—derived relaxing factor, that is, nitric oxide (NO) and reduced responsiveness to NO
- Impaired fibrinolytic activity
- Increased endothelial cell surface thrombomodulin
- Increased endothelial cell procoagulant activity
- Impaired plasmin degradation of glycosylated fibrin
- Increased levels of advanced glycosylated end products
- Increased superoxide anion generation
- NO destruction
- Increased expression of adhesion molecules

Source: Wong N, Black H, Gavdin J. *Preventive Cardiology: A Practical Approach,* 2nd ed. McGraw-Hill; 2005: Chapter 9.

Table 2.2 Abnormalities of Platelet Function in Diabetes

• Increased platelet adhesiveness
• Increased platelet aggregation
• Decreased platelet survival
• Increased platelet generation of vasoconstrictor prostanoids
• Reduced platelet generation of prostacyclin and other vasodilator prostanoids
• Altered platelet divalent cation homeostasis, that is, decreased $[Mg^{2+}]_i$ and increased $[Ca^{2+}]_i$
• Increased nonenzymatic glycosylation of platelet proteins
• Decreased platelet polyphosphoinositide content
• Decreased platelet production of nitric oxide
• Increased platelet myosin light-chain phosphorylation
• Increased platelet adhesion to endothelium

Source: Wong N, Black H, Gavdin J. *Preventive Cardiology: A Practical Approach*, 2nd ed. McGraw-Hill; 2005: Chapter 9.

The Bypass Angioplasty Revascularization Investigation trial showed the benefits (long term) of bypass surgery over stenting in diabetics with significant coronary artery disease.

Medications

Reaching goals in medical therapy to reduce the risk of cardiovascular complications in diabetics is extremely difficult. A combination of oral agents with insulin is necessary if goals are not reached. Insulin resistance and hyperglycemia increased the very LDL secretion, resulting in an expanded plasma triglyceride pool. More than 50% of diabetics have triglyceride levels that are greater than 150 mg/dl and HDL levels less than 40 mg/dl. Hence, lowering LDL, increasing HDL, and lowering triglycerides will result in a significant goal to reducing cardiovascular morbidity. Lowering

Table 2.3 Lipids, Coagulation, and Fibrinolytic Abnormalities in Diabetes

- Elevated plasma levels of VLDL, LDL, and Lp(a)
- Decreased plasma HDL-C
- Increased small dense LDL-C products
- Decreased lipoprotein lipase activity
- Elevated plasma levels of factors VII and VIII
- Increased levels of fibrinogen and PAL-1
- Elevated thrombin-antithrombin complexes
- Decreased levels of antithrombin complexes
- Decreased levels of antithrombin II, protein C1 and protein 5
- Decreased plasminogen activators and fibrinolytic activity
- Increased endothelial expression of adhesion molecules
- Increased adhesion of platelets and leukocytes to the endothelium

VLDL, very low density lipoprotein; LDL, low-density lipoprotein; Lp(a), lipoprotein(a); HDL, high-density lipoprotein; C, cholesterol; PAI-1, plasminogen activator inhibition.
Source: Wong N, Black H, Gavdin J. *Preventive Cardiology: A Practical Approach*, 2nd ed. McGraw-Hill; 2005: Chapter 9.

LDL to less than 70 mg/dl with statins will likely reduce cardiovascular events by 25%. Fibrates also help with risk reduction by lowering triglycerides. For the patients who do not have brittle diabetes or severe hyperglycemia, niacin can be effective in raising HDL levels.

The increased prevalence of hypertension is thought to be caused by reduced vascular compliance, increased sympathetic activity, sodium retention, and increased vascular wall A-II activity. Thiazides, β-blockers, calcium channel blockers, angiotensin-converting enzyme inhibitors, and angiotensin receptor blockers (ARBs) have all been demonstrated to provide an effective reduction in cardiovascular events.

Associated Conditions That May Help to Explain the Poor Outcome in Diabetes Mellitus and Insulin Resistance

- Maladaptive left ventricular remodeling of the noninfarct zone
  - Increased prevalence of silent infarct
  - Autonomic neuropathy
  - Increased collagen deposition in the myocardium
  - Increased endothelial dysfunction leading to ischemia
- Cardiomyopathy
- Associated conditions

Table 2.4 Diabetes Complications and Co-Morbidities

Complications	Pathophysiology	Signs/Symptoms
Myocardial ischemia ACS and arrhythmias	Macrovascular and microvascular atherosclerosis and endothelial function	Angina, dyspnea or no symptoms
Retinal hemorrhage	Proliferative retinopathy	Eye exam
Foot injury	Peripheral artery disease and neuropathological dysfunction	Foot ulcers, decreased peripheral pulses
Orthostatic hypotension	Autonomic dysfunction	Depressed blood pressure and heart rate to response to exercise
Peripheral artery disease	Microvascular disease	Claudication
Nephropathy	Vascular disease glomerulosclerosis	Proteinuria and hypertension

Source: Stewart K. The role of exercise training on cardiovascular disease in patients who have type II diabetes. *Cardiol Clin* 2004;22:569–586.

- Endothelial dysfunction
- Sympathovagal imbalance
- Abnormalities of coagulation, fibrinolysis, and platelet function

Exercise

Physical activity has a favorable impact against the development of cardiovascular disease, hypertension, insulin resistance, and hyperlipidemia. Exercise is extremely important in managing a patient with heart failure, previous myocardial infarction, and peripheral vascular disease. The following sections provide a brief discussion concerning body weight, insulin metabolism, hypertension, lipid

Table 2.5 Pathophysiologic Model of Development of Diabetes and Vascular Disease

Predisposing Factors	Early Metabolic Abnormalities	Currently Measured Risk Factors	Vascular Disease	Clinical Disease
Genes				
Behaviors	Hyperinsulinemia	Renal failure	Microvascular disease	CV risk factors (lipids, BP, etc.)
Central obesity	Insulin resistance	Cardiomyopathy		
Other factors (early development)	Glucose intolerance	Coronary artery disease	Macrovascular disease	Hyperglycemia
		Stroke		
		Peripheral vascular disease		

Source: Howard BV, et al. Prevention Conference VI, Diabetes and Cardiovascular Disease, Writing Group I, *Circulation* 2002;105: e132–e137.

oxidation, coagulation, pathophysiology, and epidemiology with relationship to exercise.

Exercise Affects Body Weight and Fat

Various studies have indicated that a reduction in body mass index results in a decrease in the risk of developing coronary artery disease, diabetes, peripheral vascular disease, or hypertension.

Insulin Metabolism

Regular exercise increases the sensitivity of skeletal muscles, adipose tissue, and the liver to the activity of insulin. A decrease in the basal level of plasma glucose occurs. Furthermore, there is decrease in the fasting glucose, a reduction of insulin response to glucose load, and an increase in glucose disposal rate under various conditions.

Hypertension

Regular physical activity can reduce systolic and diastolic pressures by 10 mm Hg. This decrease is not noted in all individuals who exercised but in those that reach an endurance of 40% to 60% of VO_2 max.

Lipid Oxidation

As one increases physical activity levels, more fat is oxidized as total energy expenditure increases. An increased capacity to oxidized fats occurs as a consequence of increased skeletal muscle mitochondria. Exercise is noted to increase lipolytic responsiveness to β adrenergic stimulation and to lower plasma catecholemia concentration. Vigorous exercise increases the activity of tissue lipoprotein lipase, allowing our bodies to use circulatory triglycerides as a fuel source and clearance of triglycerides at rest.

Lipid and Lipoprotein Metabolism

Regular exercise increased HDL levels (specifically HDL II subfraction) and a polyprotein A-I. Exercise is felt to be a player in the increase in lipoprotein lipase activity and the decrease in hepatic lipase activity. Furthermore, exercise increases insulin sensitivity and decreases plasma insulin levels.

Coagulation and Hemostatic Factors

Regular exercise tends to decrease plasma fibrinogen concentration and diminish antifibrinolysis activity. Further benefits include inhibition of platelet aggregability.

Pathophysiology

Exercise is directly related to cardiac performance. There is an increase in oxygen uptake resulting from increased stroke volume in widened total body arteriovenous oxygen difference. Aerobic exercise, in particular, augments peak blood flow and capillary exchange capacity. Structural vascular adaptations occur with regular exercise and result in an increase in the actual size and length of the large and small arteries and veins over time. There have been multiple studies indicating the effect of exercise training on diabetes and hypertension. In fact, the data from the *National Health Interview* survey showed that among a large spectrum of individuals who had diabetes, walking was associated with a 39% lower all-cause mortality and a 35% lower cardiovascular disease mortality. It was further postulated that one death per year could be prevented for every 61 people who walk at least 2 hours per week. The increase in regular exercise definitely plays a role in the prevention of type II diabetes and related metabolic abnormalities.

In the Insulin Resistance Atherosclerosis Study, it was revealed that increased levels of vigorous and nonvigorous exercise were associated with higher insulin sensitivities. This was also validated in the Nurses Health Study. Sedentary behavior was associated with an increased risk in obesity in type II diabetes. The Diabetes Prevention and Program Research Group study enrolled patients who had impaired glucose tolerance and had them adopt a lifestyle of intense exercise. They reduced the incidence of developing type

II diabetes by as much as 58%, whereas the pharmacological intervention of Metformin reduced the development by only 31%.

Exercise definitely plays an important role in glycemic control and in the control of elevated blood pressure. Exercise has a significant role in reducing inflammation in the microvascular and macrovascular system. Multiple studies, including data from the National Health and Nutrition Examination Survey III, showed that people who were jogging or involved in aerobic dancing were less likely to have increased cardiovascular markers such as C-reactive protein. Moreover, exercise training significantly reduced the local expression of tumor necrosis factor-α, interleukin-6 in skeletal muscles, and interleukin-1β. This was established in people with chronic heart failure who had exercised for 6 months or more.

It has been speculated that one third to one half of all U.S. adults are physically inactive, and this has been shown to be inversely associated with cardiovascular morbidity and mortality. There have been indications that physical activity at a regular level improves blood pressure, glucose tolerance, diabetes, high-density lipid protein, triglycerides, and obesity. In patients with cardiovascular disease or in symptoms suggestive of cardiovascular disease, if one is involved in a symptom limited exercise stress test, the prescription should be for them to be involved in a regular activity program (see appendix).

The American Heart Association, the Center for Disease and Prevention, and the American College of Associated Sports Medicine have all made significant recommendations for exercise and associated activities as preventive and secondary preventions for coronary artery disease. Multiple studies showed that physical activity as part of daily living is associated with a decreased risk for coronary artery disease, cardiovascular disease, strokes, diabetes, obesity, and all-cause mortality. Only 15% of Americans older than age 18 participate in regular vigorous exercise which is defined as exercising a minimum of three times a week for at least 20 minutes per session. Sixty percent of Americans report no regular exercise and 25% state that they are sedentary and participate in no formal or informal activity or exercise. This is very concerning in view of the potential for reducing cardiovascular disease in those individuals who are initially sedentary. One study, the Young Finns Study, demonstrated that the level of physical activities was associated with an overall increase in HDL-C and HDL2-C levels. It was negatively associated with triglyceride levels, anti-phospholipid (APL) lipoprotein B, and insulin levels in males. A relationship was established between increased physical activity and increased physical fitness levels with improved cardiovascular risk factors in adults. In the Pawtucket Heart study, which involved greater than 300 men and greater than 500 women, the estimated maximal oxygen consumption in self-reported physical activity was significantly improved and positively associated with blood pressure, body mass index, and levels of HDL-C. In the Post Menopausal Estrogen/Progesterone Intervention trial, self-reported physical activity was positively associated with levels of HDL and was briskly associated with decreased insulin and fibrinogen levels. Intra-abdominal adipose tissue determined by a computed tomographic angiography (CTA) appears to be negatively related to the level of physical activity. Beneficial changes in hormonal, metabolic, hemodynamic, neurologic, and respiratory functions occur with increased exercise capacity, and this is related to the increased ability to use oxygen in driving energy for work and also is related to increased oxygen uptake relating to both maximum cardiac output and the ability of the muscles that extract and use oxygen from the blood.

In summary, the mechanism through which physical activity reduces the risk for coronary artery disease is not 100% clear, but the relationship is quite substantial. Clearly, regular aerobic activity should be addressed with all individuals in prevention of coronary artery disease. A study done in 1996 showed the estimated levels of utilization risk reduction in patients who survived a myocardial infarction in the United States. It was found that cardiac rehabilitation, smoking cessation, cholesterol lowering, and the use of β-blockers, angiotensin-converting enzyme inhibitors, and aspirin were all effective in reducing the risk for subsequent morbidity and mortality for those who survived myocardial infarction. Exercise on a regular basis, whether it is low or vigorous, has a positive modification with the pathophysiology associated with inactivity. The implementation of exercise in all individuals with any notion of having risk factors for coronary artery disease or preventing risk factors for coronary artery disease should be part of the physician's plan in effective primary and secondary health maintenance programs.

Tobacco

Tobacco use accounts for more than 450,000 deaths a year. Of those deaths, 35% are cardiovascular related. It is estimated that nearly 1 billion people smoke at any one given time in the world.

Tobacco use is related to cardiovascular disease, sudden death, aortic aneurysm formation, peripheral vascular disease, and strokes. Various studies link tobacco consumption to intercranial hemorrhage and subarachnoid hemorrhage. Smoking results in an increased sympathetic tone vascular bed, accelerating atherosclerotic progression, enhanced LDL oxidation, and impaired endothelial-dependent coronary artery vasodilation.

Smoking causes dysfunctional endothelial nitric oxide biosynthesis in the acute and chronic setting. Furthermore, tobacco use is linked to increased levels of C-reactive protein, soluble intercellular adhesion molecule-1, fibrinogen, and finally homocystine. The consequence of these elevations results in increased adverse endothelial and inflammatory effects.

The following sections provide a brief discussion of smoking and its effects on peripheral artery disease, abdominal aortic aneurysm, cerebral vascular accidents, pathophysiology, and studies relating pathophysiology of exercise to clinical outcomes.

Additional adverse effects of smoking involve coronary spasm and arrhythmias. The combination of smoking and diabetes results in advanced atherosclerosis. Smoking cessation will result in a significant reduction in cardiovascular associated mortality and morbidity. In the Nurses' Health Study, there was a 61% benefit

Table 2.6 Adverse Pathological Effects of Smoking

1.	Spontaneous platelet aggregation.
2.	Increased monocyte adhesions to endothelium.
3.	Adverse alterations in the tissue type plasminogen activation.
4.	Adverse alteration in tissue pathway factor inhibition.

Source: Zipes DP, Libby P, Bonow RO. *Braunwald's Heart Disease: Textbook of Cardiovascular Medicine*, 7th ed. Philadelphia: Saunders; 2005:921–1012.

from cardiovascular disease and a 42% benefit from strokes in women who stopped smoking (after 5 years). Interestingly, fibrinogen concentration and fibrinogen synthesis are reduced after only 2 weeks of cessation. There is a further reduction in mean arterial pressure and arterial compliance.

In the Physician's Health Study, former physician smoking had a significant reduction of nonfatal strokes as well as claudication symptoms.

In the British Heart Study, there was a threefold increase of having a nonfatal myocardial infarction compared with a nonsmoker. The British Regional Heart Study found that current smokers had doubled the risk of sudden cardiac death compared with the nonsmoker.

Peripheral Vascular Disease

Tobacco use increases the risk of developing peripheral vascular disease sevenfold and progresses to symptomatic disease 10 years ahead of nonsmokers. Furthermore, smokers have twice the rate of complications for peripheral vascular disease, an increased graft failure of lower-extremity bypass surgery, and increased postoperative deaths.

Abdominal Aortic Aneurysm

Several studies, including one that was done by Lederle and Vardilaki, have shown a dose response of the number of cigarettes and the development of abdominal aortic aneurysm. There was a dose response association. For those who smoked less than one pack per day, the relative risk was three. For those who smoked three or more packs per day, the relative risk was seven.

Cerebral Vascular Accidents

In the Nurses' Health Study, there was an increased risk of stroke, both ischemic and hemorrhagic, in smokers. This risk increased with the number of cigarettes smoked. This risk was further increased with the concurrent use of oral contraceptives. Salivary damage caused by oxidation of lipids, proteins, and DNA is a key component in tobacco's effect on atherogenesis. Oxidized chemicals from tobacco include hydrogen, peroxide, and supraoxide. Tobacco causes endothelial dysfunction and increased cellular inflammation. There is an increased level of oxidized LDL, which is taken up by macrophages, leading to the development of foam cells and the atherogenic cascade. The impaired endogenous nitric oxide released deregulates platelet activation in smooth muscle cell proliferation. This results in endothelial cell injury and the deactivation of platelets. In conclusion, smoking cessation and prevention may be the most significant path leading to the reduction of heart disease. It is certainly the most preventable. Clearly, prevention is better than secondary amelioration. A tremendous amount of education must start at a young age to prevent the beginning of this terrible cascade of pathology.

Significant evidence links tobacco use to the incidence in mortality with coronary vascular disease. Over a half a million deaths attributed in the United States are related to cigarette smoking alone. It remains a significant problem in the U.S. population, as well as in other developed and developing countries worldwide. Important intervention among youth includes school-based prevention programs, community-based prevention programs, and state and federal initiatives. Behavioral treatments, self-help procedures, pharmacological therapy should all be used to help to reduce tobacco smoking. Healthcare workers and community programs, as well as physicians and other healthcare providers, should be involved informing and educating patients about using appropriate sources to help reduce the incidence of tobacco use in primary prevention of coronary vascular disease.

Links between cigarette smoking and human disease are quite convincing. Yes, cigarette smoking is linked to many cancers and is the primary factor in lung cancer and is linked to chronic pulmonary disease and chronic obstructive pulmonary disease. Tobacco smoking is one of the three major risk factors for coronary vascular disease and is linked to sudden death, myocardial infarction, and stroke. Some evidence suggests that environment tobacco smoke for nonsmokers also poses a health risk. One of the main concerns of cigarette smoking is its relationship with sudden unexpected deaths, especially among young individuals. Although it is shown to be linked to sudden death with those who have known coronary vascular disease, a study by Escobedo and Caspersen (Nathan D. Wong, Henry R. Block, Julius Garden, *Preventive Cardiology: A Practical Approach*, Chapter 5) found that smoking alone is predictive of sudden death in those who were felt not to have any known cardiovascular risks. Acute myocardial infarction in individuals in their 30s and 40s is strongly affected by association with cigarette smoking. Cigarette smoking is also linked to an increased risk with lipids, obesity, diabetes mellitus, hypertension, oral contraceptive use. Even without those factors, cigarette smoking has been known to increase the risk for cardiovascular disease. The Pathobiological Determinants of Atherosclerosis in Youth Research Group did autopsies on over 1,000 men and women aged 15 to 34 years who died of external causes, such as violence to auto accidents, and it found that there was an excess of fatty streaks in raised lesions in the abdominal aorta in these otherwise healthy individuals.

Epidemiologically, cigarette smoking has been shown to be a predictor of coronary artery disease. Most specifically, the Framingham Study showed a 10-fold increase in the relative risk of sudden death in men who smoked versus those who did not. There is also a 4.5 relative risk greater in women who smoke versus nonsmokers. Important in the assessment of risk for cardiac events related to smoking is when they started smoking, the amount they smoked, and the number of people for whom they are around who smoked. The Coronary Artery Surgery Study provided evidence that over a 5-year mortality, it was more significant for smokers than quitters (22% vs. 15%). The study done by Daly and associates followed people (for greater than 7 years after their admission) for a myocardial infarction or unstable angina. In that study, they found that the mortality for those who continued to smoke was 82% as opposed to those who stopped smoking, which was 37%.

From the pathophysiological point of view, many mechanisms are apparently involved in the relationship between smoking and cardiovascular disease. Of concern is the decreased oxygen-carrying capacity secondary to carbon monoxide and its direct effect on the hemoglobin as well as vasoconstriction, platelet hypercoagulability, and endothelial dysfunction. Nicotine and carbon monoxide seem to be the most significant components for this pathology. It has been speculated that by smoking a single cigarette the body reacts by increasing oxygen consumption, heart rate, blood pressure, peripheral resistance, and increased cardiac output. The amount of coronary blood flow in myocardial oxygen supply is decreased. Some studies have even shown that smoking enhances the platelet aggregation adhesiveness in the presence of aspirin. Other aspects of chronic smoking are decreased fibrolytic functions, further plaque formation, increased serum cholesterol, reduced high-density lipid protein, damage to blood vessels, and opportunities for exposure to lipid and thrombosis.

Conclusion

A substantial number of studies have linked cardiovascular disease to smoking, and the cost not only to the healthcare system as well as to the health of people has gone to astronomical levels. Quite a few interventions should be approached at a young age, and these involve prevention programs and understanding the pathophysiology. Clearly, the reduction in smoking and prevention of smoking itself would reduce hospitalizations from infarctions, strokes, coronary artery disease, peripheral vascular disease, and a whole spectrum of cardiovascular disease. Hopefully, in the years to come, the primary plus secondary interventions can help to reduce the incidence of coronary artery disease related to the use of tobacco.

3 ■ General Principles in Cardiac Critical Care

MATTHEW DECARO, MD

Protocols

Ample data indicate that protocol-driven care is more likely to be encompassing, evidence based, and therefore more effective. Computerized order sets where available are ideal for this reason.

Decreasing Morbidity and Mortality

Deep vein thrombosis prophylaxis

- Indicated in all situations
  - Intermittent pneumatic compression boots when anticoagulants contraindicated
  - Recent intracerebral hemorrhage—use low-dose subcutaneous heparin or low molecular weight heparin after 3 to 4 days if bleeding cessation documented

Central line infections

- This represents a large source of morbidity and mortality in the hospital, particularly in the intensive care setting. A standard set of guidelines, if adhered to, can significantly decrease this infection rate.
  - Use antibiotic impregnated catheters.
  - Use the subclavian vein.
  - Use maximal sterile barrier precautions.
  - Avoid antibiotic ointment.
  - Disinfect catheter hub at each access.
  - Remove catheters promptly.
- All catheters inserted under emergent conditions are presumed to be compromised and are immediately changed. One of the few indications for a femoral venous line is the presence of a severe coagulopathy. Although the subclavian route is preferred, ultrasound-guided placement in the

internal jugular vein is a close second. In a patient for whom permanent dialysis is on the horizon, the subclavian is best avoided.

Use of anticoagulants

- Carry significant morbidity and mortality
    - Target the lower half of the therapeutic range unless there is a life-threatening thrombotic process
        - Higher values are associated with greater morbidity, yet no greater therapeutic benefit.
        - The only down side of a lower target is a greater statistical likelihood of a downward drift to subtherapeutic values—hence the higher target in mission critical situations.
- Careful and regular monitoring of
    - Coagulation parameters where appropriate
    - Complete blood count
    - Platelets
    - Clinician signs of bleeding as well as thrombosis
- Review and adjust appropriate doses based on hepatic and renal function

General Principles

Ventilator-associated pneumonia

- Another large source of morbidity and mortality in the intensive care unit is ventilator-associated pneumonia. Several policies, both pharmacologic and nonpharmacologic, have been shown to decrease this problem.
- Nonpharmacologic
    - Effective hand washing and the use of protective gowns and gloves
    - Semirecumbent positioning of patients
    - Avoidance of large gastric volumes
    - Oral (nonnasal) intubation

  - Routine maintenance of ventilator circuits
  - Continuous subglottic suctioning
  - Type of suction catheter and its replacement
  - Humidification with heat and moisture exchangers
  - Postural changes
- Pharmacologic
  - Stress-ulcer prophylaxis
  - Administration of antibiotics
  - Combination antibiotic therapy
  - Chlorhexidine oral rinse
  - Prophylactic treatment of patients with neutropenia
  - Vaccines

Assessment of volume status

- This is one of the more challenging tasks in the critically ill patient, more so in the setting of multiorgan dysfunction. In the majority of patients, volume status is determined by the assessment of
  - Skin turgor
  - Presence of edema (distal/dependent and sacral)
  - Electrolytes, blood urea nitrogen, creatinine
  - Jugular venous pressure
  - Chest radiograph
- No single factor is adequate for this assessment; often there is a disparity in the direction of the indicators. The decision is made by judging the preponderance of the data. The key to good care is realizing that one's assessment is a starting point only, and careful observation of the response to the initial planned therapy is critical. If the expected response is not seen, a change of course, done in a timely fashion, is mandatory.
- When significant uncertainty still exists, other modalities include the use of a pulmonary artery catheter or an ultrasound assessment of the heart and inferior vena cava (IVC). It should be recalled, however, that prospective

studies on the use of the pulmonary artery catheter in the critically ill patient indicate that this modality does not have a beneficial impact on survival or duration of unit care. This applies to both medical and surgical patients, although one recent study in the most severe injured trauma patients suggested a benefit.

- By ultrasound, the size/filling of the heart chambers and also the size and collapsibility of the IVC with respiration has been suggested as an indicator of the response to fluid loading, as has the magnitude of the peak systolic pressure variation with respiration in the ventilated patient.

General principles in the management of the ventilated patient

- Criteria that suggest an individual may be able to have discontinuation of mechanical ventilation are as follows:
  - Evidence for some reversal of the underlying cause for respiratory failure
  - Adequate oxygenation (e.g., paO_2/FiO_2 ratio > 150 to 200; requiring positive end-expiratory pressure [PEEP] $\leq$ 5 to 8 cm H_2O; $FiO_2 \leq 0.4$ to 0.5); and pH (e.g., ≥ 7.25)
  - Hemodynamic stability, as defined by the absence of active myocardial ischemia and the absence of clinically significant hypotension (i.e., a condition requiring no vasopressor therapy or therapy with only low-dose vasopressors such as dopamine or dobutamine, < 5 mcg/kg/min)
  - The capability to initiate an inspiratory effort
  - Hemoglobin stable, preferably ≥ 7
  - Afebrile
  - Stable metabolic status
- The optimal weaning protocol, even in this situation, is not well established. The few well-done studies suggest that in fact there is no single best modality. If any is to be preferred, it would be the performance once every 24 hours of a spontaneous breathing trial. If successful, after 30 to 120

minutes, discontinue the ventilator; if unsuccessful, place back on a ventilation mode that provides substantial support, and do not retry for 24 hours. Objective criteria for success include the following:
  - Gas exchange acceptability ($SpO_2 \geq 85$–90%, $pO_2 \geq 50$–60 mm Hg, pH ≥ 7.32, increase in $paCO_2 \leq 10$ mm Hg)
  - Hemodynamic stability (heart rate [HR] < 120–140 beats/min, HR not changed > 20%, systolic blood pressure [BP] < 180–200 and > 90 mm Hg, BP not changed > 20%, no pressors required)
  - Stable ventilatory pattern (e.g., respiratory rate [RR] ≤ 30–35 breaths/min, RR not changed > 50%)
- Clinical indicators of failure are as follows:
  - Change in mental status (e.g., somnolence, coma, agitation, and anxiety)
  - Onset or worsening of discomfort
  - Diaphoresis
  - Signs of increased work of breathing (use of accessory respiratory muscles, and thoracoabdominal paradox)
- In the case of repeated failure to wean, the most likely causes include
  - Inadequate resolution of the underlying pathology
  - Neuromuscular insufficiency
    - Guillain-Barré
    - Critical illness polyneuropathy/myopathy
  - Excessive sedation over a prolonged period
- A dedicated respiratory therapy department whose practitioners are knowledgeable in this area and who get to know the patients in the unit is an invaluable resource.

Sedation and analgesia

- The primary focus in the critically ill patient is achieving adequate analgesia. Narcotics are the mainstay of therapy in this regard. The best compromise of ease of use, titratability and metabolic features in my opinion, is fentanyl. This may be given by intermittent intravenous boluses, but also as a continuous intravenous infusion. In the absence of contraindication, nonsteroidal agents also have a role to play in certain kinds of pain (e.g., pleuritic, arthritic, and some postoperative situations).

- Often, after ensuring appropriate pain control, especially in mechanically ventilated patients, there is a need for sedation. The most useful agents in this regard are lorazepam, midazolam, and propofol. Each can be given by intermittent bolus therapy or continuous infusion. The relative advantages and disadvantages of each include the following:
  - Midazolam
    - Positive
      - Rapid onset of action
      - Short duration of action with single dosing
    - Negative
      - Unpredictable awakening time and time to extubation if more than 48 to 72 hours
      - Accumulation of active metabolites with renal dysfunction
  - Propofol
    - Positive
      - Rapid onset, short duration
      - No change in kinetics with hepatic or renal dysfunction
      - Useful when rapid awakening is needed (e.g., neurosurgical patients)
    - Negative
      - Greater likelihood of producing hypotension
      - At high/prolonged dosing can raise triglycerides, rarely pancreatitis
      - Need for dedicated intravenous line
  - Lorazepam
    - Positive
      - Good compromise of duration and wake-up times

        - Fewer drug interactions
    - Negative
        - Slower onset, a problem in acute agitation
        - The solvent needed to solubilize can cause renal failure and acidosis at high doses
- Although much emphasis has been rightly placed on the importance of adequate sedation, inappropriately high levels of sedation are common. This can be prevented with a rigorous assessment of levels using a standardized method and a daily complete discontinuation of sedation for full awakening. The latter has repeatedly shown to decrease duration of mechanical ventilation and intensive care unit lengths of stay. After reinstitution of sedation, down titration to the minimally effective dose based on assessment of sedation level is equally important.

Hemodynamic monitoring

- The insertion of a pulmonary artery catheter (PAC) to assess and manage therapy has not been shown to improve outcomes across a wide variety of clinical situations. This has been assessed in surgical (cardiac as well as no-cardiac surgery) medical processes such as sepsis and even in the routine management of severe heart failure, and all of the trials show no benefit.
- In cardiac surgery as well as cardiogenic shock, the use of a PAC leads to more interventions, but not improved outcomes. The reason for this is unclear. To a large extent, this may be because there are two major contributing factors to the negative outcome studies. It appears that in less critically ill patients the complications of PAC insertion and use outweigh the benefits. Another factor is that the interpretation of the often-conflicting data is complex. There are many sources of error in interpretation, such that the more experienced the operator, the more reliable the information is.

- General
  - Ideally placed in West zone 3 (not difficult in the supine patient, except with high values of PEEP). An indicator of this is excessive respiratory variation in the pressures/ waveform.
  - Assess for damping—look for two to three beats of ringing when the flush pigtail is pulled and released. If there are none, it is overdamped. The most common cause is an air bubble in the tubing or catheter.
  - Beyond about 10 to 15 degrees of head elevation, the numbers are skewed.
  - Balance/calibrate/zero frequently.
  - Inflate the balloon carefully, as rupture of a pulmonary arteriole can be life threatening.
  - Read all values at end expiration. In a nonventilated patient, this is the higher pressure induced by respiratory variation. In a fully controlled ventilator patient, it is the lower pressure.
- Right atrial (RA) pressure
  - Reflects right ventricular (RV) preload, RV failure, volume status
  - Pattern of the waveform reflects right-sided compliance or tamponade (i.e., the presence and prominence of the x- and y-descents)
  - Volume (left ventricular end diastolic volume, or LVEDV) is the more precise definition of preload, not pressure
- Pulmonary artery (PA) occlusion (wedge) pressure
  - Reflects left ventricular (LV) preload, LV failure, volume status
  - Pattern of the waveform a bit less useful, except when large V-waves seen (as in severe mitral regurgitation where differentiation from PA can be difficult)
  - If close to PA mean pressure, suspect that it is not truly wedged (i.e., "overwedged")
  - May be inaccurate in the presence of severe intrinsic pulmonary disease

- Cardiac output
  - All measurements assume that the patient is in steady state
  - Fick
    - Based on O_2 content of arterial and mixed venous blood
    - Need to have true admixture, no left to right shunt
    - Accuracy depends on validity of assumed oxygen consumption—invalid in sepsis, nutritional perturbations, catabolic state, and so forth
    - Tends to give higher values in high output states
  - Thermodilution
    - Technique dependent
      - Volume of bolus
      - Speed of injection
      - Reproducible between injections and among operators
      - Need to average more beats in atrial fibrillation

Cardiovascular Specifics

Cardiogenic shock

- Definition
  - Systolic BP $\leq$ 90 mm Hg or an acute drop of 30 mm Hg
  - Low cardiac index in setting of adequate filling (LVEDP $>$ 18, RVEDP $>$ 10 to 15)
    - Confidence interval $<$ 1.8 without inotrope
    - Confidence interval $<$ 2.0–2.2 on inotrope
  - Hypoperfusion
    - Change of mental status
    - Urine output $<$ 20 ml/hr
    - Peripheral vasoconstriction marked by cool moist skin of trunk and extremities
- Common causes
  - Acute myocardial infarction with LV failure
  - Myocardial infarction complications

        - Septal rupture
        - Mitral regurgitation due to papillary muscle rupture
    - Postcardiac arrest
    - Pulmonary embolus
    - Cardiac tamponade
    - Acute myocarditis (e.g., giant cell myocarditis)
    - Predominant RV infarction in approximately 5%
    - Takotsubo cardiomyopathy (LV apical ballooning syndrome, stress cardiomyopathy)
    - Acute valvular decompensation (usually AI or MR)
        - Acute endocarditis
        - Aortic dissection
- Diagnosis
    - Echocardiogram essential
    - Right and/or left heart catheterization may be necessary
    - Evaluate for comorbid conditions
        - Hemorrhage
        - Infection
        - Pulmonary embolism
        - Bowel ischemia
- Monitoring
    - ECG
    - Urine output
    - O_2 saturation (mixed venous vs. central vein)
    - Arterial line often used
    - PAC of some value
- Treatment
    - Ischemic: prompt revascularization
    - Inotropic support
        - May increase oxygen consumption
    - Vasopressors
        - When hypotension is severe, norepinephrine is most potent.
    - Intraaortic balloon pump
    - Supportive care

    - Fluid management. In systemic inflammatory response syndrome, which often accompanies shock, there may be extravasation of tissue fluid.
    - Acidosis
      - Treat the problem not the pH
      - No clear evidence of benefit of bicarbonate therapy, although many would use it for pH < 7.10

Acute myocardial ischemic syndromes

- General
  - ECG
    - At baseline
    - Any change in clinical or pain status
    - In chest pain of unclear etiology, repeat every 15 to 30 minutes
  - Anticoagulant therapy
    - Aspirin in everyone
      - Clopidogrel if aspirin allergy and if surgery is unlikely
    - Unfractionated or low molecular weight heparin
  - β-Blocker
    - Start oral β-blocker
    - If tachyarrhythmia or hypertension, consider intravenous use
  - Analgesia
    - Morphine
  - Nitrates
    - Avoid if recent phosphodiesterase inhibitor use
    - Avoid if systolic BP < 90 or 30 mm Hg less than baseline
    - Sublingually first, intravenous infusion for ongoing symptoms
  - Arrhythmias
    - Treat as is customary for the arrhythmia
  - Other therapy
    - Statin

        - Low-flow oxygen
        - Sedation as appropriate

Acute segment of ECG meaning transmural (ST) elevation myocardial infarction (MI) (STEMI)

- Prompt revascularization with door to balloon time less than 90 minutes
    - Ideally within 6 hours of the onset of symptoms, but still reasonable for up to 12 hours
    - Can be done up to 24 hours if
        - Ongoing ischemic symptoms
        - Severe congestive heart failure
        - Electrical or hemodynamic instability
- If door to balloon time is anticipated to be greater than 90 minutes, consider lytic therapy
- Anticoagulant therapy
    - Consider GIIb/IIIa inhibitor if en route to cath lab
- Shock
    - Revascularize for up to 18 hours after the development of shock when it develops within 36 hours of the onset of myocardial infarction
- Non-ST segment elevation MI (NSTEMI) and unstable angina
    - High-risk groups
        - Elevated biomarkers
        - Greater than 0.5- to 1-mm ST segment depression in two or more leads
        - Malignant arrhythmias
        - Significant congestive heart failure, S3, new mitral regurgitation (MR) murmur
        - Age, more than 75 years
    - Some advantage demonstrated for early invasive approach, especially in highest risk patients, in terms of morbidity and possibly mortality
    - Conservative strategy may be preferred

    - Pulmonary or liver failure
    - Limited life expectancy
    - Active sepsis
    - Contraindication to anticoagulation
      - Acute central nervous system (CNS) process
        - Tumor
        - cerebrovascular accident (CVA; stroke)
        - Hemorrhage
      - Active bleeding
- Anticoagulant therapy
  - If invasive approach selected options include
    - GIIb/IIIa inhibitor or clopidogrel (with load) in addition to a heparin
    - Bivalirudin or fondaparinux instead of heparin
  - If conservative approach
    - If increased bleeding risk use fondaparinux
    - Clopidogrel (with load) in addition to a heparin

Acute decompensated heart failure

- Assess etiology, attempt to deal with the correctable aggravating or causative factors
    - Ischemia
    - Valvular heart disease
    - Arrhythmias
    - Sepsis
    - Pulmonary embolus
- Evaluate LV and RV systolic and LV diastolic function
- Assessment
    - History
      - Time course of onset of symptoms
      - Salt fluid intake
      - Characteristics of prior episodes and evaluation
        - Obtaining prior tests results is critical.
  - Physical exam
    - Edema

        - Jugular venous pressure
        - Presence of S3 gallop
        - Murmurs
        - Peripheral pulses and bruits
        - Rales
            - Useful as a reflection of the acuity of the onset of HF rather than its presence
        - Skin/extremities color and temperature
            - Cyanotic, cold clammy legs may be a sign of a low output state
    - Vital signs
        - Mean pressure
        - Pulse pressure
        - Heart rate
    - Echo
        - Systolic function
            - Regional abnormalities
            - RV and LV
        - Diastolic function
        - Valvular abnormalities
        - Pericardial fluid
    - Chest radiograph
        - Heart size
        - "Fluid status"
            - Pleural
            - Interstitial
            - Alveolar
        - Co-morbids
            - Chronic obstructive pulmonary disease
            - Infection
- Therapy
    - Restoration of euvolemic state—the cornerstone of therapy
        - Salt and water restriction
        - Diuretics
            - Usually loop diuretic

    - Often multiple daily doses intravenously
    - Continuous infusion occasionally needed
  - Supplemental thiazide diuretic when refractory
  - Proactively replace potassium commensurate with briskness of diuresis and level of renal function
- Causes of refractoriness to loop diuretics
  - Nonsteroidal antiinflammatory drug use
    - Including COX-2 inhibitors
  - Poor renal perfusion
    - Low cardiac output
    - Renal arterial disease
  - Renal insufficiency/failure
  - Excessive concern with azotemia and hypotension in the dyspneic, edematous patient
- ACE inhibitor/angiotensin receptor blocker (ARB)/ vasodilator
  - ACE preferred over ARB or vasodilator (hydralazine/ nitroglycerine [NTG]) unless a specific contraindication exists
  - Improves survival
  - Contraindications
    - Life-threatening allergic reaction history
    - Severe hypotension (less than 80 mm Hg)
    - Low BP with immediate risk of cardiogenic shock
    - Pregnancy
    - Markedly elevated creatinine (> 3)
    - Hyperkalemia (> 5.5)
    - Bilateral significant renal artery stenosis
- β-Blockers
  - Improve survival
  - Contraindications
    - Severe bronchospastic airway disease
    - Cardiogenic shock
    - Recent need for inotropic support
    - Symptomatic bradycardia or heart block
  - Start at low dose with gradual up titration
- Digoxin

        - No change in mortality, only symptomatic benefit
        - Target low serum levels (e.g., ≤ 1.0)
        - Empirically reduce dose if drugs known to interact are started (e.g., amiodarone)
    - Aldosterone antagonists (eplerenone, spironolactone)
        - Improves survival in individuals with severe heart failure (HF) or HF after myocardial infarction
        - Contraindications
            - Hyperkalemia—withhold if K > 5.0
            - Severe renal insufficiency (creatinine > 2.5)
    - Inotropes
        - Can produce an acute improvement in symptoms and promote diuresis
        - Are associated with excess mortality
        - Useful for palliative care of stage IV HF and stabilization in preparation for heart transplantation
        - Agents
            - Dobutamine
                - Occasionally associated with a drop in BP
                - Increases heart rate
                - Arrhythmogenic
                - No benefit acutely in the setting of β-blockade
            - Phosphodiesterase inhibitor (amrinone, milrinone)
                - More commonly lower systemic vascular resistance (SVR) and BP
                - A bit less arrhythmogenic
                - May be used in the β-blocked patient
    - Pressors
        - May be needed in the hypotensive patient
        - In severe systolic dysfunction, use dopamine or concomitant dobutamine

Acute endocarditis

- Diagnosis
    - History and physical

        - Symptoms of HF, infection
        - Embolic manifestations
            - Cutaneous
            - Organ specific
        - Predisposing factors
            - Immunocompromised
            - Intravenous drug abuse
            - Prior valvular pathology (e.g., rheumatic valve disease)
    - Echocardiography
        - Transthoracic
        - Transesophageal
    - Multiple blood cultures, preferably before antibiotic therapy instituted
- Therapy
    - Targeted antibiotic therapy
        - Broad coverage until a specific organism is identified
        - Narrow coverage based on sensitivity of the organism, ideally with a bactericidal agent, with attention to local patterns of antibiotic resistance
- Surgery
    - HF—most compelling indication for immediate surgery
    - Recurrent emboli
        - Large vegetations > 10 mm may be an indication
    - Persistently positive cultures
    - Local cardiac complications
        - Abscess
        - Heart block
        - Destructive penetrating lesions
    - Timing
        - There is no need to wait for bacterial response if there is a good reason for surgery.
        - In the intermediate time frame, for example, 1 to 3 weeks, maximal inflammation of cardiac tissues may make the surgery more technically challenging.

- Cautions
  - Avoid OR if prospect for meaningful recovery is poor (e.g., large cerebral emboli or severe comorbid conditions).
  - Recent cerebrovascular events increase the risk of intraoperative hemorrhage in the brain. Delaying if possible for approximately 4 to 6 weeks may be advised.

Aortic dissection

- Symptoms
  - Chest or back pain, often searing
  - Can be the symptoms of severe focal ischemia caused by specific artery compromise
    - Acute myocardial infarction
    - CVA
    - Resting limb ischemia
    - Acute abdomen
- Exam
  - Asymmetric pulses or blood pressures
  - Murmur of aortic insufficiency
  - Signs/symptoms of focal ischemia
- Testing
  - Computed tomography (CT) with contrast
  - Magnetic resonance imaging (MRI)/magnetic resonance angiography (MRA)
  - Trans-esophageal echocardiogram (TEE)
  - Evaluate for congenital syndromes that predispose (e.g., Marfans or bicuspid aortic valve)
    - Genetic counseling of relatives
- Therapy
  - Rapid diagnosis
  - Aggressive blood pressure control
    - Initially with intravenous agents
    - Target systolic BP of 110 mm Hg
    - β-Blockers are the foundation of all therapy

        - Lower the dP/dt hence shear forces, as well as BP
        - In active bronchospastic disease, consider the nondihydropyridine calcium blockers (e.g., diltiazem)
    - Surgical consultation
    - Evaluate and treat any specific organ complication (e.g., exploratory laparotomy for acute abdomen)
- Type A
    - Involving ascending aorta
    - Surgical emergency
        - Mortality approximately 2% per hour
    - Root repair possibly with aortic valve replacement/resuspension
    - Care and follow-up of the remaining aortic involvement as in type B
- Type B
    - Not involving ascending aorta
    - Medical therapy
        - Aggressive blood pressure control
        - Assessment of collateral damage
            - Rigorous follow-up schedule to follow size of aorta
    - Role of stent grafts remain to be determined

Hypertensive emergencies

- Elevated BP, usually greater than 180/110, in the setting of end organ damage
    - Cardiovascular
        - Congestive heart failure
        - Ischemia
        - Aortic dissection
    - CNS
        - Encephalopathy
        - Stroke
    - Ocular
        - Papilledema
        - Hemorrhage/retinopathy

- Renal
  - Acute tubular necrosis (ATN)
  - Rapidly progressive glomerulonephritis (RPGN)
  - Cortical necrosis
- Hematologic
  - Microangiopathic hemolytic anemia occasionally with thrombocytopenia

- Therapy
  - Intravenous titratable agents
    - β-Blockers
    - Labetalol
    - Nicardipine
    - Nitroprusside
  - Goal
    - No greater than 25% reduction in first hour
    - To 160/100 in the next 2 to 6 hours
    - To normal over the next 24 to 48 hours
    - Tighter control needed
      - Aortic dissection
      - BP control for lytic therapy
    - Less stringent reduction
      - Ischemic CVA
  - Caution
    - Adding/escalating therapy before steady state of current agents can produce subsequent hypotension
    - Continue intravenous control until signs and symptoms of end organ damage controlled or stabilized

Pulmonary embolus

- History and exam—nonspecific
  - High index of suspicion in hospitalized/susceptible patients needed
- Diagnosis
  - CT angiography
  - Ventilation/perfusion scanning

- Therapy
  - Immediate anticoagulation with a heparin product
    - Low molecular weight heparin attractive—no titration needed—avoid in severe renal dysfunction. Unfractionated heparin and fondaparinux are acceptable options.
    - Anticoagulate while waiting for diagnostic testing
  - Thrombolytic therapy
    - With hemodynamical compromise
    - In those with low risk of bleeding (i.e., no contraindications to lytic therapy) and highest risk
      - Patients who appear ill, with marked dyspnea, anxiety, and low oxygen saturation
      - Elevated troponin, indicating right ventricular microinfarction
      - Right ventricular dysfunction on echocardiography
      - Right ventricular enlargement on chest CT
    - Major contraindications to lytic therapy
      - Intracranial disease
      - Uncontrolled hypertension at presentation
      - Recent major bleeding, surgery, or trauma
  - Mechanical therapy (e.g., embolectomy)
    - Only in rare situations with severe compromise
      - Inability to receive thrombolytics
      - There is not enough time to use thrombolytics
  - IVC filter
    - Anticoagulation contraindicated
    - Severe bleeding from anticoagulation
    - Recurrent emboli despite appropriate anticoagulation
    - Start conventional anticoagulation when bleeding risk resolves
  - Start warfarin immediately

Acute valvular lesions in the cardiac intensive care unit (CCU) setting

- Aortic stenosis (AS)

    - Avoid vasodilators and an excessive drop in BP in the setting of critical AS.
    - Atrial fibrillation with rapid ventricular response (AF-RVR) is poorly tolerated.
    - I personally favor β-blockade in these patients.
- MR
    - Be mindful of the etiology regarding specific therapy
        - Acute myocardial infarction/ischemia
        - Chordal rupture
        - Destructive endocarditis
    - In severe acute MR, afterload reduction, especially with an intraaortic balloon (IABP), may be a temporizing procedure while preparing for OR
- AI
    - Be mindful of the etiology regarding specific therapy.
    - IABP is contraindicated.
- MS
    - Remember that the pressures the lungs "see" are higher than the LVEDP by approximately the mean mitral gradient. A pulmonary vein pressure of 25 (pulmonary edema range) is seen with an LVEDP of 15 (minimally increased) if the mean gradient is 10 (severe MS).
    - AF-RVR is poorly tolerated because of the decrease in diastolic filling time.

Arrhythmias

- Diagnosis
    - Complexes that are *different* from the baseline complexes are ventricular tachycardia (VT) until proven otherwise.
        - There is a 75% likelihood in the absence of structural heart disease.
        - There is a 95% likelihood in the presence of structural heart disease.
        - In a single lead strip, a "narrow complex tachycardia" may be wide on a 12-lead ECG (and vice versa)!

- Always assess for and treat exacerbating factors.
  - Myocardial ischemia
  - Hypoxemia
  - Acidosis
  - Hypokalemia, hypomagnesemia, hypocalcemia
  - Respiratory distress
- Always take the time to get a 12-lead ECG of the arrhythmia in the absence of hemodynamic collapse

- Therapy
  - The appropriate therapy for any hemodynamically compromising tachycardia is *synchronized* DC cardioversion (ventricular fibrillation is the only indication for an unsynchronized shock).
  - Amiodarone is useful for severe tachycardias regardless of mechanism (VT vs. SVT).
  - In AF-RVR, multiple agents are often needed.
  - Diltiazem based.
    - Intravenous bolus followed by an infusion
  - β-Blocker based
    - Serial intravenous doses of a β-blocker versus a continuous infusion of esmolol
  - In severe structural heart disease especially ischemia and HF, β-blockers are preferred as a first-line therapy

Assist devices

- Intraaortic balloon counterpulsation (IABP)
  - Potentially useful in almost all causes of hypotension and shock as well as myocardial ischemic syndromes
    - Refractory unstable angina
    - Ischemic malignant arrhythmias
    - Impending infarction
    - Acute myocardial infarction
    - Refractory ventricular failure
    - Complications of acute myocardial infarction (i.e., acute MR or VSD or papillary muscle rupture)

    - Cardiogenic shock
    - Support for diagnostic, percutaneous revascularization, and interventional procedures
  - Contraindications
    - Severe peripheral vascular disease
    - Significant aortic valve regurgitation
    - Aortic dissection
    - Tortuous or aneurysmal descending thoracic or abdominal aorta
    - Inability to be anticoagulated (relative contraindication)
    - Uncontrolled sepsis
    - Uncontrolled bleeding disorder
- Ventricular assist devices and extracorporeal membrane oxygenation
  - Used in situations where there is a critical decline in LV or RV function to the point of active end organ deterioration from hypoperfusion.
  - Requires a team familiar with the advanced techniques of insertion and more importantly ongoing monitoring of these devices, usually a "quaternary care" center.
  - Often serves as a bridge to cardiac transplantation.
  - Most of the contraindications for IABP apply here as well.

Therapeutic hypothermia

- Mild therapeutic hypothermia indicated in unconscious adult patients with spontaneous circulation after out-of-hospital VF cardiac arrest.
- Likely also useful in those with spontaneous circulation after out-of-hospital cardiac arrest from a nonshockable rhythm or in-hospital cardiac arrest.
- Procedure
  - Intubate and mechanically ventilate.
  - Place arterial line for monitoring. Maintain a mean pressure of approximately 90 mm Hg.

  - Obtain baseline laboratories, ABG, blood cultures.
  - As cooling is instituted, sedate with intravenous midazolam and fentanyl infusions, as well as paralysis with cisatracurium as needed to suppress shivering are used with appropriate monitoring.
  - Insert a rectal probe or pulmonary catheter to monitor core temperature.
  - Cool to 32°C to 34°C, in less than 8 hours, ideally less than 6 hours, after the arrest.
  - Start with a rapid intravenous infusion of ice-cold 0.9% saline or Ringer's lactate (30 ml/kg).
  - Devices are commercially available to facilitate ongoing cooling that surround the head, torso, and extremities with cooling "outerwear." These actively regulate the temperature.
  - Stop the paralytic when the temperature reaches 36°C.
  - Terminate active cooling after 24 hours, passively rewarm over the next 24 hours.
- Common effects
  - Increased SVR
  - Diuresis
  - Hypophosphatemia, hypokalemia, hypomagnesemia, and hypocalcemia
  - Hyperglycemia
  - Tachyarrhythmias and bradyarrhythmias
  - Impaired coagulation
  - Immunosuppression
  - Decreased drug clearance (especially sedatives)
- Contraindications
  - Major head trauma—if clinical suspicion for possible head injury with arrest, consider a noncontrast head CT to rule out intracerebral hemorrhage
  - Recent major surgery within 14 days
  - Systemic infection/sepsis

- Patients in coma from other causes (drug intoxication, pre-existing coma before arrest)
- Patients with a known bleeding diathesis or with active ongoing bleeding

4 ■ Heart Failure

Paul J. Mather, MD
Stephen Olex, MD

Definition

As defined by the American Heart Association (AHA) and the American College of Cardiology (ACC), heart failure "is a complex clinical syndrome that can result from any structural or functional cardiac disorder that impairs the ability of the ventricle to fill or eject blood."

Epidemiology

Heart failure is a major and growing health problem. There are approximately 5.2 million patients in the United States with heart failure and 23 million patients worldwide. The prevalence of heart failure increases rapidly with age, and it is projected that the prevalence in the United States will increase. In 2004, there were over 1 million hospital stays in the United States that listed congestive heart failure as the first diagnosis at discharge, and heart failure is the leading cause of admission for patients greater than 65 years old.

Approach to the Patient with Suspected Heart Failure

History

Shortness of breath, dyspnea on exertion, and paroxysmal nocturnal dyspnea suggest left-sided heart failure but are nonspecific. Orthopnea is our best history correlate of increased pulmonary capillary wedge pressure with a sensitivity of almost 90%. Peripheral edema and ascites can suggest heart failure but can also be seen in many other disease states. Fatigue and weakness at rest and with exertion are common manifestations of heart failure. Chest pain may represent true angina in ischemic heart disease but can also occur without significant coronary disease. Complaints referable to right-sided heart failure or decreased splanchnic flow initially may seem gastrointestinal in nature and may include abdominal pain, nausea, vomiting, and abdominal fullness and may be confused with gastrointestinal pathology, especially in younger patients. Historical elements associated with decreased cardiac output are less specific than those associated with elevated filling pressures. Fatigue may be present but has numerous other heart failure or nonheart failure causes. Altered mentation in the form of difficulty concentrating may be a sign of low cardiac output and may be more noticed by a patient's family.

Physical Examination

In addition to a full set of vital signs, including orthostatic blood pressure, the examination of the patient with suspected heart failure includes the following elements. An assessment should be performed as to the presence of intravascular volume overload that most reliably takes the form of jugular venous distension at rest or is evident with abdominal compression in the hepatojugular reflux. In the majority of chronic heart failure patients, elevations in jugular venous pressures correlate well with elevations of pulmonary capillary wedge pressure in the absence of pulmonary disease. A laterally displaced and enlarged point of maximal impulse suggests a dilated ventricle. The presence of valvular disease on examination suggested by pathologic murmurs suggests the possibility of structural heart disease. Auscultation revealing a pathologic S3 highly raises the suspicion for heart failure. An S4 may be heard in an ischemic or stiff ventricle (hypertension, aortic stenosis, hypertrophic cardiomyopathy [HCM]) and also may be heard in patients with significant systolic dysfunction. The fusing of an S3 and S4 at high heart rates is known as a summation gallop and has a characteristic rhythm. The lungs may reveal the presence of rales, an insensitive finding in chronic systolic heart failure because of lymphatic compensation. The examination includes palpation for an enlarged or pulsatile liver that suggests right-sided volume overload or significant TR. The presence of edema (in the extremities, scrotum, sacrum, and abdominal wall) and ascites may be seen but are not specific to heart failure.

Low cardiac output may take the form of a narrow proportional blood pressure; a pulse pressure/systolic blood pressure less than 25% has been suggested to reflect a cardiac index less than 2.2 L/min. Cool extremities, Cheyne-Stokes breathing, and agitation can occur with low cardiac output as well as a characteristic pattern of briefly appearing to be sleeping then jerking awake. In general, assessments of perfusion are not as accurate as those of volume overload.

The Electrocardiogram

The electrocardiogram should be examined for clues to the possible presence of structural heart disease such as atrial and ventricular arrhythmias, conduction abnormalities, atrial enlargement, ventricular hypertrophy, evidence of active myocardial ischemia/injury, or evidence of myocardial infarction.

The chest X-ray (CXR) may show cardiomegaly, left atrial enlargement, signs of vascular redistribution such as cephalization, interstitial edema, which takes the form of peribronchial cuffing, Kerley B lines, large hila with indistinct margins, alveolar edema (fluffy infiltrates in the hilum with a "batwing" appearance), and pleural effusions.

Computed Tomography Scan

Classic computed tomography (CT) scan findings in congestive heart failure are ground glass opacities, smooth septal thickening, pleural effusions or thickening of the fissures, vascular redistribution, peribronchial vascular interstitial thickening, and increased vascular caliber. These findings initially can appear nonspecific and can be confused with infectious etiologies or an interstitial process if a high index of suspicion for heart failure is not maintained.

Laboratory Studies

Laboratory studies are generally nonspecific; common manifestations include anemia, renal insufficiency, mild hyponatremia, and relatively minor elevations of troponin. Also, a high blood urea nitrogen/creatinine ratio is common. Liver function abnormalities can include a pattern of predominantly cholestasis from passive congestion of the liver during right-sided heart failure or a moderate transaminitis from low forward flow to the liver. Hypoalbuminemia and decreased low-density lipoprotein (LDL) from a catabolic state can also be seen in heart failure patients. An anion gap metabolic acidosis from lactic acidosis can occur with low cardiac output. The natriuretic peptides brain natriuretic peptide (BNP) and NT-pro BNP are released from ventricular myocytes and are elevated in heart failure. Generally, patients with heart failure as a cause of their dyspnea will have BNP values above 400 pg/ml, whereas a value less than 100 pg/ml has a high negative predictive value for heart failure. Natriuretic peptide levels may be increased in renal failure in the absence of clinically diagnosed heart failure and are of limited use in this setting. It has been suggested that a cutoff BNP level of 200 pg/ml should be used for patients with renal insufficiency and an estimated glomerular filtration rate (GFR) less than 60 ml/min/1.73 m^2. Both natriuretic peptides increase with age, with data suggesting the need for different cutoffs for NT-pro BNP depending on the patient's age. Cutoffs values of NT-pro-BNP values of 450, 900, and 1,800 pg/ml have been shown to yield a sensitivity of 90% and specificity of 84% for diagnosing heart failure in patients < 50, 50–75, and greater than 75 years of age. BNP and NT-pro-BNP levels may not correlate to elevated left-sided filling pressures in the intensive care unit, especially in patients with renal dysfunction. In addition, the natriuretic peptides can be elevated in patients with sepsis. BNP and NT-pro BNP can also be elevated in pulmonary embolism as well as cor pulmonale in the absence of elevations in pulmonary capillary wedge pressure. False negatives can occur in obesity, and the assay is not clinically useful in the setting of nesiritide administration. The levels can be chronically elevated in a currently well-compensated chronic heart failure patient.

Echocardiogram

The two-dimensional echocardiogram with Doppler flow is central to the evaluation of a patient with suspected heart failure and can identify structural or functional abnormalities of the left and right ventricles, atria, pericardium, valves, or vascular structures that may be causing a patient's symptoms or the clinical syndrome of heart failure.

Nuclear Imaging

The diagnosis of heart failure may be made by a calculated or estimated ejection fraction on a nuclear stress test or by use of a Multi Gated Acquisition Scan.

Cardiac Catheterization

The diagnosis of heart failure may be suggested or made during a left heart catheterization and ventriculogram or a right heart catheterization documenting low cardiac output, high filling pressures, or both.

Differential Diagnosis

Pulmonary disorders such as interstitial lung disease, pulmonary embolism, pulmonary hypertension, asthma, and chronic obstructive pulmonary disease are clinical entities that are in the differential diagnosis. Heart failure can resemble angina with chest pain and dyspnea on exertion. General deconditioning and debilitation are in the differential as well. Edema can be seen in many states, including renal failure, hepatic failure, and hypoalbuminemia from nephrotic syndrome, cirrhosis, malnutrition, and protein losing enteropathies. Dyspnea and tachypnea in a patient with possible heart failure can also be seen in anxiety/hyperventilation syndromes, and the fatigue and lethargy can be seen in depression.

Evaluation of the Patient with Newly Diagnosed Heart Failure

History

In a patient with newly diagnosed heart failure, baseline symptoms as well as functional capacity should be elicited. An assessment of functional capacity according to New York Heart Association (NYHA) class should be performed (Table 4.1), as the NYHA class is a tool that can be used to follow a patient's symptoms as well as one that has therapeutic and prognostic implications. An assessment of the patient's symptoms, including dyspnea on exertion, edema, fatigue, paroxysmal nocturnal dyspnea, and orthopnea, should be undertaken. Inquiry should be made about presyncope and syncope, which may be related to overmedication and/or overdiuresis (presyncope/syncope) or related to malignant ventricular arrhythmias (syncope). The patient should be asked about any possible ischemic symptoms, sleep disordered breathing, or other clues to an etiology (for a more complete discussion, see page 65). A full medical history is important to uncover comorbidities that may affect the course and treatment. An inquiry should be made as to symptoms suggestive of embolic events. A thorough review of the patient's medication list is in order to look for medications that may be contraindicated in heart failure.

Physical Examination

The physical examination helps to assess severity of heart failure and is used to assess the presence and degree of intravascular volume overload, the presence of left- and right-sided heart failure, and the presence of hypoperfusion (refer to the previous section on Physical Examination in Diagnosis).

Laboratory Evaluation

A baseline basic metabolic panel, magnesium, hepatic function tests, complete blood count with differential, fasting lipids, thyroid function, and urinalysis should be performed. Additional directed

Table 4.1 New York Heart Association Classification by Symptoms

NYHA Class	Patient Symptoms
Class I	No limitation of physical activity. Ordinary physical activity does not cause undue fatigue, palpitation, or dyspnea (shortness of breath).
Class II	Slight limitation of physical activity. Comfortable at rest, but ordinary physical activity results in fatigue, palpitation, or dyspnea.
Class III	IIIA: Marked limitation of physical activity. Comfortable at rest, but less than ordinary activity causes fatigue, palpitation, or dyspnea. IIIB: Marked limitation of physical activity. Comfortable at rest, but minimal exertion causes fatigue, palpitation, or dyspnea.
Class IV	Unable to carry out any physical activity without discomfort. Symptoms of cardiac insufficiency are present at rest. If any physical activity is undertaken, discomfort is increased.

Source: Adapted from Adams KF, Lindenfeld J, Arnold JMO, et al Executive Summary: HFSA 2006 Comprehensive Heart Failure Practice Guidelines. *Journal of Cardiac Failure* 2006: 12(1).

laboratory studies should be performed if needed, as described in the etiology section later here.

Electrocardiogram

The electrocardiogram (ECG) should be used to assess underlying rhythm, conduction system, and complex on ECG (QRS) duration (QRS duration has bearing on if a patient will be a candidate for a biventricular pacemaker among other factors). The ECG can also be used to assess for atrial enlargement, ventricular hypertrophy, and active ischemia and evidence of prior or current myocardial infarction. In dilated cardiomyopathy, the ECG may show left atrial or biatrial enlargement (in sinus rhythm), prominent voltage caused by left ventricular hypertrophy (LVH) or dilation, first-degree atrioventricular (AV) delay, left anterior fascicular block (LAFB), left bundle branch block (LBBB), less commonly right bundle branch block (RBBB), intraventricular conduction delay (IVCD), pathologic Q waves mimicking anterior or inferior myocardial infarction (may occur in ischemic or nonischemic cardiomyopathy), diffuse T-wave abnormalities, and supraventricular or ventricular arrhythmias. In restrictive cardiomyopathy, the ECG is usually abnormal and can show biatrial enlargement and left, right, or biventricular hypertrophy. Infiltrative cardiomyopathies may have low voltage on electrocardiogram combined with hypertrophy on echocardiogram. In amyloidosis, it is common to have low voltage and a pattern simulating an old inferior or anterior infarction, as well as disease of the conduction system. HCM most frequently demonstrates LVH on the electrocardiogram. Abnormal Q waves may be present as well as commonly primary and secondary T-wave abnormalities, including giant inverted T waves. The electrocardiogram in diastolic dysfunction may show left atrial enlargement, LVH, or possibly supraventricular arrhythmias.

A posterior to anterior (PA) and lateral chest X-ray should be performed in patients with heart failure to examine heart size, detect fluid overload, and uncover the coexistence of other disorders including pulmonary disease.

Assessment of Cardiac Structure and Function

Elements from the history, physical, electrocardiogram, and imaging studies can help to assess a patient's cardiac structure and function. The two-dimensional echocardiogram with Doppler flow studies is central to determining a patient's cardiac structure and function and allows the physician to characterize the primary abnormality as myocardial, valvular, or pericardial. It is useful to classify heart failure if myocardial as systolic or diastolic, as this has implications for etiologic mechanism as well as management; most patients with systolic heart failure will have abnormalities of diastolic function. Determination can be made by echocardiogram if the heart failure is right sided, left sided, or biventricular. Regional wall motion of the left and right ventricles, ventricular wall thickness, and ventricular geometry can be assessed, as can the atria, pericardium, valves, and vascular structures. It is useful to classify the cardiomyopathy as dilated, hypertrophic, or restrictive, consistent with arrhythmogenic right ventricular cardiomyopathy, or as an unclassified cardiomyopathy. These classifications help to narrow the etiologic differential and have implications for therapy. The dilated cardiomyopathy phenotype is often viewed as the "final common pathway" of various different types of myocardial disease and is the most common phenotype. The differential of dilated cardiomyopathy is extensive; potential causes are listed in Table 4.2.

Etiology

Elements of the history, physical, laboratory tests, electrocardiogram, echocardiogram, coronary angiography, imaging studies, and even at times endomyocardial biopsy are used to help uncover the etiology of a patient's heart failure. A search for an etiology should include an assessment for coronary artery disease (CAD) and hypertension (HTN), as these are strong risk factors for heart failure. Inquiry should be made regarding a history of hyperlipidemia, diabetes, peripheral vascular disease, and valvular heart disease. The presence of thyroid excess or deficiency should be assessed on history and physical as well as the likelihood of sleep-disordered breathing. An assessment for cardiac toxin exposure such as alcohol, cocaine, amphetamines, supplements, anabolic steroids, and chemotherapeutic agents such as anthracyclines and trastuzumab is important, as is a pregnancy history with correlation of how symptoms relate temporally. Assessment of the possibility of viral, bacterial, or parasitic disease by history and physical is needed; the diagnosis of Chagas disease should be considered for patients in or from endemic regions. Further inquiries and assessments should be made as to a history of mediastinal radiation, myopathy, rheumatic fever, heart murmur, congenital disease, or any recent major psychosocial stressors and signs or symptoms of tachyarrhythmias. Takotsubo cardiomyopathy is a recently described entity of acute cardiomyopathy secondary to profound

Table 4.2 Causes of Dilated Cardiomyopathy

Ischemia

Hypertension

Valvular disease

Tachycardia mediated

Idiopathic

Peripartum

Familial

Infection
- Bacterial—Streptococci-rheumatic fever
- Viral—HIV, adenovirus, coxsackievirus, hepatitis C
- Rickettsial
- Spirochetal
- Fungal
- Parasitic—Chagas disease (Trypanosomiasis)

Toxins
- Alcohol
- Cocaine
- Amphetamines
- Anabolic steroids

Medications
- Antichemotherapeutics—Anthracyclines, Trastuzumab
- Infiltrative disorders
- Amyloidosis
- Hemochromatosis
- Sarcoidosis

Nutritional deficiencies—protein, thiamine, selenium

Sleep apnea

Left ventricular noncompaction

Autoimmune/collagen vascular disease
- Systemic lupus erythematosus
- Scleroderma
- Rheumatoid arthritis

Endomyocardial disorders
- Loffler's endocarditis
- Endomyocardial fibrosis

Hypersensitivity myocarditis

Endocrinologic disease
- Hypothyroidism
- Hyperthyroidism
- Diabetes mellitus
- Growth hormone deficiency or excess
- Pheochromocytoma
- Arrhythmogenic right ventricular dysplasia/cardiomyopathy

End-stage renal disease associated

Neuromuscular diseases

Electrolyte related

Mitochondrial cardiomyopathies

Source: Adapted from Fuster F, O'Rourke RA, Walsh R, Poole-Wilson P eds. *Hurst's The Heart 12th edition.* China. McGraw-Hill. 2008.

psychological stress that preferentially involves the distal left ventricle causing "apical ballooning." The disease occurs in the absence of atherosclerotic disease and is rapidly reversible.

A family history of CAD, sudden cardiac death, and cardiomyopathy (up to 20% of idiopathic dilated cardiomyopathies are familial) should be uncovered. Baseline basic metabolic panel, magnesium, hepatic function tests, complete blood count with differential, fasting lipids, urinalysis, and thyroid function tests are indicated. If the etiology is not obvious, it is reasonable to focus on those diagnoses that have potential for improvement if treated. Serum ferritin and transferrin may be useful to uncover hemochromatosis as if causative then treatment may improve left ventricular function. HIV should be tested for those that are high risk, although usually patients will have other manifestations of the disease if this is the cause of the heart failure. An assessment for the risk and presence of hepatitis C may be useful, as this virus has been associated with myocarditis and cardiomyopathy. Assessment for the possibility of pheochromocytoma, Cushing's disease, and autoimmune/collagen vascular disease should be performed by history and physical, and more directed investigation should be undertaken if these diagnoses are suspected. The diagnoses of sarcoidosis or amyloidosis should be investigated in certain clinical settings. Measurement of viral titers in new-onset heart failure is generally low yield with uncertain therapeutic implications.

Assessment for CAD

Coronary artery disease is the most common cause of heart failure in the United States and is the cause for approximately two thirds of cases of heart failure in this country. Most patients with left ventricular dysfunction should have an evaluation for CAD that commonly includes coronary angiography. There may be a role for cardiac magnetic resonance imaging (MRI) or CT scanning in the assessment for CAD, although their use for this purpose is not well defined. For a full discussion of the role of assessment for CAD in a patient with heart failure please, see the ACC/AHA guidelines.

Myocarditis

Myocarditis is histologically defined as inflammation of the myocardium with cardiac myocyte injury. Myocarditis has many different causes, and many cases remain idiopathic. Although many causes go undiagnosed, care should be made to exclude potentially treatable specific causes in the initial evaluation including giant cell myocarditis. Common causes include viral/coxsackie B, acute rheumatic fever, Lyme disease, chemotherapeutic induced (doxorubicin/anthracycline), Chagas, and peripartum cardiomyopathy among others. Myocarditis typically presents as an acute or fulminant illness with new heart failure and dilated cardiomyopathy and should be considered in such patients but may also present in other ways. Treatment is controversial, and the routine use of immunosuppressive therapies is not recommended; an endomyocardial biopsy may be considered.

Role of Endomyocardial Biopsy

An endomyocardial biopsy is not routinely recommended in all cases of new-onset left-ventricular dysfunction. It may be considered in patients who have a rapid progression of their heart failure or deterioration of their ventricular function in spite of appropriate medical therapy. A biopsy should be considered in patients who may have myocardial infiltrative processes, including amyloidosis, sarcoidosis, and hemochromatosis, as well as in patients with malignant arrhythmias out of proportion to the degree of heart failure in which sarcoidosis and giant cell myocarditis would be considerations. For a full discussion of the role of endomyocardial biopsy in a patient with cardiomyopathy, see the ACC/AHA guidelines and the AHA/American College of Cardiology Foundation (ACCF)/European Society of Cardiology (ESC) scientific statement.

Evaluation and Treatment of the Patient With Acute Decompensated Heart Failure

General Principles

Approximately 1 million patients are hospitalized each year with acute decompensated heart failure (ADHF), and within 30 days, approximately 20% are rehospitalized for the same diagnosis. It is the leading cause of hospitalization in patients older than 65 years. After a patient is hospitalized for acute decompensated heart failure, the disease typically follows a different natural history course with higher mortality. Unlike chronic heart failure, there are fewer data to guide therapy and treatment is based on consensus opinion and the best available research.

Diagnosis

The diagnosis of heart failure is based primarily on signs and symptoms. For a complete discussion of the diagnosis of heart failure, see the section entitled Evaluation of the Patient With Suspected Heart Failure.

Natriuretic Peptides in ADHF

If the diagnosis is uncertain from clinical grounds, the measurement of natriuretic peptides may offer help in making the diagnosis of heart failure or help in ruling it out; however, serial BNP measurements are not recommended in the setting of ADHF. See the section on Evaluation of the Patient with Suspected Heart Failure for a more complete discussion of the diagnosis of heart failure and natriuretic peptides. BNP helps to make the diagnosis and has prognostic implications as levels correlate with in-hospital mortality in decompensated heart failure from systolic dysfunction as well as in those decompensations with a preserved ejection fraction. Furthermore, there is evidence that discharge BNP and change in BNP from admission to discharge are independent predictors for poor outcomes after an acute decompensated heart failure admission.

Precipitants of Decompensation

It is imperative to look for causes of a patient's decompensation to help prevent future exacerbations and also look for potential addressable causes that may improve a patient's clinical status. Nonadherence to diet or medication is a common cause of decompensation. The presence of cardiac ischemia, progressive myocyte dysfunction, worsening valvular disease, arrhythmias (both tachyarrhythmias and bradyarrhythmias), uncontrolled hypertension, or possibly renal artery stenosis can all precipitate decompensation. A patient that has recently had their β-blocker initiated or titrated may have a decompensation on this basis. The presence of other illnesses, including pulmonary disease, thyroid disorders, or anemia, can also cause decompensation as well. Drug use (especially stimulants and cocaine), alcohol, and anabolic steroids can also be associated with decompensation in a stable patient, as can therapeutic medications that are known to be cardiotoxic. Urinary retention or worsening renal function can contribute to volume overload as well resulting in decompensation. Drugs that may cause decompensation include non-steroidal anti-inflammatory drugs (NSAIDs) by increasing sodium retention and increasing plasma volume and negative inotropes such as nondihydropyridine calcium channel blockers. The etiology of the decompensation may be iatrogenic volume overload such as commonly occurs with blood product transfusion or intravenous fluid administration that can occur in the hospital or during surgery. The addition of AV nodal blocking agents in a patient with a right ventricular pacemaker may cause decompensation by inducing dyssynchrony if this significantly increases the percentage of right ventricular pacing.

Characterization of Decompensation

It is useful to characterize the patient's decompensation by assessing both their volume status and their perfusion status. The patient's volume status can classically be labeled as "wet" or "dry," and the perfusion status as "cold" or "warm" (see the History and Physical Examination of the section entitled Evaluation of the Patient With Suspected Heart Failure for a discussion on diagnosing volume and perfusion status). With these two variables, the patient can be placed efficiently into one of four groups: warm and wet, cold and wet, cold and dry, and warm and dry. Patients who have recent dietary indiscretion and/or medication nonadherence as the etiology for their decompensation will commonly fit into the "warm and wet" category, the most common subgroup of decompensation. The majority of ADHF patients has systemic hypertension and routinely has preserved ejection fraction, and most will have evidence of volume overload. Patients with hypotension, markedly reduced ejection fraction, and symptoms of a low flow state are in the minority. Although a physician's bedside assessment of perfusion does not correlate well to invasive measurements of cardiac index, patients assessed by physicians to have decreased cardiac output have a worse prognosis than those assessed to have better perfusion. Wet and warm patients have a twofold greater risk of death and wet, and cold patients have a 2.5-fold greater risk of death compared with dry and warm patients at 1 year. These profiles may be used not only for prognosis but also to guide therapy and monitor progress during a patient's admission for ADHF. If mild to moderate volume overload is the problem with an adequate cardiac output ("warm and wet"), then many times the patient can be "tuned up" with intravenous diuretics and may become euvolemic relatively quickly. On the other end of the spectrum, a patient with a low cardiac index from acute myocardial infarction, myocarditis, or end-stage heart failure of any etiology may fit into the "cold and dry" or "cold and wet" category. Patients may need inotropic or mechanical support to improve their cardiac output and preserve their end organ function.

Treatment

Goals of the Admission for ADHF

Per the Heart Failure Society of America (HFSA), goals of the admission for ADHF includes identification of the etiology of the patient's heart failure and treatment of any modifiable contributing factors (a full list shown previously in Precipitants of Decompensation), including notably arrhythmia, ischemia, nonadherence to diet and medications, as well as identification of those patients who may be candidates for revascularization or surgical correction of valvular lesions. Euvolemia and an adequate cardiac output should be goals of the admission if either one is not present initially. Another goal involves identification of those patients who may be candidates for orthotopic heart transplant or need mechanical hemodynamic support and those that are end stage with no further options that may be candidates for home inotropic use and/or end-of-life discussions. The admission typically provides an opportunity for optimization of the patient's outpatient oral regimen. The admission also provides an opportunity for education concerning the seriousness of the patient's disease, as well as diet, medication, and exercise. Instructions and means for the patient checking their weight at home should be provided; patients may benefit from initiation of a disease management program in which they have the added support and guidance of nurses trained in heart failure.

General Measures

A full set of laboratory tests, including a complete blood count, basic metabolic panel, magnesium, hepatic function tests, and urinalysis, is indicated, as well as an EKG and chest X-ray. Renal function should be monitored at least daily as part of a basic metabolic panel as well as electrolytes, including sodium, potassium, and magnesium. It is generally accepted that potassium should be maintained at greater than 4 mEq/L and magnesium at greater than 2 mg/dl. Patients who are diuresing greater than 2 liters per day may need more than daily electrolytes to ensure that there are no abnormalities, including especially hypokalemia. Serial troponin should be checked if the patient is suspected of having a myocardial infarction. It is reasonable to check an initial troponin, regardless of the concern for myocardial ischemia, as there is evidence that an elevated troponin, regardless of the patient's etiology for their heart failure, is predictive of increased in-hospital mortality during a heart failure exacerbation. A patient's vital signs should be monitored closely, including orthostatic blood pressure. Cardiac monitoring should generally be instituted with ADHF, and oxygen should be administered only if the patient is hypoxemic. Assessment of the patient's signs and symptoms of congestion and decreased perfusion should be assessed regularly (at least daily) and compared and reconciled with the other available data. Accurate intakes and outputs should be measured; placement of a Foley catheter may be required for more acutely ill patients. Daily weights are a useful adjunct in tracking a patient's volume status and should be performed each morning after voiding if possible. Patients in severe respiratory distress may need noninvasive positive pressure ventilation or possibly mechanical ventilation. Patients who decompensated acutely because of an atrial arrhythmia and are in severe pulmonary edema because of their arrhythmia may need emergent cardioversion. Also, patients with acute decompensation because of or complicated by malignant ventricular rhythms should be treated according to contemporary Advanced Cardiac Life Support (ACLS) guidelines.

Diuretics

Intravenous furosemide, torsemide, or bumetanide are all useful agents for treating the volume overload that can be associated with ADHF. Initial and maximum doses are seen in Table 4.3; higher initial doses may be needed depending on factors, including renal function and home dose. The dosage can generally be doubled if there is insufficient response after administration. If a patient is not adequately diuresing with 120 mg of furosemide, it may be reasonable to add a thiazide diuretic such as metolazone to diurese further the patient rather than increase the furosemide dose to minimize adverse reactions such as ototoxicity. Sodium and fluid restriction should be instituted in those patients in whom there is a level of diuretic resistance. A continuous intravenous infusion may be used, and some data show that this approach may be more beneficial with fewer side effects than bolus dosing, although this subject is not well defined. The effect of diuresis is variable, and some patients will be hypotensive with decreased cardiac output with diuretics, especially if fluid is leaving the intravascular space much faster than interstitial fluid is moving into the intravascular space. Other patients may have increased cardiac output secondary to decreased filling pressures, causing decreased myocyte stretch and decreased functional valvular regurgitation. Common adverse effects of diuretics include worsening renal function, hypotension, electrolyte disturbances such as hypokalemia and hypomagnesemia, cardiac arrhythmias from electrolyte disturbances, particularly in the setting of digitalis, and neurohormonal activation.

Renal Dysfunction in ADHF

Renal dysfunction in ADHF is a common phenomenon of likely multifactorial etiology that is associated with increased mortality. If renal function worsens despite volume overload, then diuresis

Table 4.3 Dosing of Commonly Used Diuretics for Acute Decompensated Heart Failure

Drug	Type	Dosing (Bolus)	Dosing (Continuous Infusion)
Furosemide	Loop	Typical doses 40- to 80-mg intravenous push, generally if more diuresis needed after dose of 120 mg needed may add Metolazone, 160- to 200-mg maximum single dose	Continuous infusion—40-mg intravenous load, then 10- to 40-mg/h infusion, doses of 80 to 160 mg/h have been used, but increased risk of side effects
Torsemide	Loop	Typical doses 10- to 40-mg intravenous push, maximum single dose 100 to 200 mg intravenously	Continuous infusion—20-mg intravenous load then 5 to 20 mg/h
Bumetanide	Loop	Typical dose 1- to 2-mg intravenous push, maximum single dose 4- to 8-mg intravenously	Continuous infusion 1-mg intravenous load then 0.5 to 2 mg/h
Metolazone	Thiazide	Typical dose 2.5- to 5-mg PO QD to BID 0.5 hour before loop diuretic, maximum daily dose 20 mg	N/A

Source: Adapted from Adams KF, Lindenfeld J, Arnold JMO, et al Executive Summary: HFSA 2006 Comprehensive Heart Failure Practice Guidelines. *Journal of Cardiac Failure* 2006: 12(1).

generally can be continued if the rise in creatinine is not significant. If relative or absolute hypovolemia is suspected, then a reduction or discontinuation of a patient's diuretic or vasodilator therapy should be considered. In the setting of worsening renal function, it may be reasonable to monitor hemodynamics invasively or start intravenous inotropes if the patient appears low output. Patients with significant renal dysfunction over baseline, which is probably caused by multiple mechanisms, will at times improve with diuretics. In patients resistant to diuretics because of significant renal impairment (either acute or chronic) and adequate cardiac output, then mechanical means of fluid removal by ultrafiltration should be considered. Also, if diuresis occurs but there is persistent congestion at an unacceptable level of worsening renal function and azotemia, then mechanical fluid removal may be needed.

Ultrafiltration

Potential advantages of mechanical fluid removal include decreased activation of neurohormonal mechanisms, more controlled fluid removal, and no effect on serum electrolytes. There are data to suggest the safety and efficacy of ultrafiltration in the setting of ADHF although the body of data is relatively small. Most studies used a peripherally inserted device that does not require central access. Peripheral ultrafiltration is not universally available.

Morphine

Morphine helps with preload reduction, helps relieve some of the anxiety and sympathetic drive associated with pulmonary edema, and is useful if the patient also has probable or definite ischemic chest discomfort.

Vasodilators

Vasodilators such as nitroglycerin, nitroprusside, and nesiritide may be considered in advanced heart failure patients with ADHF that have persistent severe heart failure despite treatment with diuretics and oral medications. For dosing, contraindications/cautions, and adverse effects, see Table 4.4.

Nitroglycerin

Nitroglycerin at doses of 5 mcg/min up to 200 mcg/min has beneficial hemodynamic effects for many patients in heart failure by reducing left ventricular filling pressure and minimizing

Table 4.4 Intravenous Vasodilators Used for Treatment of Acute Decompensated Heart Failure

Drug	Dosing	Contraindications/ Cautions*	Adverse Effects *
Nitroglycerin	Starting dose generally 5 mcg/min intravenously, range 5 to 200 mcg min intravenously	Hypovolemia, HOCM, phosphodiesterase-5 use	Headache, hypotension, tolerance, tachyphylaxis
Nitroprusside	Starting dose generally 0.25 to 3 mcg/kg/min, maximum is 10 mcg/kg/min for 10 minutes	Hypotension, compensatory hypertension (aortic coarctation and arteriovenous shunting), caution with renal dysfunction, hepatic dysfunction, or elevated ICP	Hypotension, cyanide toxicity, thiocyanate toxicity, methemo-globinemia, increased intracranial pressure
Nesiritide	May give bolus of 2 mcg/kg intravenously and start 0.01 mcg/kg/min, higher doses occasionally used	Hypotension, hypovolemia, HOCM, caution with renal dysfunction	Hypotension, headache, possibly effect on renal function and mortality

* Contraindications/cautions and adverse reactions listed are not conclusive and are limited to more commonly encountered and/or clinically relevant.

pulmonary congestion by promoting venodilation and decreasing preload. Nitroglycerin may also have the effect of increasing coronary blood flow and is useful for ischemia in the setting of ADHF. At higher doses, nitroglycerin may decrease afterload and increase stroke volume and cardiac output, although these effects are variable.

Nitroprusside

The venous and arterial vasodilator nitroprusside is usually used in conjunction with hemodynamic monitoring and typically produces beneficial hemodynamic effects, including decreased pulmonary capillary wedge pressure (PCWP) and increased cardiac output. Caution must be exercised in renal dysfunction, as there is an increased risk of thiocyanate toxicity. Initial doses of 0.3 to 0.5 mcg/kg/min can be titrated to a maximum of 10 mcg/kg/min minute for 10 minutes.

Nesiritide

The natriuretic peptide nesiritide is identical to human B-type natriuretic peptide and has been used for the treatment of ADHF. The peptide has been shown to have the effects of decreased systemic and pulmonary resistance, reduction in pulmonary capillary wedge pressure, inhibition of the renin-angiotensin-aldosterone system, and an increased cardiac output. At the doses currently recommended clinically of 0.01 mcg/kg/min, nesiritide decreases left ventricular filling pressure but has effects on cardiac output and sodium excretion that are variable. Some concerns were raised about worsening renal function from a meta-analysis of the available nesiritide trials; a more recent, small, randomized study has shown no effect on renal function in those patients with baseline renal dysfunction. There was an association of increased mortality that was seen in patients treated with nesiritide in a meta-analysis. Currently, there are no prospective studies or convincing data that show worsening renal function or increased mortality with nesiritide use, and more data are needed and upcoming to illustrate the effect of nesiritide on outcomes. Nesiritide is useful in the treatment of ADHF because of its beneficial hemodynamic effects and may be administered with or without a weight based bolus of 2 mcg/kg and a typical infusion rate of 0.01 mcg/kg/min.

Angiotensin-Converting Enzyme Inhibitors

In the absence of acute renal failure with significantly increased serum creatinine and hyperkalemia and in the absence of absolute or relative hypotension, it is generally reasonable to continue the patient's dose of angiotensin-converting enzyme (ACE) inhibition. In the absence of renal function that is significantly worse than baseline or other contraindications, it is generally acceptable to start ACE inhibition in the setting of ADHF with close monitoring of renal function during the hospitalization and after discharge.

Angiotensin Receptor Blockers

As with ACE inhibition, it is reasonable to continue a patient's stable angiotensin receptor blocker (ARB) dose in the absence of acute renal failure, hyperkalemia, or absolute or relative hypotension. If a patient is ACE intolerant, it is reasonable to begin ARB therapy while being treated for ADHF in the absence of contraindications. Close monitoring of renal function as described for ACE inhibition is needed during continuation, initiation, and increase.

Isosorbide Dinitrate/Hydralazine

Isosorbide dinitrate/hydralazine may be started in the setting of ADHF in the absence of contraindications and is particularly useful if ACE-I or ARB use is contraindicated. A long acting nitrate such as isosorbide mononitrate can also be considered in place of isosorbide dinitrate.

β-*Blockers*

In the absence of symptomatic hypotension or bradycardia, presumed or documented low flow state, or profound volume overload relatively resistant to diuretics, the patient's current dose of β-blockade can generally be continued as withdrawal of β-blockade may increase the risk of subsequent decompensation and possibly increase mortality. If inotropic support is needed, it may be advisable to discontinue the β-blocker dose temporarily, depending on the severity of the patient's decompensation. At times, it may be reasonable to continue the patient's β-blocker at the current or decreased dose even in the setting of inotropic use. In the setting of recent β-blocker use or especially if the β-blocker will be continued, an agent that works independently of the β-receptor such as milrinone may be more reasonable if a patient's hemodynamics will allow. If the patient is not currently on a β-blocker, the patient should be essentially euvolemic on initiation of a β-blocker. Caution should be exercised in initiating or restarting β-blockade in those patients who are thought to be recently poorly perfused, have recently required an inotropic agent, and of course, have typical contraindications to β-blockade.

Adenosine Receptor Antagonists

Adenosine receptor antagonism-inducing diuresis has shown promise in phase II trials, where a decreased need for diuretics and neutral effect on renal function have been shown. More data are needed and are coming on the role of adenosine receptor antagonism in acute decompensated heart failure.

Hyponatremia/Vasopressin Receptor Antagonism

Relatively mild hyponatremia during ADHF is associated with longer hospital stays and increased in-hospital mortality. As a result, there has been some interest in the role of vasopressin receptor antagonists in the treatment of ADHF. Currently, vasopressin receptor drugs are not included in the guidelines for ADHF, and more data are needed to define their role in treatment of acute heart failure.

Right Heart Catheterization

Routine right heart catheterization is not recommended in the setting of ADHF; however, selected patients will likely benefit from invasive hemodynamic monitoring. Right heart catheterization is generally reasonable for those patients who are hypotensive, have unclear filling pressures or perfusion state, have worsening renal function, and do not improve with initial therapy. Right heart catheterization may be useful in an end-stage cardiomyopathy patient that presents with acute decompensated heart failure that has features of low cardiac output to document an adequate hemodynamic improvement to inotropes if needed. If a patient is a transplant candidate, then an adequate response should be seen so as to ensure that a higher level of support, such as a mechanical assist device or urgent transplant, is not needed. Right heart catheterization when performed for any indication provides an opportunity to optimize a patient's oral regimen, especially if the patient has sufficient systemic vascular resistance with which to work. For transplant-eligible patients, it is important to document acceptable pulmonary pressures that are suitable for transplant (more in Chapter 5). For patients who are not transplant candidates and have features of low cardiac output, a right heart catheterization is reasonable to document response to inotropic agents if outpatient inotropes are being entertained.

Inotropes

There are data to suggest that the routine use of inotropic agents in the majority of patients who present with ADHF who have no evidence of low output state is unwarranted and associated with adverse effects. Inotropic agents are useful agents in the treatment of certain cases of ADHF from heart failure with reduced systolic function but not from heart failure with a preserved ejection fraction. Furthermore, observational analysis from the ADHERE registry suggests increased mortality with inotropes in those patients currently hospitalized for acute heart failure, most of which have normal or elevated blood pressures and are volume overload. There are concerns that in advanced heart failure inotropes may increase the heart rate, worsen ischemic disease, increase myocardial oxygen consumption, and produce symptom relief with less reduction in filling pressures, which may contribute to further myocyte loss and progressive heart failure.

Advanced heart failure patients with systolic dysfunction and left ventricular dilation and who have evidence of low cardiac output or have compromised end-organ perfusion may be candidates for inotropic use, particularly if these patients have symptomatic hypotension in the face of elevated left ventricular filling pressures or are unresponsive or intolerant of vasodilators. Similar advanced heart failure patients with low cardiac output who have worsening renal function or are unresponsive to adequate doses of diuretics may also benefit from inotropic therapy, as many times renal function will improve and urine output will be adequate with an augmented cardiac output. Patient selection for inotropes needs to be carefully considered, as does a careful assessment of risks and benefits. Inotropes are at times needed as a bridge to more definitive therapy that may be orthotopic heart transplant, mechanical hemodynamic support, including intra-aortic balloon counterpulsation or left ventricular assist device, transplant, revascularization, improvement of renal function, and control of volume status, and/or optimization of oral medical therapy. Table 4.5 shows dosing, contraindications/cautions, and adverse effects of commonly used inotropes.

Dobutamine

Dobutamine is an intravenous drug that works primarily on the β1 receptor; it is also a mild β2 agonist and a mild α1 agonist. Dobutamine is thought of as primarily an inotrope with vasodilating properties and augments cardiac output. A symptomatic improvement may occur even after infusion, which has been called a "dobutamine holiday." There is concern that if a patient were recently on β-blockers that the effect of dobutamine may be attenuated, and this attenuation may be more pronounced with carvedilol than with metoprolol. In cases of decreased cardiac output with significant hypotension, dopamine may be a better choice, as dobutamine may not raise blood pressure significantly. Tachycardia, atrial and ventricular arrhythmias, worsening of ischemic disease, an eosinophilic hypersensitivity myocarditis, especially during prolonged use, and the potential for increased mortality are all clinically relevant issues that must be considered with infusion of dobutamine. Dobutamine is commonly used at doses that range from 1 to 10 mcg/kg/min.

Table 4.5 Common Intravenous Inotropic Agents Used in the Treatment of Acute Decompensated Heart Failure

Drug	Dose	Contraindications/ Cautions*	Adverse Effects*
Dobutamine	Typical starting dose 2–3 mcg/kg/min Doses of 1–10 mcg/kg/min commonly used clinically	HOCM, caution if arrhythmia, ischemia, hypovolemia	Tachycardia, arrhythmias, hypotension, hypersensitivity myocarditis, increasing myocardial oxygen demand, possibly further myocyte loss and progressive heart failure, possibly increased mortality
Milrinone	Typical starting dose is 0.2–0.3 mcg/kg/min Doses of 0.1–0.75 mcg/kg/min commonly used clinically	Acute MI, caution if arrhythmia, hypotension, hypovolemia, or impaired renal function (may need dose adjustment)	Arrhythmias, hypotension, possibly further myocyte loss and progressive heart failure, possibly increased mortality
Dopamine	Typical starting dose is 1–5 mcg/kg/min up to maximum of 50 mcg/kg/min	Caution if arrhythmia, ischemia, post-MI	Arrhythmias, tachycardia, extravasation necrosis, gangrene

*Contraindications/cautions and adverse reactions listed are not conclusive and are limited to more commonly encountered and/or clinically relevant.

Milrinone

Milrinone is an intravenous phosphodiesterase III inhibitor that potentiates the effects of cyclic adenosine monophosphate (cAMP). It is thought of as primarily a vasodilator with inotropic properties, and it may cause hypotension. The effect of milrinone is independent of the β-receptors, and its effect is not attenuated with recent β-blockade. β-Blockade may at times be continued at the same time or usually a decreased dose with the use of milrinone. It is useful in patients with a low cardiac index, high systemic vascular resistance, and an adequate blood pressure. Milrinone is a useful tool in the patient who has pulmonary pressures that appear out of proportion to the left-sided filling pressures; many times a significant decrease in the pulmonary pressures is seen with administration. Tachycardia, atrial and ventricular arrhythmias, hypotension, and possibly increased mortality are among the concerns that must be addressed in patients who are initiated on milrinone therapy. Doses of 0.1 to 0.75 mcg/kg/min of milrinone are commonly used in clinical practice (a loading dose of 50 mcg/kg over 10 minutes has been used in the past but is no longer recommended). A bolus dose produces more rapid hemodynamic improvement with increased risk of symptomatic hypotension. Recent data show that by 2 hours the hemodynamic improvement is similar with or without a loading dose.

Dopamine is an inotrope that stimulates and activates dopamine, α-receptors, and β-receptors. Dopamine is useful for the treatment of ADHF that is complicated by significant hypotension. The arrhythmogenic potential of dopamine is thought to be more than dobutamine and milrinone, but it is considered a first-line treatment in a patient who has hypotension with decreased cardiac output. Doses of 2 to 15 mcg/kg/min are commonly used in heart failure. In doses greater than 15 mcg/kg/min, α antagonism predominates, and this level of dose may be useful in end-stage heart failure with normal or low vascular resistance states or on occasion when there is a septic component to the patient's hemodynamic picture.

IABP

In patients with cardiogenic shock unresponsive to medical treatment and also those with significant coronary disease and/or refractory ischemia intra-aortic balloon pump, counterpulsation can be considered in the absence of contraindications.

Mechanical Support

Patients who cannot be supported with inotropic agents can be considered for left, right, or biventricular mechanical support as destination therapy or possibly as a bridge to transplant.

Transplant

At selected centers in patients who are candidates, orthotopic heart transplant can be considered for patients in ADHF. (For more on mechanical support and transplant, see Chapter 5.)

Evaluation and Treatment of the Patient with Chronic Heart Failure

General Principles

The ACC/AHA classifies four stages of heart failure—A, B, C, and D—that illustrate the evolution and progression of the disorder and also provides a framework for therapy. Patients in stage A are those patients who are at high risk of heart failure and who have hypertension, diabetes, or coronary artery disease. Stage B consists of patients who have evidence of cardiac structural abnormalities or remodeling who have not yet developed heart failure. Stage C consists of those who have current or prior symptoms of heart failure. Stage D patients are those with refractory or end-stage heart failure.

Physiology of the Chronically Failing Heart

Because of cardiac dysfunction, there may be a decrease in cardiac output, arterial pressure, and subsequent baroreceptor activity. There is an adaptive increase in the sympathetic nervous system, the renin-angiotensin-aldosterone system, and the cytokine system. Arginine vasopressin (AVP) is released, and volume retention occurs that helps restore cardiac output and arterial pressure. Adaptive response becomes maladaptive as cardiac afferents send less information to the brain, which results in excessive excitatory responses from the brain to the periphery. Although the sympathetic nervous system is increased, there is a decreased response of the heart to inotropic stimuli and chronotropic stimuli because of downregulation, desensitization, and uncoupling of β-adrenergic receptors. Parasympathetic tone is decreased as is heart rate variability, and systemic vascular resistance is increased. Sustained activation of the initially adaptive systems leads to further myocyte dysfunction and remodeling of the myocardium, leading to further decompensation.

Interval History of the Patient with Chronic Heart Failure

The interval history of the patient with chronic heart failure should focus on the degree or change of symptoms such as dyspnea at rest and exertion, paroxysmal nocturnal dyspnea, orthopnea, edema, palpitations, angina, presyncope, and syncope. Medication and diet adherence and monitoring of weight and blood pressure, as well as degree and frequency of physical activity, at home should be discussed. The medication regimen should always be reviewed with attention to changes made by other physicians as well as to the presence of any vitamin or over-the-counter supplements. Serial assessment of NYHA functional class should be performed, as it helps to provide a framework for assessing response to therapy and needs for therapy.

Physical Examination

A physical examination of the chronic heart failure patient should focus on the cardiovascular and respiratory systems, with particular attention to a patient's volume status and perfusion status.

Nonpharmacological Interventions

Laboratory Assessment

Serum electrolytes and creatinine should be routinely measured, and potassium and magnesium should be repleted if necessary (generally accepted that potassium be maintained greater than

4 mEq/L and magnesium greater than 2 mg/dl). A complete blood count should be performed, as should periodic hepatic function tests, thyroid stimulating hormone (TSH), and fasting lipids.

Electrocardiogram

An electrocardiogram should be performed to assess underlying rhythm, assess QRS duration, and look for evidence of ischemia or ischemic damage.

Echocardiogram

An echocardiogram is indicated if there is a change in clinical status (deterioration or improvement) or if there has been an event or treatment that might have significantly altered cardiac function. Also, repeat assessment is warranted to document ejection fraction before possible internal cardiodefibrillator (ICD) or cardiac resynchronization therapy.

Diet

Patients should be instructed to follow a low-sodium diet (approximately 2 to 3 grams daily) with consideration of more restriction if moderate to severe heart failure.

Fluid Restriction

Less than 2 liters per day of fluid should generally be used for those with severe hyponatremia or fluid retention that is difficult to control with diuretics and sodium restriction.

Exercise

Patients with heart failure in the absence of contraindications should undergo exercise training.

Weight Monitoring

Patients should be instructed to obtain a scale for monitoring of daily weights and should be instructed to call with weight gains of typically 2 kg in 24 hours or 5 kg in 7 days.

Nutritional Support

It is important to monitor a patient's nutritional status and supplement as needed, especially in the setting of cardiac cachexia. A multivitamin should be considered.

Continuous Positive Airway Pressure

Patients with obstructive sleep apnea (OSA) and heart failure should be treated with continuous positive airway pressure ventilation (CPAP).

Referral to a Comprehensive Heart Failure Disease Management Program

Referral to a comprehensive heart failure disease management program should be considered for those recently hospitalized with heart failure or those patients at high risk; such a program allows for close follow-up with a multidisciplinary team designed to treat heart failure with a comprehensive approach. Referral to heart failure specialists can also help assess a patient's possible need and eligibility for transplant.

Pharmacologic Therapy: Systolic Dysfunction

Diuretics

Many chronic heart failure patients will need maintenance diuretics to minimize their congestive symptoms. The loop diuretics furosemide, bumetanide, and torsemide are all typically used in patients with chronic heart failure. Oral dose equivalents are approximately as follows: 1 mg of bumetanide equals 20 mg of torsemide equals 40 mg of furosemide. Bumetanide and torsemide have approximately equal bioavailability orally and intravenously; oral furosemide is generally approximately half as potent as the intravenous counterpart, although bioavailability is erratic. Patients with right-sided heart failure may have slower absorption and decreased peak concentration of furosemide because of intra-abdominal congestion; such patients may do better with torsemide, as this diuretic

Table 4.6 Oral Diuretics Used in the Treatment of Volume Overload in Systolic and Diastolic Dysfunction

Drug	Type	Dose	Maximum
Furosemide	Loop diuretic	20–40 mg QDAY or BID	600 mg/day
Torsemide	Loop diuretic	10–20 mg QDAY	200 mg/day
Bumetanide	Loop diuretic	0.5–1 mg QDAY or BID	10 mg/day
Metolazone	Thiazide diuretic	2.5 mg QDAY	20 mg/day
Ethacrynic acid	Loop diuretic	25–50 mg QDAY	200 mg/day
Spironolactone	Potassium sparing	12.5–25 mg QDAY	50 mg/day*
Eplerenone†	Potassium sparing	25–50 mg QDAY	100 mg/day

* Higher doses have been used but close monitoring is mandatory.

† Should not be with cytochrome 3A4 inhibitors.

Source: Adapted from Adams KF, Lindenfeld J, Arnold JMO, et al. Executive Summary: HFSA 2006 Comprehensive Heart Failure Practice Guidelines. *J Card Fail* 2006:12(1).

has the least variable bioavailability. The thiazide diuretic metolazone when given before the loop diuretic potentiates the effect of the loop diuretic. Ethacrynic acid is not commonly used but can be considered in cases of sulfa allergy. The aldosterone antagonists spironolactone and eplerenone are discussed later here. Oral diuretics used in chronic heart failure are seen in Table 4.6.

β-*Blockers*

The mechanism of benefit of β-blockers in heart failure is not completely understood and is likely multifactorial. β-Blockers are integral in treatment of chronic heart failure despite past concern about their negative inotropic effects and the fact that they have been shown in early studies to increase plasma volume. Chronic β-blockade (approximately 3 months) has been shown in many trials to improve symptoms, improve ejection fraction, improve exercise capacity,

Table 4.7 Beta Blockers That Have Shown Mortality Benefit in Clinical Trials of Patients with Heart Failure

Drug	Initial Dose	Maximum Dose
Carvedilol	3.125 mg BID	25 mg BID if < 85 kg 50 mg BID if > 85 kg
Metoprolol succinate	12.5–25 mg QDAY	200 mg QDAY
Bisoprolol	2.5 mg QDAY	10 mg QDAY

Source: Adapted from Hunt, SA, Abraham, WT, Chin, MH, et al. ACC/AHA 2005 Guideline Update for the Diagnosis and Management of Chronic Heart Failure in the Adult: a report of the American College of Cardiology/American Heart Association Task Force on Practice Guidelines (Writing Committee to Update the 2001 Guidelines for the Evaluation and Management of Heart Failure): developed in collaboration with the American College of Chest Physicians and the International Society for Heart and Lung Transplantation: endorsed by the Heart Rhythm Society. *Circulation* 2005; 112:e154.

reduce the risk of atrial fibrillation, have a beneficial effect on cardiac remodeling, and improve survival in patients with systolic heart failure. β-Blockers that have been shown to have a mortality benefit in heart failure include bisoprolol, metoprolol succinate, and carvedilol. Typical starting and maximum doses are shown in Table 4.7.

Contraindications

Contraindications include bradycardia (heart rate < 60), symptomatic hypotension, high-degree atrioventricular block, and possibly markedly prolonged PR interval (interval on ECG). Severe chronic obstructive pulmonary disease (COPD) is a relative contraindication, but some data suggest that cardioselective β-blockers such as metoprolol are safe in mild to moderate COPD and mild to moderate reversible airway disease. Few data suggest that the combined alpha and nonselective β-blockade of carvedilol is safe as well in COPD but not as well tolerated in asthma. Additional contraindications to initiation are presumed low flow state as well as current congestive symptoms. The subject of β-blockade in the setting of a decompensation is discussed in the acute decompensated heart failure section. Adverse reactions include hypotension, fatigue, bradyarrhythmias, worsening of heart failure, worsening of bronchospasm, worsening of peripheral vascular disease, fatigue, and depression. Some data suggest that β-blocker use with aspirin (acetylsalicylic acid) may attenuate the beneficial effects of β-blockade; however, the data are limited, and the topic is controversial. Generally, it is reasonable to use aspirin in those patients with any documented coronary disease or those at risk for coronary events. Although there are data to suggest an increased mortality with chronic administration of a phosphodiesterase inhibitor, there is some consideration of using an oral phosphodiesterase inhibitor with a β-blocker, which may decrease some of the adverse effects of survival from phosphodiesterase inhibition. There are some limited encouraging data on β-blockade and oral phosphodiesterase inhibition, but more data are needed and are upcoming on this combination of agents. An intravenous phosphodiesterase inhibitor may also allow initiation of β-blockade. The evidence-based β-blockers bisoprolol, metoprolol succinate, and carvedilol should be used in patients with systolic heart failure in the absence of contraindications, and attempts should be made to use the doses in clinical trials. Patients who have concurrent hypertension and elevated blood pressure may benefit from the α-blockade provided by carvedilol. Conversely, if there is a borderline blood pressure, metoprolol XL may be a more appropriate choice because of the absence of α-blockade. There are data to suggest that β-blockers should be initiated before discharge in stable patients. The dose should generally be doubled in the absence of contraindications at regular intervals (generally 2 weeks or more) with close monitoring for worsening of heart failure symptoms.

ACE Inhibitors

Inhibition of the angiotensin-converting enzyme (ACE) and subsequent modification of the renin-angiotensin-aldosterone axis have been shown in numerous large randomized trials to have a beneficial effect on symptoms, overall clinical status, overall sense of well being, as well as mortality in patients with heart failure (Table 4.8). ACE inhibitors may also prevent atrial fibrillation

Table 4.8 Initial and Maximum Doses of ACE Inhibitors Commonly Used for Patients with Systolic Dysfunction

Drug	Initial Dose	Maximum Dose
lisinopril	2.5–5 mg QDAY	40 mg QDAY
enalapril maleate	2.5 mg BID	20 mg BID
captopril	6.25–12.5 TID	50 mg TID
quinapril	5 mg BID	20 mg BID
ramipril	1.25–2.5 mg QDAY	10 mg QDAY
fosinopril	10 mg QDAY	80 mg QDAY
trandolapril	1 mg QDAY	4 mg QDAY
perindopril	2 mg QDAY	8–16 mg QDAY

Source: Adapted from Hunt SA, Abraham WT, Chin MH, et al. ACC/AHA 2005 Guideline Update for the Diagnosis and Management of Chronic Heart Failure in the Adult: a report of the American College of Cardiology/American Heart Association Task Force on Practice Guidelines (Writing Committee to Update the 2001 Guidelines for the Evaluation and Management of Heart Failure): developed in collaboration with the American College of Chest Physicians and the International Society for Heart and Lung Transplantation: endorsed by the Heart Rhythm Society. *Circulation* 2005;112:e154.

in patients with left ventricular dysfunction. Contraindications include hypotension, hyperkalemia, advanced renal insufficiency (although not well defined), and previous drug reaction or angioedema. Adverse effects that occur during ACE inhibitor treatment include acute renal failure, hyperkalemia, hypotension, cough, and angioedema. The drug class is contraindicated in pregnancy. There are data to suggest that aspirin attenuates some of the acute hemodynamic effects of ACE inhibition. Also, there are some data to suggest that aspirin may influence some of the survival benefit accrued with ACE inhibition, but most of the evidence does not support an attenuation of the survival benefit. It is reasonable to use aspirin in those patients with coronary artery disease and those at high risk of a vascular event and not to use it in those patients with known nonischemic cardiomyopathy and clean coronary arteries. ACE inhibition remains a cornerstone of treatment for systolic heart failure and should be used in the absence of contraindications. Doses should be initiated at low doses and increased at rates that depend on an individual's risk of adverse effects, especially hypotension, renal dysfunction, and hyperkalemia. Stopping an ACE inhibitor or angiotensin receptor blocker because of the expected small to moderate asymptomatic rises in creatinine is not routinely recommended. Although not well represented in clinical trials, there are data to suggest that the benefit of ACE inhibition extends to those with moderate renal insufficiency. The efficacy of ACE inhibition in severe renal insufficiency (GFR < 30 ml/min/1.73 m^2) is not well defined nor is the point where the benefit of ACE inhibition for the heart and the kidneys is outweighed by the risk of precipitating dialysis. Generally, patients with a GFR above 15 ml/min/1.73 m^2 should be considered for therapy with an ACE inhibitor or, if not tolerated, an ARB. Meticulous monitoring of renal function and electrolytes is necessary, as is adjustment of doses in severe renal insufficiency. The optimal target dose for ACE inhibition remains not perfectly defined; it is reasonable to strive for doses equivalent to those used in clinical trials while taking into account the need for a similar goal with β-blockade.

Initiation of Medications: β-Blockade or ACE Inhibition First?

Initially, ACE-Is were initiated first because the trials of ACE-I preceded those of β-blockers; however, it appears that outcomes may be similar if patients are started on β-blockers first.

Angiotensin Receptor Blockers

There are data to suggest that an ARB can decrease mortality compared with placebo in patients with heart failure who are intolerant of ACE inhibition (Table 4.9). The addition of an ARB to standard therapy did not produce a survival benefit in Val-Heft (and in

Table 4.9 Angiotensin Receptor Blockers Commonly Used in the Treatment of Heart Failure

Drug	Initial Dose	Maximum Dose
Candesartan	4–8 mg QDAY	32 mg QDAY
Valsartan	20–40 mg QDAY	160 mg BID
Losartan	25–50 mg QDAY	100 mg QDAY

Source: Adapted from Hunt, SA, Abraham, WT, Chin, MH, et al. ACC/AHA 2005 Guideline Update for the Diagnosis and Management of Chronic Heart Failure in the Adult: a report of the American College of Cardiology/American Heart Association Task Force on Practice Guidelines (Writing Committee to Update the 2001 Guidelines for the Evaluation and Management of Heart Failure): developed in collaboration with the American College of Chest Physicians and the International Society for Heart and Lung Transplantation: endorsed by the Heart Rhythm Society. *Circulation* 2005; 112:e154.

subgroup analysis showed increased mortality in those on an ACE inhibitor and a β-blocker), but the addition of candesartan to standard therapy, including an ACE inhibitor, reduced cardiovascular mortality in the CHARM added trial. Adverse reactions are similar to those of ACE inhibition and include hypotension, azotemia, hyperkalemia, but a much reduced rate of cough and angioedema. As with ACE inhibition, it is not clear at what point the benefit of an ARB in patients with renal insufficiency will be outweighed by the risks of precipitating dialysis. Generally, ACE-intolerant patients for reasons other than renal failure or hyperkalemia with a GFR above 15 ml/min/1.73 m^2 can be considered for therapy with an ARB in the absence of other contraindications. An ARB should be used in patients with symptomatic systolic heart failure who are ACE intolerant (for reasons other than hyperkalemia or renal insufficiency) and can be considered for patients with symptomatic systolic heart failure who are persistently symptomatic despite standard therapy, including an ACE inhibitor. Close monitoring of renal function and electrolytes is needed, especially in patients with renal dysfunction.

Aldosterone Antagonists

The mortality benefit of aldosterone antagonists was illustrated in the RALES trial, which evaluated spironolactone in patients with moderate to severe heart failure, as well as the EPHESUS trial, which evaluated eplerenone in recent post-MI patients with decreased left ventricular ejection fraction (LVEF) and evidence of heart failure or diabetes. Aldosterone antagonism should be considered in those patients in addition to standard therapy in patients with moderate to severe heart failure due to systolic dysfunction as well as those that are post-MI with EF $< 40\%$ with heart failure symptoms in the absence of contraindications. Contraindications include renal dysfunction and hyperkalemia; the creatinine should be less than 2.5 mg/dl in men and 2.0 mg/dl in women (and creatinine clearance greater than 30 ml/min/1.73 m^2), and the potassium should be below 5.0 mEq/L. Meticulous monitoring of renal function and potassium is required. Adverse reactions commonly include hyperkalemia and gynecomastia. If a patient cannot be monitored or is at risk for not following up, then the risks of aldosterone antagonism are likely outweighed by the benefits. The routine use of an ACE inhibitor, an angiotensin receptor blocker, and an aldosterone antagonist is not recommended as the risk of hyperkalemia is greater. In patients who are class III to class IV heart failure and who are reasonable candidates, spironolactone 12.5 to 25 mg once a day can be used with a maximum of 50 mg once a day. Eplerenone may have fewer endocrine effects and can be started at 25 mg once a day and increased to a maximum of 50 to 100 mg once a day. Higher doses of both agents have been used, but of course, close monitoring is mandatory.

Isosorbide Dinitrate/Hydralazine

The combination of isosorbide dinitrate and hydralazine has shown mortality benefits in patients with symptomatic systolic dysfunction. Although there is no specific mention of race in guidelines, there are data to suggest that this combination is particularly beneficial in black patients. Contraindications to Isordil include notably hypotension, HCM, and volume depletion, and an absolute contraindication is phosphodiesterase-III inhibitor use (sildenafil, etc.). Contraindications to hydralazine include hypotension and unstable angina. Adverse reactions include hypotension, headache with Isordil, and a lupus-like reaction with hydralazine. The combination is useful in those patients who have contraindications to ACE inhibitors and ARBs. Isosorbide dinitrate/hydralazine should be considered for those patients who are persistently symptomatic with systolic dysfunction despite standard therapy. The addition of this combination deserves particular consideration in patients who are black and should be included as part of standard therapy, including β-blockers and ACE inhibitors in black patients. Hydralazine is typically started at doses of 10 to 25 mg per day and increased to a maximum of 100 mg three times a day. Isordil dinitrate can usually be started at 10 to 20 mg three times a day and increased to a maximum of 40 mg three times a day. It is also reasonable to use long-acting isosorbide mononitrate at doses from 30 to 120 mg QDAY. A combination preparation (used in the A-HeFT trial described later here) is available that includes 20-mg isosorbide dinitrate and 37.5 mg of hydralazine in one pill.

Racial Differences

Data suggest racial differences in response to and outcomes with heart failure drugs. Data suggest that ACE inhibition is less efficacious in black patients; there are conflicting data regarding β-blockers in black patients, as well as data to suggest that only patients who identified themselves as black accrue a survival benefit from isosorbide dinitrate/hydralazine. These observations led to the design of A-HeFT, a trial of 1,050 patients who identified themselves as black who were randomly assigned to isosorbide dinitrate/hydralazine versus placebo in addition to standard therapy. The trial was terminated early because of a significant reduction in mortality in the isosorbide dinitrate/hydralazine group.

Digoxin

Digoxin is a drug that works by inhibiting the Na-K-ATPase pump in myocardial cells and is a positive inotrope. Digoxin has been proven to improve symptoms and decrease hospitalization in heart failure but has never been proven to improve mortality. The evidence of deleterious effects of digoxin withdrawal has been well documented. There are data to suggest that there is a correlation between digoxin levels and patient survival, with levels higher than 1.2 ng/ml being associated with increased mortality. There are also data to suggest that women have increased mortality with digoxin, although it is unclear whether this effect was due to gender differences or differences in digoxin levels. Contraindications include Wolff-Parkinson-White syndrome (WPW) with atrial fibrillation, hypertrophic obstructive cardiomyopathy (HOCM), preexisting sinus node dysfunction, and conduction disease. Significant adverse reactions include bradyarrhythmias and heart block, accelerated junctional rhythm, ventricular tachycardia or fibrillation, asystole, yellow vision, headache, dizziness, and impaired mentation. Although use of cardiac glycosides has not been shown to decrease mortality, digoxin can be considered in addition to β-blockers and ACE inhibitors for symptomatic patients to treat symptoms and reduce admissions in those with systolic heart failure. Also, digoxin is useful for rate control in patients with atrial fibrillation with inadequate ventricular rate control. If added, the dose should be adjusted for renal insufficiency, and the level should likely be kept on the lower end of therapeutic (< 1.0 ng/ml).

Statins

Statins may be beneficial in heart failure for possible effects on ventricular remodeling; however, to date, there have been no prospective studies documenting a mortality benefit.

Atrial Fibrillation/Flutter

Patients with chronic left ventricular dysfunction and atrial fibrillation/flutter may benefit from the hemodynamic improvement noted with restoration of atrial kick. Patients commonly revert to atrial fibrillation and may need repeated cardioversion to sinus rhythm and possibly amiodarone or dofetilide to maintain sinus rhythm. Digoxin is useful in rate control in patients with atrial fibrillation and heart failure, especially when β-blockade therapy cannot be quickly titrated for rate control secondary to concerns of worsening heart failure. Patients may experience significant increases in ejection fraction when their ventricular rate is controlled.

Anticoagulation therapy should be instituted in heart failure patients in the absence of contraindications for patients with atrial fibrillation or atrial flutter or a previous thromboembolic event. Anticoagulation is also typically used for those patients who have a left ventricular thrombus, and some physicians may use anticoagulation for those in sinus rhythm with a markedly reduced ejection fraction, although there is a lack of supportive evidence for these approaches.

Calcium Channel Blockers

Amlodipine and felodipine are the only two calcium channel blockers that have been shown to have no adverse effects on mortality in systolic heart failure, and these calcium channel blockers can be used for the treatment of hypertension or angina in heart failure.

Drugs That Have at Least Relative Contraindications in Heart Failure

NSAIDs should be used with caution because of their effects of hypertension and fluid retention. Thiazolidinediones cause fluid retention and may precipitate heart failure, whereas patients who are taking metformin may be at increased risk of lactic acidosis. The phosphodiesterase inhibitor cilostazol for the treatment of peripheral vascular disease is contraindicated, as it has positive inotropic properties and as such unknown effect on mortality. Similarly, the phosphodiesterase inhibitor sildenafil for the treatment of erectile dysfunction should be used with discretion, as this drug may have inotropic effects and unknown effects on mortality. Class I antiarrhythmic drugs, as well as the class III agents ibutilide and sotalol, should be avoided. Amiodarone is generally the preferred antiarrhythmic in heart failure; dofetilide can be used as well. Calcium channel blockers other than those described previously here should be avoided in patients with systolic dysfunction.

Asymptomatic Left Ventricular Dysfunction

A mortality benefit for ACE inhibition has been demonstrated in NYHA class I heart failure. Although there are no randomized trials specifically evaluating the effect of β-blockers on cardiovascular outcomes in patients with left ventricular dysfunction who are not post-MI, the benefit of β-blockade is thought to extend to this group. As such, both β-blockers and ACE inhibition should be used in NYHA class I patients in the absence of contraindications.

Heart Failure with a Preserved Ejection Fraction

A significant amount of patients with symptoms of heart failure have a normal or near-normal ejection fraction. Many different disease processes fall under the umbrella of heart failure with a preserved ejection fraction and include conditions in which diastolic function is impaired, such as hypertensive cardiomyopathy, HCM, restrictive cardiomyopathy, pericardial constriction, and aortic stenosis. This group also includes other valvular processes such as mitral regurgitation and aortic regurgitation, right ventricular dysfunction, high output heart failure, and diseases of mitral obstruction. HCN, restrictive cardiomyopathy, and pericardial constriction are discussed individually. Hypertensive LVH is the most common cause of heart failure with a relatively preserved ejection fraction. Unlike the large body of data for patients with systolic dysfunction, there are less data to guide therapy heart failure patients with a preserved ejection fraction. The syndrome is a failure of the cardiovascular system with a major component of left ventricular stiffness causing impaired diastolic filling and subsequent increased left ventricular end diastolic, left atrial, and pulmonary capillary wedge pressures. Hypertension with abnormal ventricular–vascular interaction also may play a significant role in this disorder. Patients with diastolic dysfunction tolerate tachycardia as well as elevated blood pressure poorly. Diastolic filling can also be worsened or caused by myocardial ischemia.

Diagnosis

Based on the 2007 consensus statement of the Heart Failure and Echocardiography Society Associations of the European Society of Cardiology, three conditions are required for the diagnosis of diastolic heart failure: (1) signs or symptoms of heart failure, (2) normal or mildly abnormal LV systolic function, and (3) evidence of diastolic dysfunction by invasive or noninvasive methods. In addition, left atrial enlargement is commonly present. A detailed discussion of the echocardiographic features of diastolic dysfunction is outside the scope of this chapter.

Treatment

Control of systolic and diastolic hypertension remains vital in the treatment of heart failure with a preserved ejection fraction. There are data to suggest that various antihypertensive medications provide benefit in heart failure with preserved ejection fraction, but there are no data suggesting improved mortality. Per HFSA guidelines, ACE inhibitors or ARBs should be considered for patients with heart failure and preserved ejection fraction. β-Blockers are recommended for patients with heart failure with preserved ejection fraction that have prior myocardial infarction and hypertension or need rate control in atrial fibrillation. Calcium channel blockers should be considered in patients with uncontrolled atrial fibrillation failing β-blockade (diltiazem or verapamil), symptom limiting angina, and hypertension (amlodipine). There are data to suggest that aldosterone antagonism has beneficial effects on diastolic function and that statins have a beneficial effect on mortality in patients with diastolic dysfunction without known coronary artery disease. Treatment of heart failure with a preserved ejection fraction also involves decreasing pulmonary congestion and peripheral edema with diuretics and salt restriction and control of ventricular rate in atrial fibrillation. Volume overload can be treated with salt restriction, diuretics, and ACE inhibition to reduce the effects of the renin-angiotensin-aldosterone axis. The ventricular rate in atrial fibrillation should be controlled. If a patient is in acute pulmonary edema because of intolerability to atrial fibrillation, then emergent cardioversion should be considered. There is not consensus for maintenance of sinus rhythm in stable patients with atrial fibrillation to improve symptoms but can be considered if the patient is symptomatic. Evaluation for the possibility of coronary disease is recommended for patients with heart failure with a preserved ejection fraction. Exercise may be a beneficial adjunct to treatment as well.

HCM

The most common genetic cardiovascular disorder is a disease typically affecting the sarcomere in which hypertrophy occurs in the absence of another systemic or cardiac condition that is capable of causing the magnitude of hypertrophy present (systemic hypertension, aortic stenosis, some expressions of the athlete's heart). The disorder has a heterogeneous clinical expression and can present in infancy or in older persons. HCM may cause heart failure at virtually any age and sudden death in young patients. The clinical presentations result from varying components of diastolic dysfunction, arrhythmias (most commonly atrial fibrillation), left ventricular outflow obstruction, mitral regurgitation, and autonomic dysfunction. Severe heart failure is less common and occurs in only 10% to 15% of patients; end-stage HCM with systolic dysfunction occurs in approximately 3%.

Diagnosis

Clinical presentations vary widely; the diagnosis can be made in an asymptomatic patient who has a heart murmur and an abnormal ECG, or patients can be symptomatic. Clinical manifestations include the triad of dyspnea, angina, and presyncope or syncope. Palpitations may be experienced from arrhythmia; the heart failure symptoms of orthopnea and PND can occasionally occur. Prominent physical examination signs include a localized but sustained apical impulse that may be bifid (the "triple ripple" is classic with outflow obstruction but rarely observed), a harsh systolic ejection murmur that increases with maneuvers that decrease left ventricular end-diastolic volume, possibly a mitral regurgitation murmur, an S4 (may be palpable), and also an S3. The electrocardiogram is usually abnormal and most frequently demonstrates LVH as well as commonly primary and secondary T-wave abnormalities, including giant inverted T waves. Abnormal Q waves as well as atrial and ventricular arrhythmias may be present. The echocardiogram shows a small or normal-sized left ventricle and may show asymmetric septal hypertrophy (although asymmetric septal hypertrophy is most common the disease can present as concentric, apical, or free wall hypertrophy). An outflow gradient may be seen that is demonstrated on Doppler echocardiography as a late-peaking signal that has a typical dagger shape. If outflow tract obstruction is present, then SAM of the mitral valve is frequently seen. Echocardiography can also characterize abnormalities of diastolic function. Cardiac catheterization will typically show vigorous systolic function and may show a dynamic left ventricular outflow tract gradient. The Brockenbrough response is a classic hemodynamic pattern in HCM that demonstrates increased left ventricular systolic pressure, decreased aortic pressure, and increased gradient because of more severe obstruction after a postextrasystolic beat secondary to increased ventricular contractility.

Treatment for obstructive HCM includes avoidance of competitive athletics and strenuous activity (patients may participate in low level aerobic exercise), avoidance of dehydration, screening of first degree relatives, and avoidance or cautious use of high-dose diuretics, pure vasodilators, and inotropes such as digoxin. Screening for ventricular arrhythmias and risk stratification with Holter monitoring may help determine who will benefit from a defibrillator. Large doses of β-blockers (generally first choice) and/or nondihydropyridines (typically verapamil) should be used in symptomatic patients, although care must be used when prescribing nondihydropyridines for patients with large outflow tract obstructions, as the peripheral vasodilation may cause acute hemodynamic deterioration. The class I antiarrhythmic with negative inotropic properties, disopyramide, may also be used. Surgical myomectomy is the primary treatment strategy for severe disabling symptoms and offers good results. Alcohol septal ablation is an alternative to surgery for HCM but has some limitations and associated complications. Dual-chamber pacing may be beneficial for some patients but is reserved for those that cannot undergo surgical myomectomy or alcohol septal ablation. A risk assessment for sudden cardiac death and consideration for an ICD implantation is warranted as well. Treatment of nonobstructive HCM involves diuretics if needed and is aimed at treating the diastolic function of the left ventricle with inhibition of the renin-angiotensin-aldosterone axis.

Restrictive Cardiomyopathy

Restrictive cardiomyopathy is a disease of the myocardium that impairs ventricular filling with normal or near-normal systolic function of the heart and wall thickness that is usually secondary to increased stiffness. Small increases in volume increase the pressure substantially in the ventricles. Systolic function may be normal initially, but deterioration of systolic function typically occurs. Restrictive cardiomyopathy has numerous etiologies; the disease can be idiopathic or secondary to infiltrative diseases of the myocardium, such as amyloidosis and sarcoidosis, or secondary to storage diseases, such as hemochromatosis among many other causes.

Diagnosis

Dyspnea and fatigue, as well as symptoms of right-sided heart failure, are common. Signs and symptoms of systemic disease may be present, including amyloidosis or iron storage disease. Physical examination may reveal an elevated jugular venous pulsation, Kussmaul's sign (an inspiratory increase in venous pressure), a palpable apical impulse, and an S3 or S4. The ECG is nonspecific and may show ventricular hypertrophy, conduction disease, or atrial fibrillation. In amyloidosis, it is common to have low voltage and a pattern simulating an old inferior or anterior infarction, as well as disease of the conduction system. The echocardiogram can show normal or increased left ventricular wall thickness and mass, small or normal left ventricular cavity, biatrial enlargement, typically preserved systolic function, and abnormal diastolic function with restrictive diastolic filling and other Doppler characteristics. A characteristic granular sparkling texture of the myocardium may be seen with amyloidosis. Cardiac catheterization may variably show the "square root" sign in ventricular pressure recordings (a rapid early diastolic pressure decline followed by a rapid rise and plateau in early diastole, which is also seen in constrictive pericarditis), preserved systolic function, and elevated left- and right-sided filling pressures.

Treatment other than addressing the underlying disease if present involves minimizing pulmonary and systemic congestion with careful titration of diuretics to achieve the desired effects without reducing ventricular filling pressures and decreasing cardiac output. Maintenance of sinus rhythm is important, as the atrial contribution may be needed for ventricular filling. Digoxin should be used with caution, especially in amyloidosis, as these patients have increased sensitivity to digitalis preparations. Dual-chamber pacing may be beneficial to help ensure synchronization between the atria and ventricle to aid in diastolic filling in patients who have a high-degree atrioventricular block. Anticoagulation is frequently warranted for atrial fibrillation and atrial thrombus formation.

Constrictive Pericarditis

Constrictive pericarditis is a disorder in which there is restricted filling of the ventricle caused by an inelastic pericardium (thickened or calcified). Common etiologies include idiopathic or viral, postcardiac surgery, postradiation therapy, connective tissue disorders, infections, including tuberculosis, and miscellaneous etiologies, including, trauma, sarcoidosis, asbestosis, malignancy, drug induction, and uremia-associated complications.

Diagnosis

Constrictive pericarditis can be a difficult diagnosis to make. The main clinical features are dyspnea and signs of marked systemic venous congestion such as edema, ascites, and hepatomegaly. Patients may undergo evaluation for primary liver disease before the diagnosis is made. On physical examination, the Kussmaul's sign is usually present. The apical impulse is not palpable, and a pericardial knock may be present. The ECG is nonspecific and may show nonspecific T-wave changes, low voltage, left atrial abnormality, and atrial fibrillation. An echocardiogram may show normal wall thickness, pericardial thickening, and prominent early diastolic filling with abrupt displacement of early diastolic filling during early diastole ("septal bounce") and certain Doppler study findings. Cardiac catheterization typically shows the square root sign described previously here. A CT or MRI can be used to demonstrate pericardial thickening and help to make the diagnosis in the right clinical settings.

Treatment

Medical therapy is limited and involves treatment of edema with diuretics and salt restriction. Definitive treatment of constrictive pericarditis involves pericardiectomy if the patient is a suitable candidate; this can have good results. Ultrasound or laser debridement also may be used as an adjunct or as primary therapy for high-risk patients.

Differentiating Constrictive Pericarditis From Restrictive Cardiomyopathy

Differentiating constrictive pericarditis from restrictive cardiomyopathy is difficult, and a complete discussion is outside of the scope here. In the right clinical setting, findings of pulsus paradoxus, a pericardial knock, pericardial thickening or calcification, and a "septal bounce" favor pericardial constriction, whereas the absence of a pericardial knock and normal septal motion favor restrictive cardiomyopathy. Doppler echocardiography can also be used to help make the distinction. In addition, cardiac catheterization can be used to differentiate the two, although the distinction can be difficult to make.

Right Ventricular Failure and Pulmonary Hypertension

Right ventricular failure secondary to left-sided heart failure is a common entity and carries a worse prognosis than isolated left ventricular dysfunction. Right ventricular failure secondary to pulmonary hypertension also commonly occurs; isolated right ventricular failure from RV infarct is less common. Other than the judicious use of diuretics to minimize signs and symptoms of right-sided heart failure while preserving left ventricular filling, treatment should be individualized to the underlying condition. If the patient has intrinsic pulmonary hypertension in the absence of left-sided heart disease, then the pulmonary hypertension should be addressed. If the right-sided heart failure is secondary to left-sided heart disease, then optimization of the patients' heart failure regimen is warranted. The treatment of pulmonary hypertension that is likely in proportion to left-sided heart disease involves treating the underlying left-sided heart disease. Optimal medical management, correction of valvular lesions, and revascularization for coronary disease if appropriate can help minimize the degree of pulmonary hypertension. If the patient is a transplant candidate, reversibility of the pulmonary hypertension should be documented (discussed in more detail in Chapter 5). Mechanical assist devices have been used in an attempt to reverse a patient's pulmonary hypertension so as to allow transplant, but they are controversial. The treatment of pulmonary hypertension that is thought to be out of proportion to a patient's left-sided heart disease is less well defined. The phosphodiesterase inhibitor sildenafil has shown some promise with symptoms in the setting of pulmonary hypertension and left heart disease, but long-term safety and efficacy data are lacking.

Anemia and Heart Failure

There are no large randomized trials documenting the benefit of treating anemia in heart failure, but more data are forthcoming on this topic.

The Cardiorenal Syndrome

Cardiorenal syndrome can be defined as the presence or development of renal dysfunction in patients with heart failure during treatment (GFR < 60 ml/min/1.73 m^2) or worsening renal function limiting diureses despite obvious clinical volume overload. The treatment of patients with kidney disease and heart failure is challenging, as the two processes contribute to each other; additionally, the renal insufficiency can limit treatment for the heart failure. The presence of renal dysfunction in a heart failure patient confers a worse prognosis.

Prognosis

The onset of symptomatic heart failure is associated with a high morbidity and mortality. It has been shown that patients admitted to the hospital for decompensated heart failure have a worse prognosis than stable outpatients. Many other factors contribute to prognosis in heart failure, including etiology of the cardiomyopathy (with ischemic cardiomyopathy having a worse prognosis) and extent of CAD in ischemic cardiomyopathy. Other factors contributing to a worse prognosis include decreased left ventricular ejection fraction and other echocardiographic findings, decreased cardiac index, advanced NYHA class, decreased peak VO_2 (peak oxygen consumption) and other exercise variables, right ventricular dysfunction and pulmonary hypertension, renal insufficiency, diabetes, hypotension, increased heart rate, hyponatremia, BNP levels, diastolic dysfunction, QRS duration and LBBB, and other variables. Patients with NYHA class IV heart failure have 6-month and 1-year mortality rates of 44% and 64%, respectively. There have been predictive models developed that help to assess an individual patient's prognosis based on numerous variables. Although these prognostic models have potential benefits, they also have significant limitations. Honest discussions with patients regarding prognosis should be undertaken at all stages of heart failure. In end-of-life discussions, consideration must be made with regards to turning of a patient's defibrillator if the device is implanted, as an arrhythmic death may be preferable to repeated shocks or a death from pump dysfunction.

Device Therapy

Cardiac Resynchronization Therapy

Those patients with an ejection fraction of less than 35% and a QRS duration on an electrocardiogram of greater than 120 ms that are NYHA class III or class IV may benefit from biventricular pacing and the addition of a left ventricular lead (placed as a coronary sinus or epicardial lead). In selected patients, biventricular pacing has shown improved contractile function and reverse remodeling among numerous other benefits. Most of the patients included in the studies had left bundle branch block, and the need for biventricular pacing in right bundle branch block is not currently fully defined; however, the current guidelines recommend the use of biventricular pacing based on QRS duration and not morphology. The issue of biventricular pacing in NYHA class II patients is further defined by upcoming data, but as of the most recent guidelines, it is not universally recommended. Biventricular pacing may be considered for NYHA class I and class II patients who are receiving a permanent pacemaker or ICD and have an anticipated frequent dependence on right ventricular pacing. For a detailed discussion of the indications for biventricular pacing, refer to the guidelines.

ICD

Many patients with chronic heart failure will be candidates for an implantable cardioverter-defibrillator for primary or secondary prevention of sudden cardiac death, as these devices have shown a mortality benefit in patients with heart failure. Patients who have left ventricular dysfunction, who meet certain ejection fraction criteria (generally less than 35%), and who are NYHA class I to class III heart failure (and selected NYHA class IV) that are on optimal medical therapy may be considered for an implantable cardioverter-defibrillator for primary prevention. For a detailed discussion of the indications for primary and secondary prevention with respect to the etiology of cardiomyopathy and the presence of prior myocardial infarction, see the guidelines.

Surgical Options

Coronary Artery Bypass Surgery

Determining which patients with coronary artery disease and depressed ejection fraction will benefit from surgical revascularization is a difficult management dilemma. Large observational studies suggest that mortality is improved in patients with significant CAD and heart failure; subsequent studies have illustrated that the benefit is limited to those with viable myocardium. Coronary revascularization should be considered in those patients with significant coronary disease who have viability in regions with significant obstructive disease and those with inducible ischemia. More data are upcoming on the role of coronary revascularization in ischemic cardiomyopathy.

Repair of Valvular Lesions

Some degree of mitral regurgitation is common in patients with dilated cardiomyopathy and helps to precipitate further dilation. It is at times difficult to distinguish whether a patient with a dilated ventricle and severe mitral regurgitation had the dilation of the ventricle or the mitral regurgitation as the inciting pathologic event. Repair or replacement of the mitral valve for those patients who have mitral regurgitation secondary to ventricular dilation is not generally recommended. There has been some success in mitral valve repair in patients with reduced ejection fraction, but it remains unclear which patients will benefit, which patients will not, and ultimately when it is futile to attempt to fix the regurgitant valve. Consideration of repair of valvular lesions, including mitral regurgitation, should be considered with respect to the ACC/AHA guidelines and HFSA guidelines.

Other Surgical Techniques

Other surgical techniques involve reducing the volume of the left ventricle. The Batista procedure removes part of the left ventricular free wall in dilated cardiomyopathy and has generally lost favor in the heart failure community and has little or no application today. The Dor procedure involves exclusion of the dyskinetic or akinetic apical and septal components of a dilated left ventricle when other walls have retained reasonable function. Data evaluating this procedure in patients undergoing coronary artery bypass graft (CABG) are forthcoming.

Mechanical Assist Device

In selected patients that are candidates, a mechanical assist device is an option for chronic heart failure as a destination therapy or as a bridge to transplant (see Chapter 5 for more on this topic).

Orthotopic Heart Transplant

In selected patients who are candidates, an orthotopic heart transplant is an option for patients with chronic heart failure (see Chapter 5 for more on this topic).

Possibly Emerging Therapies

Possibly emerging therapies for heart failure may include immunosuppressive therapy in patients with chronic inflammation as sequelae of acute myocarditis, intravenous immune globulin, immunoadsorption, thalidomide, and interferon. Also, vasopressin receptor antagonism as well as sildenafil may have more of a role to play in the treatment of heart failure in the future. There may be a role for enhanced external counterpulsation, a treatment for intractable angina, in heart failure. An implantable hemodynamic monitoring device that allows hemodynamic data to be provided has shown some promise in assisting management. Continuous aortic flow augmentation is a system for delivering continuous flow to the aorta by removing blood from a peripheral artery, circulating this blood through a pump outside the body, and returning this blood through a second arterial site. There has been some promise shown in a small series of 24 patients, but more data are needed.

5 ▪ Evaluation and Treatment of Patients Who Are Candidates for and Are Undergoing Orthotopic Heart Transplant

Paul J. Mather, MD
Stephen Olex, MD

General Principles

Heart failure is a major and growing health problem in the United States and worldwide. Despite the advances in medical, device, and surgical techniques in the treatment of heart failure, some patients will have a high rate of mortality with their native heart in the absence of intervention. For certain patients within this group that are candidates, an orthotopic heart transplant (OHT) may be an option for treatment of their heart failure. The International Society for Heart and Lung Transplantation (ISHLT) estimates that 5,000 transplants are performed worldwide annually.

The number of people eligible for transplant each year is greater than the amount of transplants done; the limiting factor is the availability of donor organs.

Indications

Generally accepted indications for transplant include New York Heart Association class III–IV heart failure with severe functional limitations or refractory symptoms despite maximal medical therapy; angina refractory to medical, interventional, and surgical treatment; and ventricular arrhythmias not responding to treatment and severe hypertrophic or restrictive cardiomyopathy.

Candidate Selection

Deciding when a heart failure patient will benefit from transplant is at times challenging and involves identifying the sickest patients who are likely to have a higher mortality with their native heart than after OHT. Significant mortality occurs in the first 6 months after transplant; after this time, the survival curve drops at a fairly linear rate of approximately 3.4% per year. The survival at 1 year for OHTs is greater than 80%. The half-life of a heart transplant (the time when 50% of the patients are still alive) is 10 years, and a conditional half-life (for those that survived the first year) is 13 years.

The current treatment of heart failure has progressed, and the prognosis for heart failure has improved because of the advances in treatment, including neurohormonal blockade with β-blockers, angiotensin-converting enzyme inhibitors, and aldosterone antagonism, as well as device therapy with cardiac resynchronization therapy, as well implantable cardioverter-defibrillators. With the survival from heart transplant being improved but still with significant mortality in the first year and improved survival from the current treatment of heart failure, it is important to recognize correctly who will benefit from heart transplant. Some of the factors that are taken into consideration when making this decision are discussed here.

VO_2

Measurement of peak oxygen consumption during cardiopulmonary exercise is a useful tool to help prognosticate and to help with the timing of transplant for a heart failure patient. Those patients with a severely depressed VO_2 (< 10 ml/kg/min) are most likely to experience a benefit from transplant. Those with a VO_2 of between 10 and 14 ml/kg/min are in an intermediate area where continued therapy may offer similar outcomes as transplant. In this intermediate level of VO_2, other factors may contribute, such as the ability to tolerate a β-blocker, the presence of an ICD, and possibly the patient's Heart Failure Survival Score (HFSS; discussed later here). Patients with a VO_2 of greater than 14 ml/kg/min generally have better outcomes with continued medical therapy and should be managed appropriately with close follow-up, including serial exercise testing. If a patient tolerates a β-blocker, 12 ml/kg/

min have been proposed as an appropriate cutoff for the need for transplant.

Predictive Models

To aid in predicting a patient's prognosis, risk scores have been developed based on factors validated in a statistical analysis. These scores are used and may be helpful when the VO_2 is ambiguous.

HFSS

A tool used by some to help prognosticate a patient's survival from heart failure is the HFSS. The score separates patients into low, medium, and high risk based on variables of the patient. A limitation to this score is that it may not be applicable currently, as its inception was before medical and device advances that improve survival in heart failure.

Seattle Heart Failure Model

A newer tool that incorporates current medical and device therapy is the Seattle Heart Failure Model. This model helps to estimate 1-, 2-, and 3-year survival and also the likely mode of death as well.

Possibility of Other Options

At times, other options may be more attractive than transplant and may save the patient from having to undergo lifelong immunosuppression. A thorough consideration as to whether there is a role for percutaneous interventions for coronary disease, high-risk bypass surgery, or valvular surgery should be undertaken, preferably with a multidisciplinary team, including, of course, cardiothoracic surgeons. There are times when these options may be possible, but transplant remains the best long-term approach for the patient. Although high-risk coronary artery bypass graft (CABG) or valve surgery may be technically feasible, if the procedure does not allow the patient a good possibility of meaningful intermediate-term survival, then the patient may still need a transplant in a relatively short time and would be higher risk because of a previous sternotomy.

Contraindications

Pulmonary Vascular Resistance

Fixed irreversible pulmonary hypertension is a contraindication to transplant, as the donor heart's right ventricle will likely not be able to handle the increase in afterload and the recipient will be at high risk for right-sided heart failure and death. Generally, the pulmonary vascular resistance and the transpulmonary gradient (mean pulmonary artery pressure–wedge pressure) are used for assessment of the purpose. A pulmonary vascular resistance that is greater than 4 to 6 Wood units is at the concerning level. The ISHLT guidelines use a cutoff of 5 Wood units as a relative contraindication to transplant. Transpulmonary gradients greater than 13 are concerning as well; the ISHLT uses greater than 16 to 20 as a relative contraindication. If the pulmonary pressures and pulmonary vascular resistance are elevated, then attempts should be made to show reversibility if possible. Treatment with nesiritide, nitroprusside, milrinone, nitric oxide, or prostacyclin may acutely reduce the pulmonary pressures to an acceptable range. If the pressures are not reduced, then short-term treatment with the previously mentioned vasoactive agents combined with milrinone, dobutamine, and possibly diuretics may reveal reversibility of the pulmonary pressures and allow a patient to be listed for transplant. Mechanical devices such as intra-aortic balloon counterpulsation (IABP) or left ventricular assist devices (LVADs) can be considered when medical therapy fails to reduce pulmonary pressures. Serial right heart catheterization (RHC) (hemodynamics) should be performed in patients to ensure the reversibility of the pulmonary hypertension, the frequency of which is likely dependent on how severe and difficult it was to reverse the patient's pulmonary pressures initially.

Age

Age is a factor that contributes to a patient's candidacy for transplant. Patients should generally be less than 70 years old to be considered for OHT, although the ISHLT recognizes that carefully selected patients older than 70 years may be considered, possibly using an alternate-type program with older donors. Although the absolute number is a factor, the patient's physiologic age and end-organ function are important factors as well.

Diabetes Mellitus

Diabetes mellitus is a relative contraindication, particularly if the patient has evidence of significant end-organ damage, including neuropathy or nephropathy, or nonhealing diabetic ulcers on the patient's extremities.

Lung Disease

Advanced restrictive or obstructive lung disease is a contraindication to transplant, as lung disease will increase the risk of postoperative complication as well as increase the complications seen with immunosuppressive therapy.

Renal Disease

A creatinine clearance of less than 40 ml/min is concerning, as the immunosuppressive therapy after transplant is nephrotoxic. A heart–kidney transplant is an option in patients who meet the criteria for a double-organ transplant.

Noncardiac Vascular Disease

Significant noncardiac vascular disease is a relative contraindication to transplant.

Hepatic Disease

If advanced, hepatic disease will be a contraindication, as the operative risk will be increased and long-term survival will be compromised.

Infection

Active infection is typically an absolute contraindication to transplant, as immunosuppressive therapy will worsen the patient's underlying condition.

Malignancy

Active malignancy is generally an absolute contraindication to transplant, with the exceptions of nonmelanoma skin cancers, some prostate cancers, and some cardiac tumors. If the patient has had a malignancy, then detailed records of the involvement as well as consultation with an oncologist regarding risk of tumor recurrence are warranted.

Pulmonary Embolisms with Infarcts

A pulmonary embolism with infarct is generally a temporary contraindication to transplant, as the infarct has a high chance of becoming an abscess after transplant.

Body Mass Index

Those with a very high or very low body mass index (BMI) may not have good outcomes with transplant, and this should be considered in the decision to proceed, as should the potential for weight loss or nutritional improvement, as is appropriate.

Substance Abuse

Patients who are actively using alcohol, tobacco, or drugs are generally not considered to be transplant candidates. If a patient has ever abused substances of any kind, then a thorough assessment of his or her use and risk of reusing should be undertaken.

Psychosocial Factors

The patient undergoing a heart transplant should be assessed for the ability to adhere and understand a complex medical regimen and follow-up, the adequacy of social support (more is needed if the patient's understanding is somewhat lacking), psychological health, and his or her ability to handle physiologically stressful circumstances.

Combined Organ Transplants

Heart–Kidney

A heart–kidney transplant is an option for patients who have significant renal disease.

Heart–Lung

A heart–lung transplant is possible for patients who are candidates and are generally younger than 55 years old. This is a possibility for the heart failure patient who has irreversible pulmonary hypertension or the patient with significant lung disease that would preclude heart transplant alone.

Heart–Liver

Although not common, heart–liver transplants have been performed in appropriate candidates.

Mechanical Support Devices

Extracorporeal Membrane Oxygenation

As a form of cardiopulmonary support that can be used for respiratory support alone or respiratory and hemodynamic support, extracorporeal membrane oxygenation can be used in venovenous (respiratory support) and venoarterial configurations (respiratory and hemodynamic support). Bleeding, vascular complications, and thromboembolism are complications of extracorporeal membrane oxygenation use.

Cardiopulmonary Assist Device

The Bard CPS is a device that can provide full cardiopulmonary support to a patient, and it can be placed percutaneously. The catheters reside in the right atrium and the aorta, and the system is able to provide oxygenization of venous blood as well as hemodynamic support for those in cardiogenic shock or high-risk percutaneous intervention. Local vascular and neurological complications are common complications of the CPS.

Centrifugal Pumps

An extension of cardiopulmonary bypass, centrifugal pumps use rotating impellers or pumps to create nonpulsatile flow. The devices can be used in left ventricular assist device (LVAD), right ventricular assist device (RVAD), and bi-ventricular assist device (BIVAD) configurations but have the limitations of the patient not being able to ambulate when the device is in place, the need for intravenous anticoagulation, and significant hemolysis.

Axial Flow Pumps

Axial flow devices work on the principle of the Archimedes screw, which consists of a screw inside of a hollow pipe. The Impella microaxial flow device is an example and can be used in LVAD, RVAD, and BIVAD configurations.

Percutaneous Left Atrial to Left Femoral Device Tandem Heart PTVA System

As a percutaneous device designed for short-term use, the Tandem Heart involves a left atrial cannula placed by a trans-septal method as well as an arterial cannula placed in the femoral artery. The pump is capable of augmenting a patient's cardiac output by up to 4 liters per minute.

Abiomed Biventricular System

An extracorporal pump that can be used as BIVAD, RVAD, and LVAD configurations and was designed as an alternative to the centrifugal pumps, the Abiomed Biventricular System is pneumatically powered and is capable of providing short-term support to a failing heart.

Thoratec VAD

A device that uses suction drainage with pulsatile flow, the Thoratec VAD, has the versatility of left, right, or biventricular support. It is available in paracorporeal (pump outside the body) as well as an implantable version known as the Thoratec Implantable Assist Device, which was approved by the Food and Drug Administration in 2004 as a bridge to transplant.

Thoratec Heartmate

The Heartmate LVAD comes in two versions—the implantable pneumatic and the vented-electric—and is a device that has been implanted frequently since 1986. The device allows rehabilitation and hospital discharge. Patients with the device do not need full-dose anticoagulation and can be maintained on aspirin. Common complications include infection and inflow valve incompetence. A survival benefit with the Heartmate for those with class IV heart failure that were ineligible for transplant was seen in the REMATCH trial in which 129 patients who were class IV heart failure but transplant ineligible were assigned to the Heartmate device versus medical therapy. The device group had a survival benefit and also an improved quality of life. Furthermore, patients who received the Heartmate may have better outcomes after transplant than those maintained on intravenous inotropic therapy. The Heartmate XVE has been approved by the Food and Drug Administration for destination therapy of patients with class IV heart failure that fulfill certain characteristics.

Heartmate II

The Heartmate II axial flow rotary pump is a newer and smaller device that offers nonpulsatile flow as support for the end-stage heart failure patient. The device has been studied as a bridge to transplant and can offer prolonged mechanical support in this setting.

Baxter Novacor

The Novacor Left Ventricular Assist System (LVAS) is an electromagnetically driven pump that is implanted below the diaphragm. The pump is connected to a controller outside the body through a percutaneous drive line and is battery powered. The device provides pulsatile flow to the patient and is able to give adequate output to sustain life independent of the patient's left ventricular function. Common complications include thromboembolism (anticoagulation is required) and infection.

Jarvik 2000 FlowMaker

As an intracardiac axial flow impeller pump that is compact and provides continuous flow support, the Jarvik 2000 has been studied as a bridge to transplantation, in limited patients as a destination therapy, and in those that were initially transplant ineligible.

Debakey Pump

The Debakey pump was the first long-term axial flow pump that was implanted as a bridge to transplant and has also been implanted as destination therapy.

Cardiowest Total Artificial Heart

A device that is inserted orthotopically (it is inserted where the patient's heart is with removal of the patient's ventricles) is the Cardiowest Total Artificial Heart. The device has been studied and been successful as a bridge to transplantation.

Abiomed Total Artificial Heart

This is a device that involves total excision of the patient's heart and uses low-viscosity oil and a rotary pump to provide circulatory support to the end-stage heart failure patient. The device is currently being studied for its role in end-stage heart failure.

Waiting List

Organs for transplant are allocated by an agency licensed by the federal government known as United Network for Organ Sharing. Factors that contribute are severity of the patient's disease and time accrued waiting for an organ. Status 1A patients are those with a right heart catheter in place and who are receiving one inotrope at a certain dose, two inotropes at any dose, or mechanical support such as an IABP or mechanical ventilation. Patients that have an LVAD are allowed to have 30 days for status 1A time as well. Status 1B patients are those who are requiring inotropes but do not have a right heart catheter in place and those who have a mechanical assist device and are not currently using their status 1A time. Status 2 patients are those that are relatively stable outpatients, and status 7 patients are those that are currently not transplantable.

Donor Selection and Management

The procurement process is initiated by the local or host organ procurement organization. The process involves a history and physical, including past medical and surgical history, a social history and substance abuse history, donor height and weight, and information about the cause of death and the clinical course. Basic laboratory studies are ordered, and in addition, hepatitis B and hepatitis C, HIV, Epstein-Barre virus (EBV), cytomegalovirus (CMV) titers are sent off. A potential donor will get a chest X-ray, an electrocardiogram, and an echocardiogram as well. Males more than 45 years and females more than 55 years will undergo cardiac catheterization, as will younger patients with significant risk factors. Electrocardiogram may show deep t-wave inversions ("cerebral t waves"). An echocardiogram will look for potential factors that would make the heart less desirable, including left ventricular hypertrophy, significant valvular defects, or congenital heart disease. Coronary angiography will, of course, be looking for obstructive coronary artery disease; there are times when a patient with coronary artery disease will be used as a donor. The patient should have an adequate blood pressure and adequate hemodynamic parameters if measured and should not be requiring high-dose inotropes. Furthermore, the patient should generally be hepatitis B, hepatitis C, and HIV negative and free of overwhelming infection or malignancies (with certain exception, including some primary brain tumors). HIV is an absolute contraindication to transplant, whereas hepatitis B and hepatitis C may be offered to selective higher risk patients or matched to those that have the same disease. HLA prospective cross-matching is reserved to presensitized heart transplant recipients and those with greater than 10% to 20% reactivity to a panel of common donor antigens. A retrospective cross-match is routinely done, the significance of which is unclear.

A full discussion on donor management is outside the scope of this chapter. General principles include maintaining hemodynamic parameters, including blood pressure, cardiac output, and systemic vascular resistance, and maintaining oxygenization and volume status. To accomplish this, many times pressor and inotropic support as well as triiodothyronine replacement (which may be depleted in the brain-dead patient) is administered.

Surgical Technique

The donor heart is usually excised by the transplant team of the recipient hospital after it is arrested with cold cardioplegia. The team members working with the recipient will generally proceed with final preparation, including intubation, after the donor heart is visualized by the other team members and known to be a suitable selection. The biatrial technique for heart transplantation was the original technique described by Lower and Shumway in 1960. In this technique, the donor and the recipient's hearts are excised at the midatrial level, and the aorta and pulmonary artery are transected above the aortic and pulmonic valves. Currently, the bicaval technique is used, which leaves the donor atria intact and transects the superior and inferior vena cava to remove the donor heart. This technique allows for improved atrial and ventricular function, improved valvular function, less atrial arrhythmias, and less sinus node dysfunction and heart block after implantation.

Postoperative Care

Postoperative care is similar in many ways to routine open heart surgery cases. Notable exceptions are the need for immunosuppression, as well as the careful attention that must be given to the right ventricle. There is often the need for significant inotropic and pressor support to maintain cardiac output and blood pressure. There must be careful consideration given to the preload and afterload of the right ventricle after transplant. This is always important, but particularly so when the recipient's pretransplant pulmonary pressures were borderline or elevated. The central venous pressure should not be allowed to be significantly elevated so as to cause distension and mechanical disadvantage of the right ventricle. If the central venous pressure is significantly elevated, diuresis is usually needed, even if the patient's renal function is not optimal so as to prevent right ventricular dilation and failure. The transplanted heart may have sinus node dysfunction postoperatively and may need support with pacing (with epicardial leads placed in the operating room) or pharmacologic support with isoproterenol. At times, this sinus node dysfunction persists, and there is need for permanent pacing.

Immunosuppression

The risk of rejection is generally increased in the first few months after transplant and subsequently decreases. The regimen for immunosuppression since the 1980s has consisted of a calcineurin inhibitor such as cyclosporine or tacrolimus, an antimetabolite (azathioprine or mycophenolic acid), and corticosteroids. Some transplant programs use induction therapy with antilymphocyte antibodies during the postoperative period to give augmented immunosuppression during that time. Induction therapy may allow delayed administration of nephrotoxic immunosuppression in patients with compromised renal function. The anti-interleukin antibodies daclizumab or basiliximab are also used and are useful when a patient's immune system may be more activated, such as in multiparous women, patients who have had an LVAD, and those with a high percentage on a test of reactive antibodies. Mammalian target of rapamycin (mTOR) inhibitors such as sirolimus and everolimus block interleukin (IL)-2– and IL-15–driven proliferation of T, B, and smooth muscle cells.

Common side effects of the immunosuppression used in heart transplant include nephrotoxicity from the calcineurin antagonists, cytopenias and increased risk of viral infections with the antimetabolites, and the well-known problems with chronic steroids, including problems with glucose tolerance, hypertension, and osteoporosis.

Immuknow

A test known as the Immuknow by Cylex is designed to help measure cell-mediated immunity in transplant patients and provide information regarding a patient's immune status and help guide therapy.

Posttransplant Care

Frequent right heart catheterization and biopsies are needed soon after transplant and decrease thereafter, the exact frequency of which varies by center. Left heart catheterization is typically performed at a baseline soon after transplant and then every year as part of an annual assessment.

Complications

Infection

Infection remains the major cause of death in the first year after transplant and can be caused by many sources. Common sources initially are those that arise from the surgical wound, pneumonia, urinary tract infections, indwelling catheters, and involve nosocomial organisms commonly seen in the intensive care unit. After the immediate postoperative period, the infections are more diverse and can be donor acquired, as in the case of CMV or toxoplasmosis. The transplant patient is also susceptible to fungi including *Aspergillus*, Candida, and *Pneumocystis*, as well as Mycobacteria, Nocardia, and Legionella species.

Rejection

Rejection of the donor heart is classified as hyperacute, acute cellular, acute antibody mediated (humoral), or chronic. Hyperacute rejection usually occurs in the setting of circulating preformed antibodies against the ABO blood group or as a result of antibodies against major histocompatability antigens in the donor. This relatively rare phenomenon occurs within the first few minutes to hours after transplantation and requires immediate action in the form of significant hemodynamic support, plasmapheresis, and emergent retransplantation.

Acute cellular rejection is a common phenomenon, with between 50% and 80% of patients having at least one episode in the first year. The incidence is greatest in the third to sixth months after transplant, with the incidence decreasing after that. Table 5.1 illustrates the ISHLT grading system for heart transplant rejection; the older system, because it is well established, is used as well. The presence or absence of antibody mediated rejection is denoted as AMR 0 (no antibody mediated rejection) or AMR 1 (presence of antibody mediated rejection) based on the results of the biopsy.

Malignancy

A sequela of chronic immunosuppression malignancies is common after transplant. Nonmelanotic cutaneous malignancies are common, and lymphomas are as well and are known as posttransplant lymphoproliferative disorder.

Hypertension

Although the mechanism is not completely understood, many patients will have posttransplant hypertension. The mechanism may be related to preglomerular vasoconstriction in the kidney.

Table 5.1 ISHLT Standardized Grading for Presence of Rejection in Heart Biopsies Based on Cellular Rejection

Evidence of Rejection (Cellular)	Grade (1990 system)	Grade (2004 system)
No rejection	0	0
Interstitial and/or perivascular infiltrate with up to one focus of myocyte damage	1A 1B 2	1r (mild)
Two or more foci of mononuclear cell infiltrate with associated myocyte damage	3A	2r (moderate)
Diffuse infiltrate with multifocal myocyte damage with or without edema, hemorrhage, or vasculitis	3B 4	3r (severe)

Adapted from Stewart S, Winters GL, Fishbein MC, et al. Revision of the 1990 working formulation for the standardization of nomenclature in the diagnosis of heart rejection. *J Heart Lung Transplant* 2005;24(11):1710–1720.

Diabetes

Chronic steroids often disrupt a patient's ability to handle glucose, and blood sugars elevate. This provides another motivation to get a patient off chronic steroids if possible.

Posttransplant Vasculopathy

Although the pathogenesis is not fully known, posttransplant vasculopathy or transplant coronary artery disease commonly occurs in the transplanted heart and happens regardless of the patient's original need for transplant. Classically, the disease appears as pruning of the distal vessels on coronary angiography. Some data suggest that the antiproliferative immunosuppressive agents sirolimus and everolimus may help to prevent or decrease the rate of progression of transplant vasculopathy.

6 ■ Pathophysiology of the Failing Heart—Basic Mechanisms: Cellular and Subcellular Abnormalities

Risto Kerkela, MD, PhD
Thomas Force, MD

A large number of cellular and subcellular abnormalities characterize the failing heart, and although these processes often do not initiate the onset of heart failure, they are critically important in the progression of disease to advanced failure. In the cell membrane of the cardiomyocyte, two major abnormalities are prevalent: (1) downregulation and desensitization of the β_1-adrenergic receptor (AR) and (2) activation of receptors for various neurohormonal mediators, most importantly angiotensin II and aldosterone. Within the cardiomyocyte, alterations in activity of various signaling pathways lead to abnormalities of calcium handling and to activation of proapoptotic programs. The latter leads to myocyte loss, and this, together with the abnormal calcium handling, leads to contractile dysfunction. Remodeling of the extracellular matrix (i.e., increased interstitial fibrosis) is also central to the progression of heart failure, although the mechanisms driving this remain poorly understood.

Herein, we examine the contributions that abnormalities of β-AR signaling, calcium handling, and apoptosis make to heart failure progression. We also discuss strategies to manipulate these responses to potentially retard the progression of heart failure. The latter is critical because very few novel approaches to prevention of heart failure progression are in the offing, and outcomes are still extremely poor in this patient population. Although this cannot be a thorough look at the molecular pathophysiology of heart failure, it will serve as an introduction. Interested readers are referred to the references at the end of this book.

Abnormalities of β-Adrenergic Receptors

There are three types of β-ARs in the human heart—β_1, β_2, and β_3—with β_1 accounting for 75% to 80% of the total. Appropriate responsiveness to catecholamine stimulation, mediated primarily by activation of β_1-ARs, is critical for the heart's response to stressors. Similarly, there must be a way to deactivate β-receptors to avoid overstimulation. This is accomplished by a process called desensitization, which results when a molecule called β-arrestin binds to the receptor and prevents further interactions with downstream mediators. In addition, β-arrestin internalizes the receptor, leading to downregulation (i.e., a decrease in receptor number). Surprisingly, given the increased levels of circulating catecholamines in patients with heart failure, it has been known for over 20 years that β_1-adrenergic signaling is reduced. This is due to the fact that receptor density and responsiveness are depressed in the failing human heart (caused by receptor downregulation and desensitization). This mechanism underlies part of the reason for the failure of β-AR agonists in patients with heart failure because when used chronically they lead to further desensitization and downregulation. Multiple studies in various mouse models of heart failure have demonstrated that restoration of β-AR levels and responsiveness, achieved by blocking β-arrestin's function, have beneficial effects on the heart. Currently, the only available therapeutic approach to re-storing β-AR responsiveness is the use of β-receptor antagonists or β-blockers. Although this sounds antithetical, this is necessary to counteract the downregulation and to restore some level of expression of the receptor; however, the dysregulation of this system also points out the problem with β-blockers in the acute decompensated heart failure patient. In these patients, β-receptors are typically markedly downregulated, and inhibiting the few remaining receptors with β-blockers can cause a profound deterioration in hemodynamic status. As one can see, too little or too much β-AR signaling in the failing heart is detrimental, and it is necessary to attempt to optimize this—a difficult task in the heart failure patient.

Abnormalities of Calcium Handling

Proper Ca^{2+} handling is essential for efficient excitation-contraction coupling, the backbone of heart function. With cell depolarization, Ca^{2+} enters through the voltage-dependent Ca^{2+} channel (target of commercially available "calcium channel blockers"). This Ca^{2+} entry activates the ryanodine receptor (RyR2), the major calcium release channel of the sarcoplasmic reticulum (SR; the storage pool for Ca^{2+}), which then releases calcium, leading to myocyte contraction. Cardiac relaxation occurs when Ca^{2+} is removed from the system by being taken up by the SR Ca^{2+}-ATPase, SERCA2a. A number of abnormalities in this system characterize the failing heart and are currently the focus of much investigation, including clinical trials. One classic abnormality is a decrease in the amount of SERCA2a in the failing heart. This leads to impaired reuptake of Ca^{2+}, increased diastolic [Ca^{2+}], and alterations in diastolic relaxation. In addition, the SR becomes partially depleted of Ca^{2+} such that insufficient amounts of Ca^{2+} are released during systole, leading to systolic dysfunction. Numerous studies by Hajjar and coworkers have demonstrated improvement of cardiac function in various animal models of heart failure after adenovirus-mediated gene transfer of SERCA2a, and a clinical trial of SERCA2a gene therapy is now recruiting.

Another abnormality involves RyR2. Increased sympathetic tone activates the β_1-AR, and this leads to the dissociation of an inhibitory factor from the RyR2. This can lead to excess diastolic leak of Ca^{2+}, which together with the already increased diastolic [Ca^{2+}] caused by dysfunctional SERCA2a, can lead to delayed after-depolarizations, triggering ventricular tachyarrhythmias. Small molecule drugs are currently in development to block the RyR2 leak.

Apoptosis

The decline in left ventricular function in heart failure has been associated with a reduction in the total myocyte number. This is mainly due to increased cell death, but there *may* also be a component of insufficient myocyte regeneration. Cell death can occur by apoptosis or necrosis, but both often coexist in the diseased heart. An additional type of cell death, autophagy, which shares several features with apoptosis, has been recognized more recently in the failing heart, but the significance of this is entirely unclear at this time. Necrosis appears to be the main type of cell death in the ischemic heart (although apoptosis is also clearly present), whereas apoptosis predominates in chronic heart failure.

Apoptosis is an energy-requiring process that is characterized by cell shrinkage, caspase activation, and DNA fragmentation. It can be triggered by two different mechanisms: extrinsic and intrinsic. The extrinsic pathway is activated by binding of death ligands to tumor necrosis factor receptor family members on the cell surface. This recruits procaspase-8 into the death-inducing signaling complex. Activated caspase-8 then cleaves and activates the common executioner caspase, procaspase-3, leading to cell death.

Activation of the intrinsic, or mitochondrial, pathway can be triggered by the extrinsic pathway but more importantly by a number of different cellular stresses, such as energy or nutrient deprivation, hypoxia, radiation, DNA damage, toxins, or reactive oxygen species. In human heart failure, there is evidence of increased myocardial oxidative stress. Not only is reactive oxygen species production increased in the failing heart. There is also a decrease in the activity of antioxidant enzymes, and markers of oxidative stress are increased in the blood.

Studies have reported apoptosis rates of 0.08% to 0.25% in patients with end-stage dilated cardiomyopathy compared with 0.001% to 0.002% in controls. One nagging question has concerned whether these low rates of apoptosis contribute substantially to the progression of heart failure. Although this is a difficult question to answer, the general consensus, based on animal models and calculations based on explanted hearts, is that apoptosis does contribute significantly to the progression of heart failure. Because caspases in the apoptotic machinery can also cleave contractile proteins, including actins, myosin, and troponins, it is possible that activation of apoptotic pathways could also contribute to contractile dysfunction, independent of effects on cell death.

Abnormalities of Intracellular Signaling Pathways

A number of intracellular signaling pathways have been identified as critical transducers in many of the pathological conditions of the heart, and dysregulation of these pathways is associated with both maladaptive cardiac remodeling and end-stage heart failure. In this section, we briefly highlight two critical signaling pathways that are dysregulated in heart failure and therefore that may play a role in the progression of heart failure. This is not a thorough examination of this issue, because of space constraints, but we attempt to simply describe how signaling pathways regulate various aspects of hypertrophy and heart failure.

Prosurvival Pathways: Phosphoinositide-3-Kinase Pathway

The dominant prosurvival pathway in the heart is the phosphoinositide-3-kinase (PI3K) pathway. This pathway leads to the activation of the canonical prosurvival kinase, Akt (also known as protein kinase B, or PKB, in Europe). This pathway is typically activated by growth factors, including insulin, insulin-like growth factor-1, platelet-derived growth factor, and so forth. Activation of either PI3K or Akt/PKB has been shown to protect from ischemic injury in animal models. This is accomplished in part by blocking activation of proapoptotic pathways (Bad, FOXO, GSK-3, etc.) and also by enhancing glucose uptake into cells by increasing activity of glucose transporters in the cardiomyocyte membrane. This pathway also regulates physiologic cardiac hypertrophy (i.e., an athlete's heart), but does not appear to be important in the development of pathologic hypertrophy such as one sees with extreme pressure loads on the heart or after a large myocardial infarction. Interestingly, activity of Akt appears to be significantly increased in failing human hearts. Obviously, the survival benefits that this may confer on the failing heart are inadequate to prevent progression of heart failure.

Prohypertrophic Pathway: Calcineurin

Calcineurin is a protein phosphatase (i.e., it removes phosphate groups from other proteins, altering their activity or cellular distribution). It is the target of tacrolimus (Prograf), although inhibition of calcineurin in heart transplant patients is aimed at the immune system, not calcineurin's effects on hypertrophy. Calcineurin has been shown to play a central role in the development of pathologic hypertrophy in experimental models. Calcineurin physically interacts with and dephosphorylates members of the NF-AT (nuclear factor of activated T-cells) family of transcription factors. Once dephosphorylated, NF-ATs translocate to the nucleus, where they trigger expression of genes involved in the immune response in T cells. In cardiomyocytes, NF-ATc4 has been shown to associate with the transcription factor GATA-4 to activate transcription of a number of genes driving myocyte growth. Although there are a number of signaling pathways implicated in the development of cardiac hypertrophy, calcineurin is one of the few factors consistently activated in hypertrophied human hearts. Calcineurin is also increased in failing human hearts, and enzymatic activity of calcineurin is significantly increased in these hearts. Increased calcineurin activity also contributes to decreased SERCA2a activity and impaired calcium reuptake in the failing human myocardium. Finally, calcineurin has been reported to activate apoptosis in some settings. Thus, hypertrophic growth, altered calcium handling, and increased apoptosis are consequences of calcineurin activation.

Gene Expression

The initial response of cardiomyocytes to increased load is to hypertrophy, and the first genetic response is classical activation of a pattern of early response, or immediate early genes: *c-fos*, *c-myc*, and *c-jun*. This is followed by induction of the so-called fetal gene program, that is, increased expression of genes encoding fetal isoforms of sarcomeric proteins and the natriuretic peptides, atrial natriuretic peptide (ANP) and brain natriuretic peptide (BNP). The time line for activation pattern in the human heart is not clear, but long-term stress leads to induction of ANP and BNP, as well as the sodium calcium exchanger (NCX), which is hypothesized to compensate for impaired calcium reuptake secondary to decreased SERCA2a activity. BNP expression is triggered by atrial stretch, which is in most cases secondary to increased filling pressure in the left ventricle (LV). This accounts for its utility as a biomarker of heart failure.

Conclusions

Much remains to be discovered about the signaling networks that regulate processes as diverse as β-AR expression/desensitization, apoptosis, calcium handling, hypertrophic responses, and so forth. Ultimately, discoveries related to these pathways will drive new drug development and offer the hope of being able to halt, or even reverse, the inexorable progression of heart failure.

7 ▪ Hemodynamics

Anish Koka, MD
David L. Fischman, MD

Right Heart Catheterization

- Right heart catheterization allows direct measurement of pressures on the right side of the heart, including the right atrium, right ventricle, pulmonary artery, and pulmonary occlusive pressure.
- Access to the right heart is typically obtained through the right internal jugular vein, the right subclavian vein, or the femoral veins.
- Bedside floatation of a balloon-tipped catheter from the right atrium to the right ventricle to the pulmonary artery to measure right heart hemodynamics was pioneered by Swan and Ganz, and thus, the catheter used is often called the Swan-Ganz catheter.
- The right atrial pressure waveform consists of the following:
  - *a* Wave—atrial contraction, which immediately follows the p wave on the ECG
  - *c* Wave—onset of right ventricular systole
  - *x* Descent—atrial relaxation and ventricular contraction that pulls the floor of the right atrium towards the apex
  - *v* Wave—passive filling of the right atrium when the tricuspid valve is closed
  - *y* Descent—passive ventricular filling from the atria after the tricuspid valve opens
  - Right atrial pressure is generally considered the mean of the *a* wave, as this approximates right ventricular end diastolic pressure
  - Normal RA pressures range from 2 to 8 mm Hg

- Right ventricular pressure waveform consists of the following:
  - Sharp rapid upstroke and a rapid down stroke that approximates the baseline before rising slightly
  - Normal right ventricular pressures range from 15 to 30 mm Hg systolic and 2 to 8 mm Hg diastolic
- Pulmonary artery pressure waveform consists of the following:
  - A rapid upstroke and down stroke
  - A dicrotic notch that marks closure of the pulmonary valve
  - Smooth, progressive runoff (diastole)
  - The peak of the pulmonary artery (PA) wave usually comes *before* the T wave, which helps distinguish pulmonary artery pressure from the wedge pressure tracing
  - Normally PA systolic pressures are equal to right ventricular systolic pressures
  - Normal PA pressures range from 15 to 25 mm Hg systolic and 4 to 12 mm Hg diastolic
- Pulmonary artery occlusion pressure
  - Floatation of a balloon-tipped catheter into the pulmonary artery and continued advancement results in "wedging" of the catheter in the interlobar arteries of the pulmonary artery.
  - This creates a hydrostatic column of fluid from the pulmonary artery all of the way to the left atrium and thus approximates left atrial pressure in the absence of mitral valve disease.
  - The normal wedge waveform is similar to the right atrial waveform, except it is delayed:
    - *a* Wave—left atrial contraction, which usually occurs right after the QRS complex
    - *c* Wave—closure of the mitral valve, usually not very prominent on wedge tracings

- *x* Descent—atrial relaxation and ventricular contraction that pulls the floor of the left atrium towards the apex of the heart
- *v* Wave—passive filling of the left atrium when the mitral valve is closed, typically occurs *after* the T wave, which often helps distinguish a significant *v* wave from the pulmonary artery pressure
- *y* Descent—passive filling of the left ventricle from the left atrium after the mitral valve opens
- Normal wedge pressure—5 to 12 mm Hg

Factors That Influence the Magnitude of Wave Forms

- A number of factors can augment or diminish the pressure wave forms.
    - Heart failure
    - Hypertension
    - Vasoconstriction
    - Vascular disease

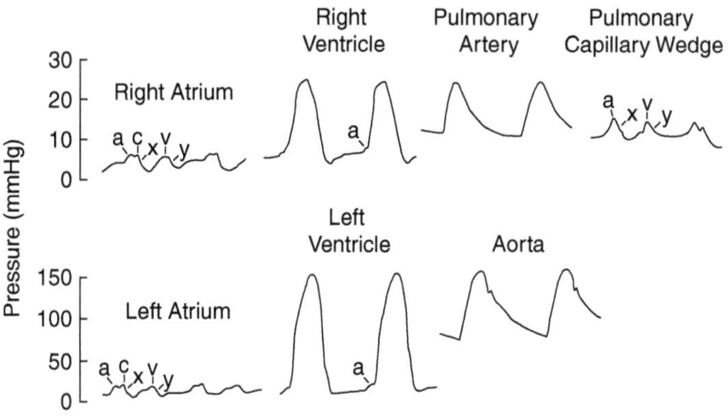

■ **Figure 7.1** Normal Pressure Waveforms

Table 7.1 Normal Hemodynamic Measurements

Pressures	Normal Values (mm Hg)
Right atrial pressure	2–8
Right ventricular systolic pressure	15–30
Right ventricular diastolic pressure	2–8
Pulmonary artery systolic pressure	15–25
Pulmonary artery diastolic pressure	4–12
Pulmonary artery occlusion pressure (wedge)	5–12
Left atrium	4–16
Left ventricle peak systolic	90–140
Left ventricle end diastolic	5–12
Central aorta peak systolic	90–140
Central aorta end diastolic	60–90
Vascular resistance	Mean (dyne-sec-cm –5)
Systemic vascular resistance	1,170 ± 270
Pulmonary vascular resistance	67 ± 30
Cardiac output	6–8 L/min

  - Valsalva maneuver
  - Vasodilation
  - Hypovolemia
  - Hypotension
- Pathological changes of the atrial pressure wave form
  - Large *a* wave
    - Hypervolemia
    - Valvular stenosis
    - Pericardial disease/effusion
    - Congestive heart failure/infarction
    - Poor compliance
  - Missing *a* wave

    - Atrial arrest
    - Atrial fibrillation
    - Atrial flutter
  - Giant *a* wave
    - AV dissociation
    - Complete heart block
    - Premature atrial beats
  - Elevated *v* wave
    - Increased flow
    - Valvular insufficiency (regurgitation)
    - Myocardial ischemia/infarction
  - *x* Descent
    - Absent *x*—descent: valvular regurgitation interrupts *x* descent (*c-v* wave)
    - Steep *x*—descent: constrictive pericarditis
  - *y* Descent
    - Rapid, deep descent occurs with severe tricuspid regurgitation (TR), constrictive pericarditis
    - Slow *y* descent—valvular stenosis, atrial myxoma, and pericardial tamponade all delay ventricular filling

Indications for Right Heart Catheterization

- Differentiation between cardiogenic and noncardiogenic pulmonary edema
- Differentiation between causes of shock
- Management of patients with cardiomyopathy and congestive heart failure
- Evaluation of pulmonary hypertension
- Diagnosis of pericardial tamponade
- Evaluation and management of complications of myocardial infarction
- Pretransplant evaluation
- Evaluation of congenital heart disease
- Evaluation of valvular heart disease

Left Heart Catheterization

- Allows direct measurement of pressures of the left side of the heart (left ventricle) as well as central aortic pressure. Left atrial pressure cannot be directly measured without transversing the mitral valve in a retrograde fashion. More commonly, when necessary, it can be obtained via a transseptal approach from the right side of the heart.
- Access to the left side of the heart is usually through the femoral or brachial artery.
- The best approximation of left ventricular filling pressure (preload) is left ventricular end diastolic pressure.

Cardiac Output

- The volume of blood pumped by the ventricle into the systemic circulation per minute is usually measured in liters by the Fick Principle or Thermodilution technique.
- The Fick Principle assumes that the rate at which oxygen is consumed is a function of the rate of blood flow and the rate of oxygen pickup by the red blood cells.
  - The total uptake or release of any substance by an organ is the product of the blood flow to the organ and the arteriovenous (AV) concentration difference of the substance.
  - Cardiac output equals the oxygen consumption by lungs/ AV oxygen difference across pulmonary vascular bed.
  - Oxygen consumption can be measured by metabolic rate meters, but is usually assumed to be 125 ml/m^2.
  - Measuring oxygen content in the pulmonary artery and systemic arterial bed provides the AV oxygen difference across the pulmonary vascular bed.
  - Cardiac output (CO) equals oxygen consumption/ (arteriovenous O_2 difference $\times$ Hgb $\times$ 1.36 $\times$ 10)
- Pulmonary artery thermodilution
  - This also uses Fick's general principle.

  - Cold saline is injected in a proximal port of the right heart catheter.
  - A temperature sensor (thermistor) in a distal port of the catheter measures the temperature change after injectate given.
  - An algorithm is used by the computer to measure cardiac output.
  - It is unreliable in the presence of significant tricuspid regurgitation.

Vascular Resistance

- Resistance = mean pressure drop across a vascular circuit/flow across the vascular circuit
  - Systemic vascular resistance = (mean systemic arterial pressure – right atrial pressure)/cardiac output
  - Pulmonary vascular resistance = (mean pulmonary arterial pressure – pulmonary artery wedge pressure)/cardiac output
  - These equations give units of mm Hg/liters per minute = hybrid resistance units or Wood units.
  - Hybrid resistance units $\times$ 80 = dynes-sec-cm^{-5}

Intracardiac Shunts

- Right heart catheterization can be used to identify abnormal communications between the right and left sides of the heart by performing a "shunt run" or an "oximetry run."
  - In an oximetry run, the oxygen content (or percent saturation) of blood is measured in blood samples drawn sequentially from the pulmonary artery, right ventricle, right atrium, superior vena cava, and inferior vena cava.
  - Normally, oxygen saturation should not vary much in these right-sided structures, as they sample blood that has not been oxygenated by the lungs.
  - A left-right shunt may be detected and localized if a significant increase (step-up) in oxygen saturation is found in one of the right heart chambers.

Table 7.2 Detection of Left-to-Right Shunts (Criteria for Significant Step Up)

Level of Shunt	O_2 % Sat	Possible Causes
Atrial (SVC/IVC to RA)	≥ 7	ASD, partial anomalous pulmonary venous return
Ventricular (RA to RV)	≥ 5	VSD, primum ASD, coronary fistula to RV
Great Vessel (RV to PA)	≥ 5	PDA, aorta–pulmonary window

Valvular Pathology

- Mitral stenosis (see Figure 7.2)
  - Stiff mitral valve leaflets result in a diastolic pressure gradient between the left atrium and left ventricle.

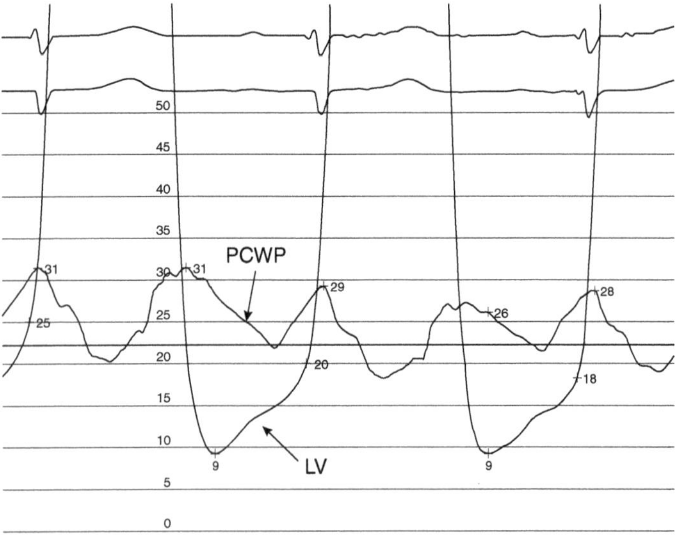

■ **Figure 7.2** Mitral Stenosis

- The Gorlin formula allows an estimation of valve area based on the diastolic pressure gradient and cardiac output.
- Mitral regurgitation
  - Giant *v* waves are typically seen in acute mitral regurgitation, although this is not at all specific.
  - A large *v* wave on a left atrial pressure tracing suggests mitral regurgitation.
- Aortic stenosis (see Figure 7.3)
  - Noncompliant aortic valve leaflets result in a systolic pressure gradient between the left ventricle and the aorta.
  - The Gorlin formula can be used to estimate valve area based on the systolic pressure gradient and the cardiac output.

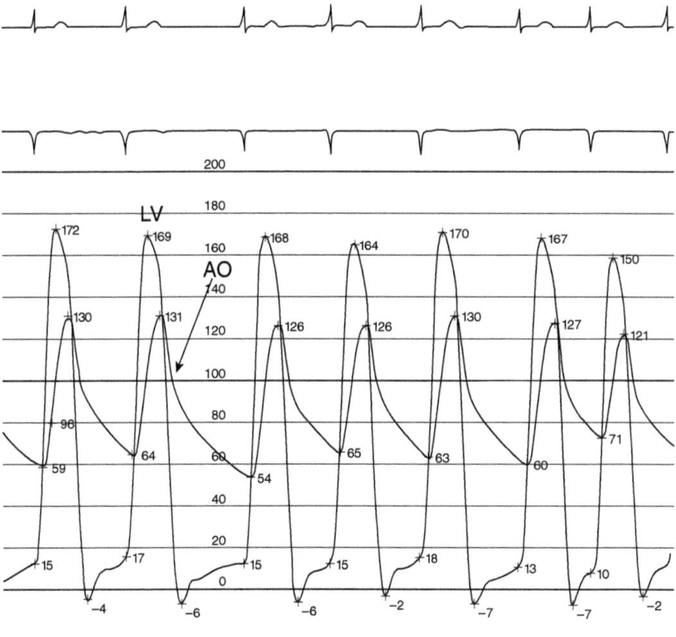

■ **Figure 7.3** Aortic Stenosis

$$\text{Valve area} = \frac{\text{Cardiac Output}}{\text{HR} \times \text{SEP} \times 44.3 \times \sqrt{\Delta P}}$$

$$\text{SEP} = \text{Systolic ejection period}$$
$$\text{HR} = \text{Heart rate}$$
$$\Delta P = \text{Pressure gradient}$$

- A simplified formula for calculating valve area is the Hakki equation:

$$\text{Valve area} = \frac{\text{Cardiac Output}}{\Delta P}$$

$$\Delta P = \text{Pressure gradient}$$

- Aortic regurgitation
  - Blood leaks into the left ventricle during diastole because of incompetence of the aortic valves.
  - A large stroke volume enters the aorta and raises systolic blood pressure, but subsequent regurgitation during diastole lowers diastolic blood pressure leading to a widened pulse pressure.
  - Blood flowing into the left ventricle during diastole raises left ventricular pressure and may cause premature closure of the mitral valve.
  - Hemodynamic waveforms are characterized by decline in aortic pressure through diastole and late diastolic rise of left ventricular pressure.
- Tricuspid regurgitation
  - Large systolic *v* wave in the right atrial pressure tracing
  - With increasing regurgitation, right atrial waveform resembles right ventricular wave form, with rapid upstroke and rapid runoff

Pericardial Diseases

- Pericardial effusion/tamponade
  - Normally the pericardial space has a minimal amount of fluid in it that is hemodynamically significant.

- Instillation of fluid into the pericardial space results initially in a reduction of pulmonary arterial stroke volume that is followed soon after by a reduction in aortic stroke volume.
- Thus, pericardial fluid exerts much of its effect by decreasing right ventricular filling, which secondarily results in a lower left ventricular output.
- As fluid accumulates in the pericardial space and pericardial pressures increase, diastolic filling pressures in the cardiac chambers begin to equalize because they are now dependent on pericardial pressure.
- Examination of the jugular venous pulsation or right atrial pressure waveform during catheterization demonstrates a preserved *x* descent and an attenuated *y* descent. The mechanism is explained here:
  - Blood can only enter the heart when blood that is in the heart leaves the heart.
  - The right atrial *y* descent normally begins with opening of the tricuspid valve.
  - Because there is equalization of diastolic pressures in the right atrium and right ventricle, there is no gradient for flow.
  - There is also no blood leaving the right ventricle.
  - Thus, no blood can enter the heart, and the *y* descent is lost.
  - In contrast, the *x* descent occurs during ventricular systole, and thus, blood from the right atrium can flow into the right ventricle to replace the blood that was just ejected during systole.
- Pulsus paradoxus is evident in tamponade.
  - There is exaggeration of the normal variation in pulse that occurs with respiration.
  - Normally during inspiration, negative intrathoracic pressures increase venous return and thus increase filling of the right ventricle.

    - Because the right ventricle (RV) and left ventricle (LV) share a wall (the septum), an increase in RV filling causes an increased LV diastolic pressure, which reduces the gradient to flow from the pulmonary veins and left atrium into the left ventricle.
    - This reduces preload on the left ventricle and results in a lower stroke volume, causing a drop in systemic arterial pressure.
    - In the presence of a significant pericardial effusion, the right ventricle can not bow out into the pericardial space and thus has a much bigger impact on the left ventricle.
    - The exaggerated rise in left ventricular diastolic pressure that is affected results in an exaggerated drop in stroke volume and systemic pressures during inspiration.
    - The exaggerated drop in systemic arterial pressure (> 10 mm Hg) with inspiration is referred to as pulsus paradoxus.
  - Pulsus paradoxus is not specific for pericardial tamponade and can also be seen in
    - Pulmonary embolism
    - Cardiogenic shock
    - Tension pneumothorax
    - Asthma
    - Anaphylactic shock
    - Superior vena cava obstruction
- Constrictive pericarditis
  - This is the end stage of an inflammatory process involving the pericardium.
  - The pericardium becomes dense, fibrotic, and often calcified.
  - This results in restricted filling of the ventricle.
  - Abnormally high atrial pressures and accentuated early diastolic ventricular suction result in rapid early filling, which ceases abruptly when ventricular volume reaches the limits of the stiff pericardium.

- The stiffened, thick pericardium serves to insulate the cardiac chambers from changes in intrathoracic pressures during respiration.
- A reduction in pulmonary venous pressures causes a reduction in the small pulmonary vein to left atrial gradient that normally determines left ventricular filling.
- Reduced filling of the left ventricle results in a leftward shift of the interventricular septum and augmentation of right ventricular filling.
- The opposite phenomenon occurs during expiration.
- Examination of the jugular venous pulse or a right atrial waveform during right heart catheterization demonstrates the following:
  - A prominent *y* descent because of the increased gradient between the left atrium and left ventricle in early diastole
  - Simultaneous measurement of right and left ventricular pressures during diastole demonstrates the "square root" sign—a rapid early dip in right and left ventricular pressures that abruptly ceases
- Kussmaul's sign

Table 7.3 Differentiating Tamponade from Constrictive Pericarditis

	Tamponade	Constrictive Pericarditis
Paradoxical pulse	Usually present	Present in ≈ 1/3
Equal left/right filling pressures	Present	Present
Systemic venous wave morphology	Absent *y* descent	Prominent *y* descent (M or W shape)
Inspiratory change in systemic venous pressure	Decrease (normal)	Increase or no change (Kussmaul sign)
"Square root" sign in ventricular pressure	Absent	Present

    - Lack of a decrease or an increase in the jugular venous pulse with inspiration
    - Present in approximately one third of patients with constrictive pericarditis
    - Absent in pericardial effusion/tamponade

Restrictive Cardiomyopathy

- Restrictive cardiomyopathy is a disease of the heart in which the major pathophysiologic process is diastolic dysfunction.
- The diagnosis is made by the finding of elevated filling pressures out of proportion to systolic dysfunction or valvular abnormalities.
- Hemodynamic findings include the following:
  - High filling pressures in all four chambers of the heart
  - A "dip and plateau" pattern in ventricular pressure waveforms during early diastole
  - Rapid *x* and *y* descents in atrial pressure waveforms
- Differentiating restrictive cardiomyopathy from constrictive pericarditis can be difficult (Table 7.4).
  - Processes resulting in restriction affect the left ventricle more than the right ventricle, resulting in a difference in end diastolic pressures of the left and right ventricle.

Table 7.4 Differentiating Restrictive Cardiomyopathy from Constrictive Pericarditis

Restrictive	Constrictive
LVEDP 5 mm HG > RVEDP	LVEDP – RVEDP < 5 mm Hg
Pulmonary artery pressure > 50 mm Hg	Pulmonary Artery Pressure < 50 mm Hg
Ratio of RVEDP to RV systolic pressure < 1:3	Ratio of RVEDP to RV systolic pressure > 1:3

  - Severe pulmonary hypertension is associated with restrictive cardiomyopathy.
- Common causes of restrictive cardiomyopathy include amyloidosis, sarcoidosis, and hemochromatosis.

Hypertrophic Obstructive Cardiomyopathy

- Hypertrophic cardiomyopathy is a common autosomal dominant genetic disorder resulting in severe hypertrophy of the left ventricle with obstruction to left ventricular outflow.
- Typically, a systolic pressure gradient exists between the left ventricle and the central aorta because of outflow tract obstruction caused by extensive hypertrophy of the interventricular septum.
- The pressure gradient is made worse by maneuvers that reduce intracavitary ventricular volume or increase cardiac contractility.
- Hemodynamic findings observed with hypertrophic cardiomyopathy (HOCM) include the following:
  - Diastolic dysfunction with elevated left ventricular end diastolic pressure (LVEDP) is seen.
  - A dynamic pressure gradient across the aortic valve is dependent on preload, afterload, and contractility with a characteristic spike and dome configuration of the aortic pressure waveform.
  - Valsalva and extrasystoles both increase the dynamic gradient.
  - An increase in the gradient and a decrease in the pulse pressure after a premature contraction are hallmark findings and are known as the Brockenbrough-Braunwald sign (see Figure 7.4).
  - The fall in pulse pressure is believed to be due to worsening obstruction in setting of augmented contractility because of increased calcium loading and increased preload after a premature beat.

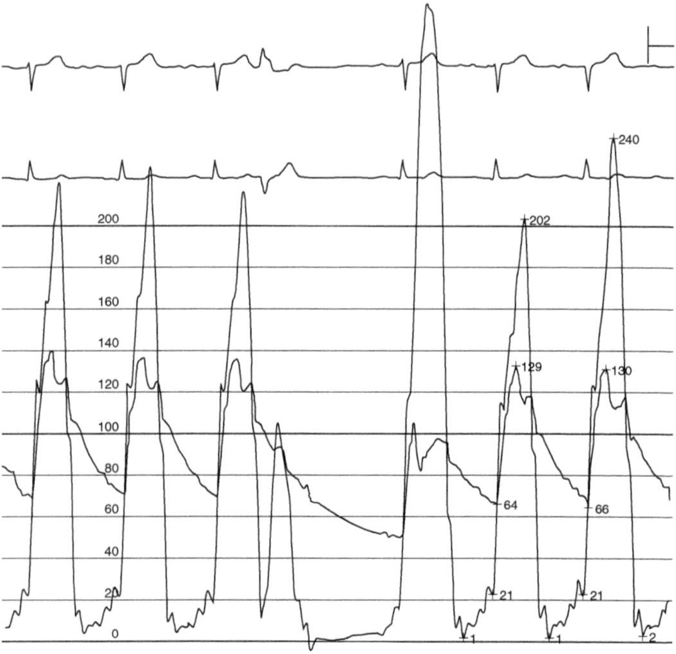

■ Figure 7.4 Brockenbrough-Braunwald sign

Complications of Right Heart Catheterization

- A number of complications can occur during the course of a right heart catheterization. These include the following:
  - Vascular injury during insertion of the catheter
  - Knotting of catheter within the vasculature
  - Pneumothorax
  - Pulmonary perforation
  - Tamponade
  - Infection
  - Atrial and ventricular arrhythmia
  - Complete heart block

- If the patient has an underlying left bundle branch block, a complete heart block may result in injury to the right bundle branch during catheter passage through the right ventricle.
- If right heart catheterization is absolutely necessary, perform this under fluoroscopy.
- Emergent transvenous pacer placement may be necessary if complete heart block results.

8 ■ Coronary Interventional Techniques

Nicholas J. Ruggiero II, MD, FACC, FSCA
Thomas J. Kiernan, MD
Michael P. Savage, MD

In 1977, the late Swiss radiologist Andreas Gruentzig first performed balloon angioplasty as an alternative to coronary artery bypass surgery for patients with coronary artery disease. Since this landmark procedure, the field of interventional cardiology has grown considerably, and the use of interventional techniques after diagnostic angiography for the treatment of ischemic heart disease is now commonplace. This chapter provides a basic foundation for the indications, techniques, contraindications, and complications of coronary artery interventions.

Percutaneous coronary intervention (PCI), commonly known as coronary angioplasty or simply angioplasty, is a therapeutic procedure to treat the stenotic (narrowed) coronary arteries of the heart found in coronary artery disease.

Figures 8.1 and 8.2 show a generalized schematic of a coronary angioplasty:

1. A guiding catheter is seated in the ostium of the target coronary artery.
2. A thin, steerable guidewire is manipulated through the guide into the coronary artery and placed across the stenosis into the distal portion of the vessel.
3. An angioplasty balloon is then passed over the guidewire across the lesion.
4. Once positioned correctly, the balloon is inflated several times for various periods of time (from 10 seconds to several minutes, with the average being approximately 30 seconds).

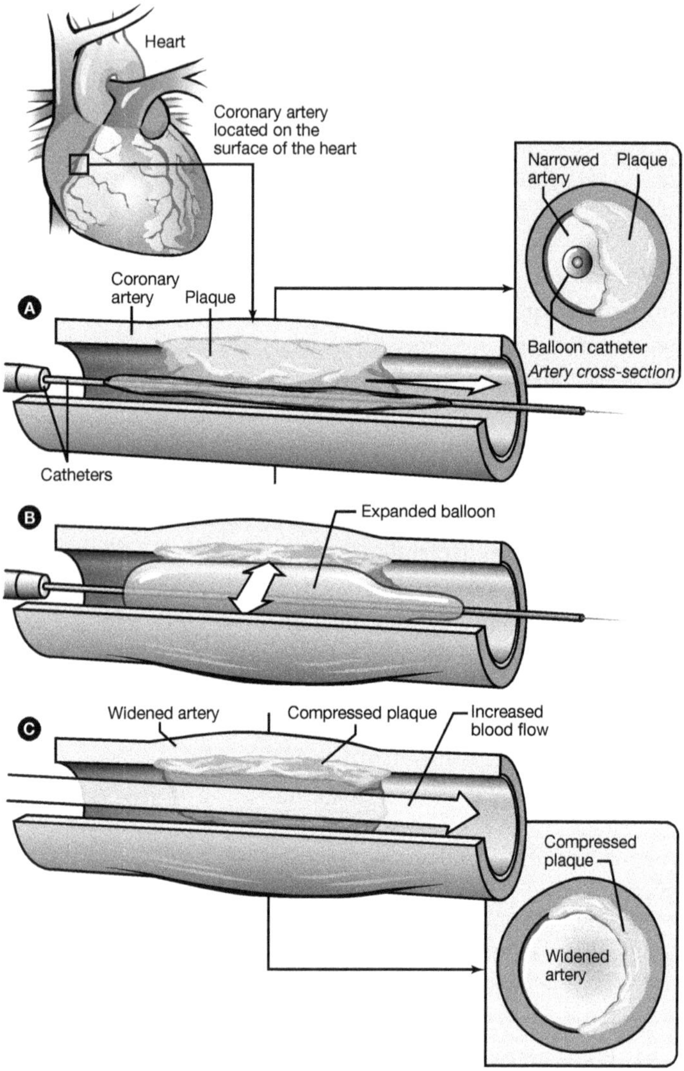

■ **Figure 8.1** Schematic of percutaneous transluminal coronary angioplasty

Source: US Dept of Health and Human Services. NIH. NHLBI. http:www.nhlbi.nih.gov/health/dci/Diseases/Angioplasty/Angioplasty_All.html

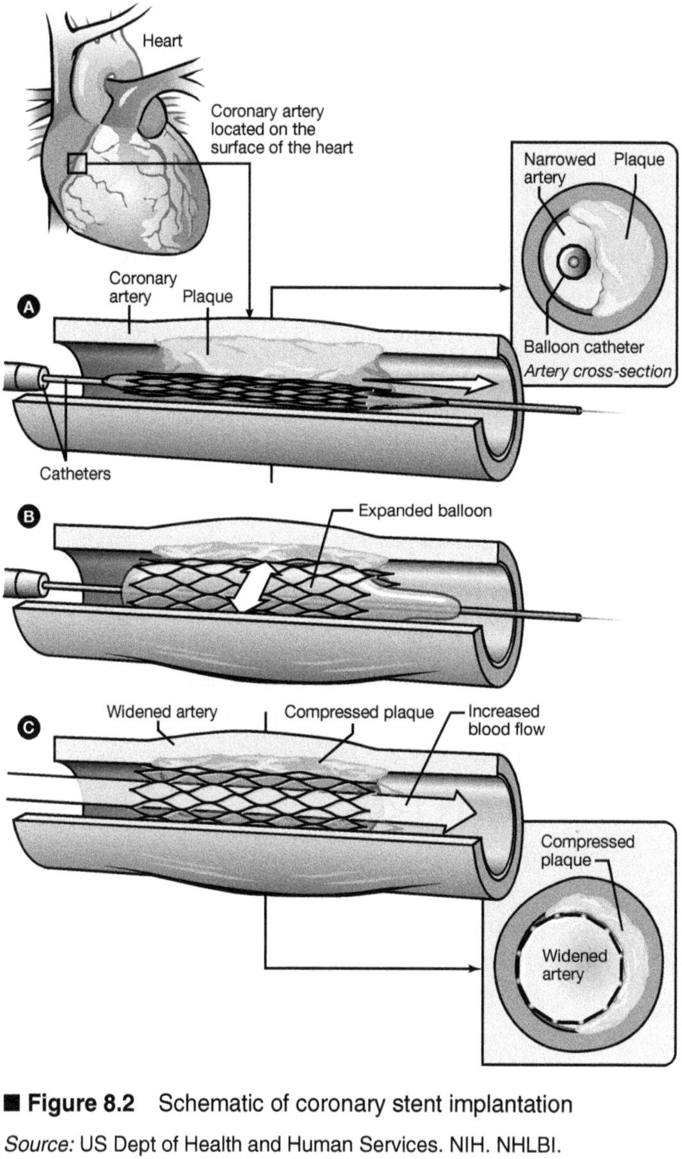

■ **Figure 8.2** Schematic of coronary stent implantation

Source: US Dept of Health and Human Services. NIH. NHLBI. http:www.nhlbi.nih.gov/health/dci/Diseases/Angioplasty/Angioplasty_All.html.

5. The inflation and deflation of the balloon compress the lesion and restore blood flow to the distal vessel. This is known as predilation.
6. After the vessel is opened, a metallic stent mounted on an inflation balloon is place across the lesion and expanded to maintain patency, as seen in Figure 8.2.

Theories of How Balloon Angioplasty Works

- The balloon inflation exerts pressure against the plaque and arterial wall, accounting for fracture of the plaque. This typically occurs at the thinnest/weakest point of a concentric lesion and at the junction of the plaque and the arterial wall in eccentric lesions. This dissection or separation of the plaque from the medial wall releases the narrowing effect and results in a larger lumen.
- The balloon inflation causes stretching/thinning of the medial wall and loss of elastic recoil; however, over time (1 to 6 weeks), there may be a renarrowing of the artery because of elastic recoil, which is prevented by stent placement.
- The shear stress of the balloon inflation accounts for stripping of endothelial cells and an extrusion of plaque components.

Indications for PCI

- Symptomatic angina pectoris despite optimal medical therapy
- Angina pectoris with objective evidence of ischemia
    - Abnormal stress test
    - Fractional flow reserve (FFR) < 0.75
    - High-grade lesion more than 70% in a vessel supplying a large area of myocardium
- Unstable angina
- Primary therapy of acute myocardial infarction or secondary therapy in patients with persistent or recurrent ischemia after failed thrombolytic therapy

- Angina pectoris after coronary artery bypass graft (CABG)
- Restenosis after a prior successful PCI

Contraindications for PCI

- Unsuitable coronary anatomy
- High-risk coronary anatomy in which closure would result in patient death
- Contraindication to CABG (unless PCI is the only alternative)
- Bleeding diathesis
- Patient noncompliance with the procedure and post-PCI instructions
- Multiple PCI restenoses
- Patients who cannot give informed consent, unless it is an emergency procedure

Complications

- Death (< 1%)
- Myocardial infarction (< 3% to 5%)
- Emergency CABG caused by abrupt vessel closure (0.8%)
- Complications associated with normal cardiac catheterization
  - Bleeding
  - Infection
  - Acute renal failure/hemodialysis
  - Stroke
- Restenosis (intimal hyperplasia at the site of PCI)
  - Occurs in approximately 10% to 30% of patients after bare metal stent placement
  - Less than 10% after drug-eluting stent placement
  - Typically occurs in the initial 6 months after PCI and presents with recurrence of anginal symptoms
- Stent thrombosis
  - Acute—occurs within 24 hours of stent implantation

- Early—occurs within 30 days of stent implantation. The risk is highest within the first 48 hours and occurs in approximately 0.9% of cases. The risk factors are as follows:
  - Significant untreated dissection
  - Poor or inadequate stent deployment
  - Compromised outflow distal to the stented segment
  - Residual thrombus
  - Length of stented segment
  - Cessation of dual antiplatelet therapy
- Late—occurs after 30 days of stent implantation. This was seen in observational studies up to 1.3% of drug-eluting stents placed. The major risk factor for this was cessation of dual antiplatelet therapy and thus accounted for extending the duration to a minimum of a year. Many operators will leave their patients with drug-eluting stents on dual antiplatelet therapy lifelong as long as it can be tolerated. Stopping of therapy for any type of invasive procedure must be discussed with the cardiologist; this point cannot be stressed enough.

Angioplasty Equipment

- Guiding catheter
  - Used to engage the coronary ostium and guide the PCI equipment to the target lesion
  - Have thinner walls and larger lumens to allow for contrast injections and pressure monitoring to be performed while the guidewire and balloon catheters are in place
  - Stiffer than diagnostic catheters to provide support for delivering the PCI equipment
  - Typically are 6 Fr or greater in size without a tapered tip, which may account for pressure dampening. If pressure dampening occurs, a guide with side holes may be used to maintain perfusion.

  - Come in various shapes to allow for proper backup (stable support position to allow for advancement of the wire and balloon catheter across the stenosis)
- Balloon catheter
  - Dual-lumen catheter 145 to 155 cm in length with a pre-mounted balloon
  - Central lumen for guidewire
  - Second lumen for balloon inflation
  - Three different types
    - Over-the-wire balloon (Figure 8.3)
    - Monorail or rapid exchange (Figure 8.3)
    - Fixed wire (not commonly used)
- Angioplasty guide wires
  - Small-caliber (0.014 to 0.018) steerable wires are used that allow for crossing the lesion to be dilated.
  - A small J-tip is made by the operator to allow for negotiation through vessel angulations and side branches.
  - These come in two lengths:
    - 300 cm, which allows for over-the-wire catheters to be used

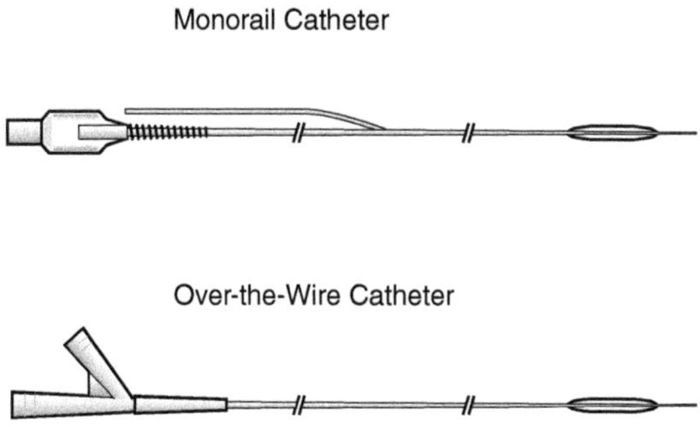

■ **Figure 8.3** Monorail catheter and over-the-wire catheter

        - 190 cm, which allows for monorail or rapid exchange catheters to be used
        - The torque control, flexibility, and stiffness of the wires are variable and should be chosen based on the vessel and lesion, which is being addressed.
- Other equipment
    - Tuohy Borst, which is a Y connector hemostasis valve, allows for the passage of equipment through the guiding catheter without significant bleeding while minimizing the introduction of air into the system.
    - Inflation device, which is used to inflate the balloon and allow for stent placement. It is numbered to allow for a precise atmospheric pressure to be produced.
    - A torque device is a small cylindrical device that is placed over the wire to allow for fine manipulation of the coronary angioplasty guidewire.
- Accessory procedures
    - The fractional flow reserve can be used to determine the hemodynamic significance of a lesion or the end point of PCI. To measure the translesional pressure, a pressure wire is placed across the lesion. Hyperemia is induced using either intracoronary injections or intravenous infusion of adenosine. The distal to proximal pressure ratio is measured at maximal hyperemia, which is the FFR. An FFR < 0.75 is consistent with inducible ischemia and therefore warrants intervention. An FFR that is greater than 0.75 is considered to not be hemodynamically significant. Although recent studies indicate that 0.75 to 0.8 can be hemodynamically significant and are left to the discretion of the operator, an FFR > 0.9 is indicative of a successful angioplasty procedure.
    - Coronary atherectomy is a procedure to debulk percutaneously a plaque prior to angioplasty and stent implantation. Three devices have approval for this: rotablation, directional coronary atherectomy, and transluminal extraction catheter.

- Directional coronary atherectomy is a cylindrical chamber at the tip, which houses a cutting device to shave the plaque within a coronary artery prior to angioplasty and stent implantation; however, studies such as Coronary Artery versus Excisional Atherectomy Trial (CAVEAT) and Canadian Coronary Atherectomy Trial (CCAT) showed no benefit to this procedure, and its utilization has been significantly reduced to only a few sites.
- Rotablator is an olive-shaped steel burr (1.25 to 2.5 mm) that is embedded with microscopic diamond chips, which is rotated at high speeds to allow for debulking of calcified coronary lesions. The abrasive surface performs selective ablation, which pulverizes hard plaque but does not affect soft plaque. Several passes are typically made to make a channel to allow for subsequent angioplasty and stenting. Randomized comparisons indicate no change in restenosis rates but a higher procedural success. Specific complications are no reflow, bradycardia, and heart block, which is why a temporary venous pacer is always placed prior to the procedure.
- Thrombus aspiration catheters can be used to perform manual extraction with a syringe at the catheter base, which is used to aspirate thrombus typically in the setting of acute myocardial infarction. There is also an automated AnjioJet Rheolytic Thrombectomy system, which uses a high-pressure water jet to produce a vacuum and therefore allowing for effective thrombus aspiration. The use of AnjioJet in the coronary arteries has been surpassed by manual extraction catheters because of ease of use and similar efficacy.

Clinical Procedure

- Preprocedure preparation
  - The patient must have a functional intravenous line to allow for medication administration.

  - The patient must be completely informed about the procedure, including the procedural aspects and possible results. He or she must also be formally consented to the possible risks of the procedure, which were covered earlier in the chapter.
  - Appropriate laboratories must be ascertained and reviewed, including complete blood count with platelets, metabolic panel (including electrolytes, blood urea nitrogen, and creatinine), prothrombin time, partial thromboplastin time, type, and screen (especially if patient has a low hemoglobin or high-risk procedure).
- Patient preparation in the catheterization suite
  - Use ECG (inferior and anterior leads), 12-lead with radiolucent leads if necessary.
  - The inguinal area is shaved and sterilized with an approved agent (the wrist for a radial approach or brachial region).
  - The patient should receive aspirin 325 mg orally, Benadryl 25 mg (intravenous or orally), and Plavix 600 mg prior to proceeding.
  - Versed and Fentanyl are used for sedative and analgesic purposes.
  - Arterial access should be obtained (and venous access as well) if the patient is at high risk, or is hemodynamically unstable, having an acute myocardial infarction (MI). Also, if a patient has left bundle branch block, or a right coronary artery (RCA) intervention, rotablation or thrombus aspiration is planned, then arterial and venous access is needed.
  - After access is obtained, the patient should be anticoagulated with heparin 40 to 70 μg/kg bolus for an activated clotting time of more than 250 seconds; if used in conjunction with a IIb/IIIa blocker, a smaller bolus can be used, and the activated clotting time can be greater than 200 seconds. The use of argatroban for PCI is increasing because of very reliable anticoagulation and rapid

metabolism allowing for earlier sheath withdrawal and less chance of bleeding. An infusion of Argatroban should be started at 25 mcg/kg/min and a bolus of 350 mcg/kg administered via a large bore intravenous line over 3 to 5 minutes. Activated clotting time should be checked 5 to 10 minutes after the bolus dose is completed. The procedure may proceed if the activated clotting time is greater than 300 seconds.

- Guiding catheter angiograms
  - The guiding catheter is used to perform coronary arteriograms, which allow for vessel sizing, definition of anatomy/collaterals, and balloon-stent position.
  - Guiding catheter sizes are variable (8 F = 2.87 mm, 7 F = 2.3 mm, 6 F = 2 mm).
- PCI procedure
  - The proper guiding catheter is used to allow for coaxial alignment with the vessel ostium.
  - The guidewire is advanced into the vessel and manipulated beyond the stenosis in the target vessel.
  - The balloon and stent are advanced through the hemostatic valve and advanced into the center of the lesion.
  - The balloon and subsequent stent are subsequently inflated to allow for resolution of the lesion.
- PCI results
  - Enlarged artery lumen (≤ 20% residual lesion).
  - Good angiographic flow (Thrombolysis in Myocardial Infarction [TIMI] grade 3)
  - Evaluate for adverse angiographic markers such as thrombus or dissection
  - No residual ischemia (ECG changes with or without chest pain)
  - If there is recoil, a dissection or slow TIMI flow, then additional balloon angioplasty or stenting may be required.
  - If there is doubt about the results of the procedure, then intravascular ultrasound (IVUS) or FFR should

be performed to assure that the optimal result has been achieved.

- After procedure
  - The guidewire is removed, and final angiograms are taken in orthogonal views to assure satisfactory results.
  - A femoral angiogram can be performed to evaluate the groin for closure device.
  - If the groin is not going to be closed, then the sheaths are sutured in place and remain in place until an activated clotting time < 180 or a partial thromboplastin time (PTT) < 60 is achieved. The sheaths are then removed, and manual pressure is held until complete hemostasis is obtained.
  - The groin is evaluated for bleeding, hematoma, ecchymosis, pulse, and bruit. Distal pulses are evaluated to assure no compromise to distal blood flow.
  - A postprocedure ECG, laboratories, including complete blood count with platelets, metabolic panel (including electrolytes, blood urea nitrogen, and creatinine), prothrombin time, partial thromboplastin time, and cardiac markers should be obtained.
- Postprocedure medications
  - The patient should be maintained on aspirin 325 mg orally daily and Plavix 75 mg daily. For bare metal stents, dual-antiplatelet therapy should be used for at least 1 month and for drug-eluting stents for at least 1 year.
- Patient follow-up
  - The patient should follow-up within 2 weeks to evaluate the site of the procedure and any recurrence of anginal symptoms.

Stent Implantation

The use of stents in the treatment of coronary disease has been shown to improve long-term results compared with balloon angioplasty alone, as reflected by the reduction of restenosis as seen in the BENESTENT, STRESS, and SAVED trials. Many different types of stents are available, but they all perform essentially three roles:

1. Function as a metal scaffold to hold the lumen and plaque open
2. Hold dissection flaps against the arterial wall
3. Stop arterial elastic recoil and narrowing of the lumen

Compared with angioplasty alone, stenting provides a larger minimal lumen diameter, maintains arterial patency, and reduces restenosis at 6 months. Some general principles can be used to determine which patients should receive a stent.

The indications are as follows:

1. Those eligible for balloon angioplasty.
2. Those with symptomatic ischemic heart disease and a flow-limiting stenosis.
3. Those with de novo or restenotic lesions, coronary artery lesions with a vessel diameter $\geq$ 2.5 mm.

The contraindications are as follows:

1. An inability to take antiplatelet therapy.
2. A history of bleeding or other conditions that preclude anti-coagulation during the stent procedure or the maintenance of dual antiplatelet therapy after.
3. Noncardiac surgery within the next month after the stent procedure.

The decision to implant a drug-eluting stent or a bare metal stent is left to the discretion of the operator; however, in general, drug-eluting stents are best implanted in patients who

1. Can take dual antiplatelet therapy for at least a full year.
2. Have no upcoming surgical procedures that necessitate a cessation of dual antiplatelet therapy.
3. Have no bleeding issues and/or are not high risk for bleeding.

4. Have a lesion in a smaller vessel diameter, to decrease the incidence of restenosis.
5. Are at high risk of restenosis, such as diabetic patients, and so forth.

With each generation of coronary stents that are manufactured, the efficacy has been improving and the side-effect profile decreasing. The frontier includes stents that can elute different drugs at different time intervals to reduce restenosis but promote endothelialization. Bioabsorbable stents, which will perform a scaffolding role and then be completely absorbed by the body, have already been implanted in humans, the results of which, although preliminary, look very promising.

In 2007, the world of interventional cardiology was challenged by the COURAGE trial, which concluded an initial management strategy in patients who have stable coronary artery disease. PCI did not reduce the risk of death, myocardial infarction, or other major cardiovascular events when added to optimal medical therapy. Although this was initially thought to go against the practices of interventional cardiology, it simply reinforced that PCI is best used for symptomatic relief in medically refractory patients. In subsequent subgroup analysis, patients who underwent PCI had a better quality of life and were less hindered by their angina than those who received medical therapy alone. There were no significant differences in death, myocardial infarction, or major adverse cardiac events (MACE) in the subgroup analysis.

In conclusion, the field of interventional cardiology has come a long way from the first balloon inflation by Gruentzig in 1977; however, as we get better equipment, better techniques, and more data from large randomized trials, we also will get more complex patients. With these complex patients we must always evaluate each patient and clinically decide the best approach for them. Just because a procedure can be done, it does not necessitate that it should be done. A good interventionalist is a good doctor first.

9 ▪ Stress Testing and Nuclear Cardiology

Gregary D. Marhefka, MD
Christopher L. Hansen, MD

I. Exercise stress testing
   A. Anatomic versus physiologic test
      - Unlike cardiac catheterization and coronary computed tomography angiography, which demonstrate normal or pathologic anatomy, stress testing is a physiologic test.
      - Stress testing demonstrates a normal and pathologic physiology.
   B. Normal physiology of coronary blood flow
      - Myocardial oxygen extraction is near maximal at rest (coronary sinus oxygen saturation ≤ 30%).
      - Therefore, the only way to increase oxygen delivery is to increase blood flow.
      - Measures of myocardial oxygen consumption
        - Heart rate—simple to measure
        - Wall stress—more difficult to measure
          - Roughly dependent on preload and afterload
          - Contractility
      - In healthy hearts, there is linear relationship between myocardial oxygen consumption and coronary blood flow.
      - Autoregulation at coronary arteriole smooth muscle level allows for maintenance of perfusion over certain range of aortic pressures.
      - Coronary flow reserve is the ability to increase coronary flow above resting levels.
      - The maintenance of coronary blood flow involves metabolic, autonomic, and mechanical factors.

- Adenosine, prostaglandins, nitric oxide, and endothelin
- Oxygen and carbon dioxide tensions, ATP-sensitive potassium channels

C. Pathophysiology of coronary blood flow

- "Clogged pipe" paradigm
  - The model of coronary blood flow describes stable angina, not acute coronary syndromes.
  - Arteries are conduits ("pipes") with obstructive atheroma ("clogs").
  - This is a simplistic but workable model for stable angina and stress testing.
  - Effect of obstructing atheroma dependent on
    - Degree of stenosis
    - Amount of blood flow
  - At resting blood flow, there is no effect on coronary blood flow until stenosis reaches 85% to 90% (Figure 9.1A).
  - At peak blood flow, the effect can be seen when stenosis is greater than about 50% (Figure 9.1B).

D. Implications for physiologic test

- Rarely able to detect stenoses $< 50\%$ (no physiologic effect)
- Ability to detect stenoses dependent upon increasing coronary blood flow
  - Ability to detect borderline stenoses greater at higher blood flows
  - Ways to increase blood flow
    - Exercise
      - Exercise hemodynamic response and tolerance important prognostically
    - Pharmacologic
      - Inotropic stimulation or coronary vasodilation
- Surrogate markers of coronary blood flow
  - Used to assess reliability of test

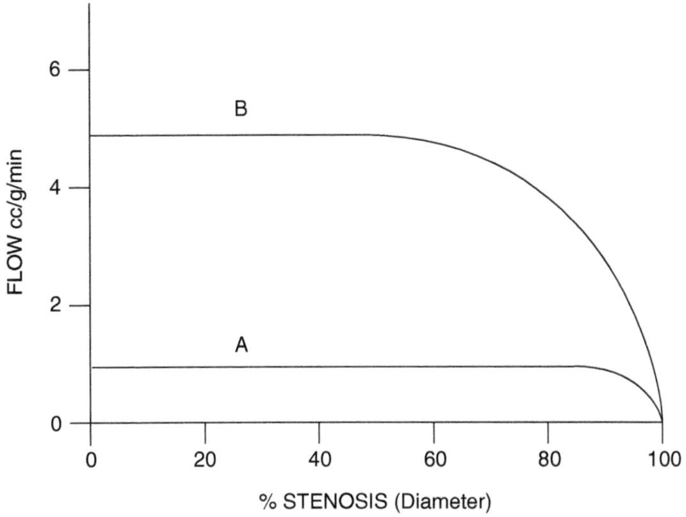

■ **Figure 9.1** Coronary Blood Flow. **(A)** Under resting conditions, no effect on coronary blood flow unless stenosis > 85–90%. **(B)** At peak blood flow, effect on coronary blood flow seen when stenosis > 50%.

- Heart rate (> 85% maximum predicted heart rate [220 – age] most often used)
- Heart rate and afterload (rate pressure product)
  - HR × SBP
  - > 20–25,000 preferred

E. Graded exercise testing

- Exercise tolerance measured by a metabolic equivalent (MET) (Table 9.1)
  - Surrogate for myocardial oxygen consumption and functional capacity
  - 1 MET = 3.5 ml O_2/kg/min (which is equal to average O_2 consumption of individual at rest)
  - VO_2 is total amount of oxygen consumed (measured in ml O_2/kg/min)

Table 9.1 Metabolic Equivalent (MET) Estimates Based on Activity

METs/Hour of Activity	Activity
1	Resting
2	Light housework
3–4	Gardening
4–5	Heavy housework Walking upstairs
6	Hiking
9–11	Jogging
10	Soccer
4–10	Cycling
5–19	Rowing

MET refers to amount of oxygen consumed at rest (volume of O_2 in mL/kg/min or VO_2).

Source: Adapted from Jette M, Sidney K, Blumchen G. Metabolic equivalents (METS) in exercise testing, exercise prescription, and evaluation of functional capacity. *Clin Cardiol* 1990;13:555–565.

- Number of METs: VO_2 divided by 3.5 ml O_2/kg/min
- For typical activities of daily living, exercise intensity of at least 4 METS used

- Exercise protocols
  - Bruce protocol most widely adopted (Table 9.2)
    - Three-minute stages, with incremental increases in speed and incline
  - Others: Naughton, Cornell, Weber, Asymptomatic Cardiac Ischemia Pilot (ACIP)
  - Stationary bicycle ergometer
- Hemodynamic response
  - Heart rate response
    - Heart rate normally rises in gradual fashion with increasing levels of exercise

Table 9.2 Bruce Protocol: Standard Exercise Protocol Using 3-Minute Stages of Incrementally Increased Speed and Incline

Bruce Protocol				
Stage	**Minutes**	**% Grade**	**MPH**	**Approximate METs**
1	3	10	1.7	4
2	6	12	2.5	7
3	9	14	3.4	10
4	12	16	4.2	13
5	15	18	5.0	16

F. Chronotropic incompetence: failure to achieve ≥ 85% maximum predicted heart rate (HR)
   - Causes: medications, sick sinus syndrome, heart failure, advanced age
   - In absence of medication effect, independently predicts higher mortality

G. Rapid rise in HR at low exercise level
   - Causes: deconditioning, atrial fibrillation, hypovolemia, anemia, hyperthyroidism
   - Target HR met in less than 1 minute suggests that HR may be uncoupled from VO_2 and therefore may not be accurate surrogate of myocardial oxygen consumption

II. Heart rate recovery

A. Decrease in HR on completion of exercise in recovery is due to parasympathetic reactivation

B. Failure to decrease HR ≥ 12 beats during first minute of recovery is abnormal and independently predicts higher mortality

III. Blood pressure response
   A. Systolic blood pressure normally rises and diastolic blood pressure normally remains unchanged or falls slightly.
   B. Exercise induced hypotension (systolic blood pressure decrease ≥ 10 mm Hg) or failure of systolic blood pressure rise is a potential marker of significant disease.
      - Causes: multivessel, left main or severe coronary artery disease (CAD); left ventricular (LV) outflow tract obstruction; LV dysfunction, medication
   C. Exercise-induced hypertension (systolic blood pressure ≥ 210 mm Hg) is abnormal.
      - Causes: underlying hypertension, poorly controlled hypertension, holding antihypertensive medications
      - In absence of significant epicardial stenoses, may lead to subendocardial ischemia and false-positive ST segment depression
      - In nonhypertensive patient, associated with increased risk developing hypertension

IV. Pathophysiology of electrocardiographic changes
   A. During exercise, the subendocardium has a higher myocardial oxygen demand than subepicardium, in part because of increased wall tension, and therefore is most vulnerable to ischemia.
   B. Normally, repolarization occurs from epicardium (shorter action potential) to endocardium (longer action potential).
   C. In presence of significant epicardial stenoses, perfusion to subendocardium cannot be increased, substantially leading to ischemia during exercise.
   D. Subendocardial ischemia leads to shortened action potentials in subendocardium with resulting spatial electrical gradient during repolarization and ST segment depression and T-wave inversion.

V. Electrocardiographic application and interpretation
   A. Mason-Likar lead system—extremity leads moved to torso to minimize movement artifact

B. Arm electrodes in lateral infraclavicular fossa
C. Leg electrodes above anterior iliac crests
D. Results in axis shift, increased inferior voltage, loss of inferior Q waves

VI. Normal ECG changes during exercise
A. P-wave amplitude increases
B. R-wave amplitude decreases
C. J-point depression
D. ST segment becomes sharply upsloping
E. QT interval shortens
F. T-wave amplitude may decrease

VII. Interpreting ST segment displacement (Table 9.3)
A. PQ junction is considered isoelectric point (TP segment vanishes with increasing HR).
B. When analyzing raw tracings, measurements are taken from three consecutive beats with stable baseline.
C. Use of computer averaged beats and corresponding measurements requires inspection of raw tracings to exclude artifact and agreement with marker placement for PR segment, J point, and ST segment.
  - Types of ST segment depression
    - Nonischemic
      - Rapidly upsloping: normally J point can depress with exercise
  - Ischemic
    - Horizontal: ≥ 0.1 mV (1 mm) J point depression and ST segment depression 80 ms after the J point
    - Downsloping: ≥ 0.1 mV (1 mm) J point depression and ST segment depression 80 ms after the J point
      - Slowly upsloping: ≥ 0.15 mV (1.5 mm) J point depression and ST segment depression 80 ms after the J point
      - Less specific
      - Not universally accepted as marker of ischemia

    - At higher HR may measure ST segment changes 60 ms after J point (at 80 ms ST segment may be upsloping into T wave).
    - If resting < 0.1 mV (1 mm) ST segment depression, abnormal response is ≥ 0.1 mV (1 mm) beyond the original ST segment depression.
    - ST segment depression does not localize to corresponding coronary territory.
- ST segment elevation: ≥ 0.1 mV (1 mm) J-point elevation and ST segment elevation 60 to 80 ms after the J point
    - In Q-wave lead, not considered ischemia
    - In non–Q-wave lead indicates severe ischemia
    - ST-segment elevation localizes to corresponding coronary territory

Table 9.3 **Ischemic ST Segment Depression:** Horizontal ≥ 0.1 mV (1 mm) J point depression and ST segment depression 80 ms after the J point; downsloping ≥ 0.1 mV (1 mm) J point depression and ST segment depression 80 ms after the J point; upsloping ≥ 0.15 mV (1.5 mm) J point depression and ST segment depression 80 ms after the J point.

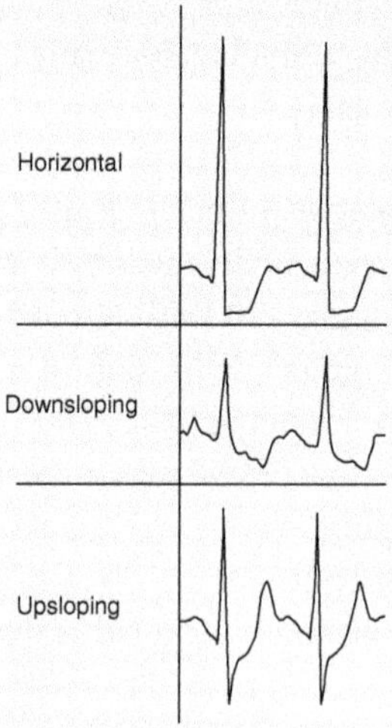

- T-wave changes unreliable
  - Influenced by body position, respiratory pattern, medications, hypertrophy, ischemia, and pH
  - Pseudonormalization of T-wave inversion
    - Could indicate ischemia, but not reliable marker
- U-wave changes—anterior U-wave inversion during exercise reportedly associated with significant left main or left anterior descending stenoses
- Electrocardiographic changes unreliable for ischemia in presence of specific baseline abnormalities or while patient is on certain medication; therefore, stress testing should be performed with imaging (in some cases, vasodilator nuclear stress imaging is preferred over exercise).
  - More than 0.1 mV (1 mm) resting ST segment depression
  - Pre-excitation (Wolff-Parkinson-White) syndrome
  - Left bundle branch block (vasodilator nuclear stress imaging preferred)
  - Paced ventricular rhythm (vasodilator nuclear stress imaging preferred)
  - Left ventricular hypertrophy
  - Patient is on digoxin

D. Exercise stress testing to diagnose obstructive CAD
- The Bayes' theorem includes pretest probability with result of test to determine predictive value of result.
- Pretest probability for CAD can be estimated for age, gender, and nature of symptoms (Table 9.4).
  - Typical angina defined as
    - Substernal chest pain or discomfort
    - Provoked by exertion or emotional stress and
    - Relieved by rest and/or nitroglycerin
  - Atypical angina consists of only two of these three characteristics.

Table 9.4 Pretest Probability of Coronary Artery Disease by Age, Gender, and Symptoms*

Age (y)	Gender	Typical/ Definite Angina Pectoris	Atypical/ Probable Angina Pectoris	Nonanginal Chest Pain	Asymptomatic
30–39	Men	Intermediate	Intermediate	Low	Very low
	Women	Intermediate	Very low	Very low	Very low
40–49	Men	High	Intermediate	Intermediate	Low
	Women	Intermediate	Low	Very low	Very low
50–59	Men	High	Intermediate	Intermediate	Low
	Women	Intermediate	Intermediate	Low	Very low
60–69	Men	High	Intermediate	Intermediate	Low
	Women	High	Intermediate	Intermediate	Low

*No data exist for patients <30 or >69 years, but it can be assumed that prevalence of CAN increases with age. In a few cases, patients with ages at the extremes of the decades listed may have probabilities slightly outside the high or low range. High indicates >90%; intermediate, 10%–90%; low, <10%; and very low, <5%.

Source: Reprinted from J Am Coll Cardiol 2002; 40: Gibbons, Raymond J, et al. ACC/AHA 2002 guideline update for exercise testing: summary article: A report of the American College of Cardiology/American Heart Association Task Force of Practice Guidelines (Committee to update the 1997 exercise testing guidelines), 1531–1540, 2002, with permission from Elsevier.

- Nonanginal chest pain consists of only one of these three characteristics.

- Exercise testing is most useful diagnostically when there is intermediate pretest probability of coronary artery disease
- Requires interpretable electrocardiogram, including those with complete RBBB or less than 0.1 mV (1 mm) of resting ST segment depression

E. Assessment of risk and prognosis in patients with suspected or known CAD
   - Exercise capacity very powerful predictor of mortality
     - CAD patients exercising ≥ 10 METs have better prognosis.
     - CAD patients able to exercise ≤ 5 METs have increased cardiac events.
   - Reassess patients with suspected or known CAD, with a significant worsening in symptoms or clinical status
   - Assess lower risk chest pain syndrome patients 8 to 12 hours after onset of symptoms (without active symptoms or objective markers of ischemia)
   - Assess intermediate-risk chest pain syndrome patients after 2 to 3 days of stabilization of symptoms (without active symptoms or ischemia)

F. Exercise stress testing after myocardial infarction
   - Assess risk to categorize patients as low risk for conservative medical management or high risk for more aggressive invasive evaluation
   - Submaximal stress testing before discharge to assess prognosis, activity limitations, and adequacy of medical therapy (at 4–6 days)
   - Symptom limited stress testing after discharge to assess prognosis, activity limitations, and adequacy of medical therapy (14–21 days)

G. Exercise stress testing in special populations
   - Asymptomatic patient: exercise stress testing less defined role
     - May be used as guide to risk factor treatment in presence of multiple risk factors
     - May be used prior to initiating exercise program in men more than 45 years old and women more than 55 years at high risk for CAD
     - May be used to evaluate patients with certain occupations where public safety is concern

- Valvular heart disease
  - Aortic stenosis
    - Exercise stress testing generally contraindicated in severe symptomatic aortic stenosis
    - Sometimes performed carefully in asymptomatic severe aortic stenosis patients to unmask signs and symptoms
  - Chronic aortic regurgitation
    - Exercise stress testing reasonable for assessment of functional capacity and to unmask symptoms when history of equivocal symptoms related to aortic regurgitation
- Before or after revascularization
  - Demonstration of ischemia before revascularization
  - Evaluation of patients after revascularization with recurrent symptoms that suggest ischemia
  - Not recommended (without imaging) for localizing regions of ischemia before revascularization
  - Not recommended for routine screening after revascularization in absence of specific clinical indication

H. Confounders of stress ECG interpretation

- Medication
  - Digitalis can produce resting and/or exercise induced ST segment depression, resulting in nondiagnostic test
  - Anti-ischemic therapy can prolong time to ischemic response or normalize exercise ECG (decision to stop such therapy before stress testing should be individualized)
  - Beta-blocker and calcium channel blocker therapy can lead to failure to achieve target heart rate (decision to stop such therapy before stress testing should be individualized)
- Resting ST abnormalities

  - If < 1 mm resting ST segment depression, in absence of LVH or digitalis, still reasonable to use exercise stress testing alone
  - If > 1 mm resting ST segment depression, imaging stress test recommended
- Severe hypertension can lead to subendocardial ischemia and therefore abnormal ECG response even in absence of significant epicardial stenoses
- Women
  - Higher false-positive rates possibly because of the effect of estrogen
  - If suspected CAD, able to exercise and normal resting ECG, should perform exercise stress testing alone
  - If unable to exercise adequately and/or abnormal baseline ECG, should perform imaging stress test
- Conduction abnormality
  - RBBB—ST segment and T wave changes are nondiagnostic in V1–V3 (can still do exercise stress testing alone)
  - Left bundle branch block (LBBB)—ST segment and T wave changes are nondiagnostic throughout (should not do exercise stress testing, vasodilator stress testing preferred, see Pharmacologic Stress Testing on pp. 198–203).

I. Symptoms or arrhythmias with stress testing
- Chest discomfort
  - Typical angina during or after exercise associated with greater extent of CAD and ischemia
- Arrhythmias
  - Supraventricular
    - Atrial premature depolarizations, atrial fibrillation, atrial flutter, and supraventricular tachycardia

        - Not diagnostic for CAD
    - Ventricular
        - Frequent ventricular premature depolarizations, nonsustained ventricular tachycardia, and sustained ventricular tachycardia
        - Possibly predicts higher mortality, particularly on completion of exercise in recovery

J. Safety

- Risks
    - Rate of serious complication such as myocardial infarction or death about 1 in 10,000 (0.01%)
    - Rate of ventricular tachycardia or fibrillation 1 in 5,000
    - Advanced cardiac life support (ACLS) equipment and ACLS trained supervising personnel must be present
- Internal cardiodefibrillator (ICD)
    - Lower programmed detection rate for therapy should be known
    - Exercise can be terminated at least 10–20 beats/min below detection rate
- May need to reprogram ICD to higher detection rate
- Contraindications (from American College of Cardiology [ACC]/American Heart Association [AHA] 2002 Guideline Update for Exercise Testing)
    - Absolute
        - Acute myocardial infarction (within 2 days)
        - High-risk unstable angina
        - Uncontrolled cardiac arrhythmias causing symptoms or hemodynamic compromise
        - Symptomatic severe aortic stenosis
        - Uncontrolled symptomatic heart failure
        - Acute pulmonary embolus or pulmonary infarction
        - Acute myocarditis or pericarditis
        - Acute aortic dissection

- Relative
  - Left main coronary stenosis
  - Moderate stenotic valvular heart disease
  - Electrolyte abnormalities
  - Severe arterial hypertension (> 200/110 mm Hg)
  - Tachyarrhythmias or bradyarrhythmias
  - Hypertrophic cardiomyopathy and other forms of outflow tract obstruction
  - Mental or physical impairment leading to inability to exercise adequately
  - High-degree atrioventricular block
- Indications for terminating exercise testing (from ACC/AHA 2002 Guideline Update for Exercise Testing)
  - Absolute
    - Drop in systolic blood pressure > 10 mm Hg from baseline blood pressure despite an increase in workload, when accompanied by other evidence of ischemia
    - Moderate to severe angina
    - Increasing nervous system symptoms (e.g., ataxia, dizziness, or near syncope)
    - Signs of poor perfusion (cyanosis or pallor)
    - Technical difficulties in monitoring ECG or systolic blood pressure
    - Subject's request to stop
    - Sustained ventricular tachycardia
    - ST elevation (≥ 1.0 mm) in leads without diagnostic Q waves (other than V1 or a VR)
  - Relative
    - Drop in systolic blood pressure of ≥ 10 mm Hg from baseline blood pressure despite an increase in workload, in absence of other evidence of ischemia
    - ST or QRS changes such as excessive ST depression (> 2 mm of horizontal or downsloping ST segment depression) or marked axis shift

- Arrhythmias other than sustained ventricular tachycardia, including multifocal PVCs, triplets of PVCs, supraventricular tachycardia, heart block, or bradyarrhythmias
- Fatigue, shortness of breath, wheezing, leg cramps, or claudication
- Development of bundle-branch block or intraventricular conduction delay (IVCD) that cannot be distinguished from ventricular tachycardia
- Increasing chest pain
- Hypertensive response (> 250/115 mm Hg)

K. Prognostic parameter: Duke Treadmill Score
- Prognostic marker of exercise tolerance combining objective and subjective markers of ischemia
- Exercise time in minutes (Bruce protocol)—5 × ST segment depression in mm—4 × exercise angina (0 is no angina, 1 angina occurred, 2 angina was reason for stopping exercise)
  - High-risk score ≤ –11, average annual cardiovascular mortality ≥ 5 %
  - Intermediate-risk score –10 to 4
  - Low-risk score ≥ + 5, average annual cardiovascular mortality 0.5%

L. Exercise testing with ventilatory gas analysis
- Direct measure of myocardial oxygen consumption and functional capacity
- Adjunctive tool in assessment of cardiovascular and/or pulmonary diseases
- Measures respiratory oxygen uptake (VO_2), carbon dioxide production (VCO_2), minute ventilation, and ventilatory/anaerobic threshold (VAT)
- VAT is point during exercise where oxygen supply does not meet oxygen demand and anaerobic glycolysis results in lactate production
  - Lactate is buffered by HCO_3^-, resulting in increased CO_2 and therefore markedly increased ventilation

Table 9.5 Classification of Exercise Capacity in Patients with Heart Failure, Based on Peak Oxygen and Ventilatory Anaerobic Threshold

Class	Impairment	Peak VO_2 (mL/kg/min)	VAT (mL/kg/min)
A	None to mild	>20	>14
B	Mild to moderate	16–20	11–14
C	Moderate to severe	10–16	8–11
D	Severe	<10	<8

VO_2 indicates oxygen uptake; and VAT, ventilatory anaerobic threshold.

From Gibbons, RG, Balady, J., Bricker, Timothy J., et al. ACC/AHA 2002 guideline update for existing testing. *Circulation.* 2002;106:1883. © 2002 American Heart Association, Inc.

Source: Reprinted from J Am Coll Cardiol 2002; 40: Gibbons, Raymond J, et al. ACC/AHA 2002 guideline update for exercise testing: summary article: A report of the American College of Cardiology/American Heart Association Task Force of Practice Guidelines (Committee to update the 1997 exercise testing guidelines), 1531–1540, 2002, with permission from Elsevier.

- Used in heart failure patients to assess exercise capacity response to treatment and to assess heart transplant candidacy (Table 9.5)

VIII. Nuclear imaging

A. Myocardial Perfusion Imaging (MPI)

- Determining relative regional distribution of coronary blood flow throughout myocardium by detecting injected myocardial tracer emitted photons
- Planar
  - Raw two-dimensional images typically recorded with patient supine in three standard views, one of which is best septal view at about 45° left anterior oblique
  - Largely replaced by single photon emission computed tomography (SPECT)

- SPECT
  - Raw two-dimensional images are acquired at multiple points around 180° or 360° arc, reconstructed, and then reoriented into cardinal planes of heart in tomographic slices (short axis, horizontal long axis, vertical long axis)
- Instrumentation
  - Anger (Gamma) camera
    - Collimator—functions as a lens
      - Allows photons of certain trajectory to travel through
      - Controls scatter and resolution
    - Sodium iodide crystal
      - Photons strike sodium iodide crystal, converted to visible light
    - Photomultiplier tubes
      - Amplifies light and converts to electrical signal
  - Multicrystal camera
    - Contains several sodium iodide crystals with separate photomultiplier tubes
    - Generally allows for higher count sensitivity but lower spatial resolution
    - Used in first pass imaging
- Electrocardiogram (ECG) gating
  - Counts acquired are placed into frames or bins according to time acquired in cardiac cycle
  - Allows evaluation of wall motion, ventricular volumes, and ejection fraction
  - Assists in differentiation of fixed defects from attenuation artifact and perfusion defects by assessing regional wall motion (improved specificity)
  - Gating rate set at eight frames per cycle most commonly; however, minimum of 16 cycles for equilibrium radionuclide angiocardiography
  - Apply acceptance windows to reject cycle lengths (i.e., due to PVCs) that fall out of range to improve

accuracy and reliability (may prolong acquisition time or decrease counts)

- Attenuation correction
  - Hardware and software methods used to reduce artifact
  - Improves specificity
- Exercise SPECT: sensitivity 87%, specificity 73%
- Vasodilator SPECT: sensitivity 89%, specificity 75%

B. Radiopharmaceuticals

- Thallium-201 (Thallous Chloride Tl 201) (Tl-201)
  - Cyclotron produced and decays by electron capture to mercury (Hg) 201
  - Potassium analogue—active and passive membrane transport
  - Energy detected for myocardial imaging: primarily 68–80 keV from mercury (Hg) 201 X-rays; also to lesser extent 167 and 135 keV
  - Half-life of Tl-201 is 73.1 hours
  - Accumulates in myocytes early after injection reflecting regional myocardial perfusion, maximal at about 10 minutes with high first-pass extraction of 85%
  - Tracer washes out depending on regional myocardial perfusion
    - Regions of normal myocardial perfusion: rapid washout evenly throughout
    - Regions with significantly reduced myocardial perfusion: slow washout resulting in "redistribution" or "normalization" of myocardial defects
- Technetium-99m (Tc-99m) based perfusion agents
  - Produced in generator (colloquially called "cow") by beta decay of parent compound molybdenum-99 (Mo-99)
    - By-product of nuclear reactor
    - Mo-99 has half-life 66 hours

- Decays by isomeric transition to Tc-99, emitting gamma ray
- Gamma ray energy detected for myocardial imaging: 140 keV
- Half-life of Tc-99m is 6.02 hours
- Higher energy and shorter half-life allows higher dose and improved specificity compared with thallium
  - Particularly for women in whom false-positive thallium results were caused by breast attenuation
  - Tc-99m based perfusion agents have largely replaced Thallium-201 as myocardial tracer of choice
- Technetium-99m-sestamibi and Tc-99m-tetrofosmin are cationic lipid soluble compounds with hepatobiliary excretion
  - Retained in mitochondria, with negligible washout ("redistribution")
- Technetium-99m-teboroxime is neutral lipophilic compound with affinity for myocellular membrane
  - Less practical due to rapid washout

C. Myocardial perfusion imaging interpretation
- Raw data—assess technical adequacy of acquired data
  - Sufficiency of myocardial activity
  - Patient motion during image acquisition
  - Overlying breast attenuation in females
  - Diaphragmatic attenuation in males
  - Hepatic activity interfering with interpretation
  - Artifacts
  - Lung uptake assessment particularly with Tl-201 as poor prognostic sign
  - Abnormal extracardiac focal tracer uptake—may represent malignancy
- Standard views
  - Planar (Figure 9.2)

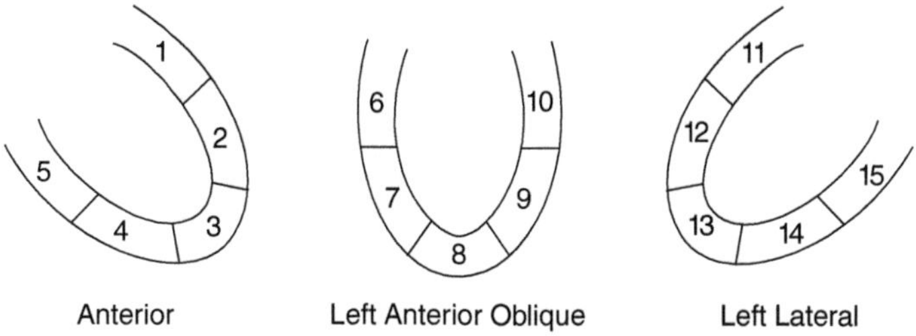

■ **Figure 9.2** Three standard views for planar imaging. [1] Basal anterolateral. [2] Mid anterolateral. [3] Apical. [4] Mid inferoseptal. [5] Basal inferoseptal. [6] Septal. [7] Inferoseptal. [8] Inferoapical. [9] Inferolateral. [10] Lateral. [11] Basal anterior. [12] Mid anterior. [13] Apex. [14] Mid inferior. [15] Basal inferior.

- Three standard views
  - Anterior
  - Left anterior oblique
  - Left lateral
- SPECT
  - Splash view (Figure 9.3)
    - Cardinal planes of heart with stress above resting images
      - Short axis: slices from apex to base
      - Vertical long axis: slices from septal to lateral walls
      - Horizontal long axis: slices from inferior to anterior walls
  - Bull's eye view (Figure 9.4)
    - Orients short axis slices with base at perimeter and apex at center
    - 17-Segment model proposed as standard for myocardial perfusion imaging (MPI), echocardiogram (ECHO), computed tomography (CT), and magnetic resonance imaging (MRI)
  - Coronary artery supply (Figure 9.5)

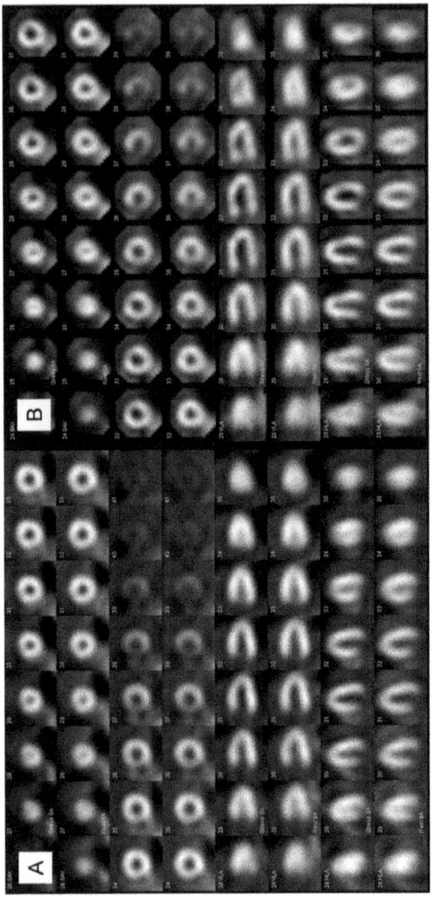

■ **Figure 9.3** Splash Images. Stress images are above rest images. Short axis (SA) at top displayed left to right from apex to base, vertical long axis (VLA) in middle from septum to lateral wall, horizontal long axis (HLA) at bottom from inferior to anterior wall. A) Normal perfusion study. B) Abnormal perfusion study from 57 year old male with typical angina at peak exercise with ischemic ECG response. There is medium sized, moderate intensity reversible defect in anterolateral and lateral walls, with mild transient ischemic dilatation (TID). Cardiac catheterization confirmed medium sized first diagonal vessel with 90% ostial stenosis with non-obstructive disease elsewhere.

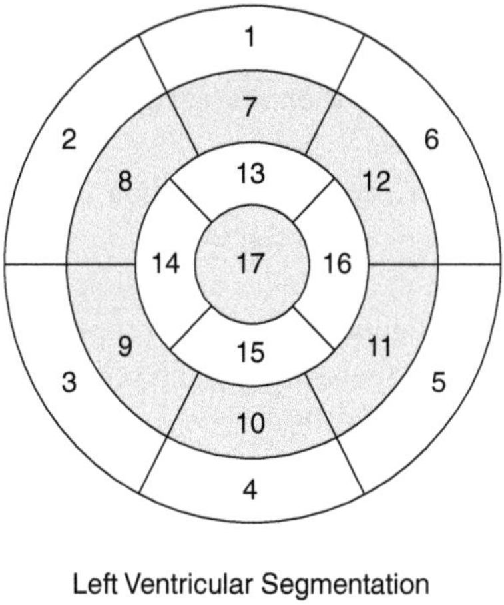

■ **Figure 9.4** [1] Basal anterior. [2] Basal anteroseptal. [3] Basal inferoseptal. [4] Basal inferior. [5] Basal inferolateral. [6] Basal anterolateral. [7] Mid anterior. [8] Mid anteroseptal. [9] Mid inferoseptal. [10] Mid inferior. [11] Mid inferolateral. [12] Mid anterolateral. [13] Apical anterior. [14] Apical septal. [15] Apical inferior. [16] Apical lateral. [17] Apex.

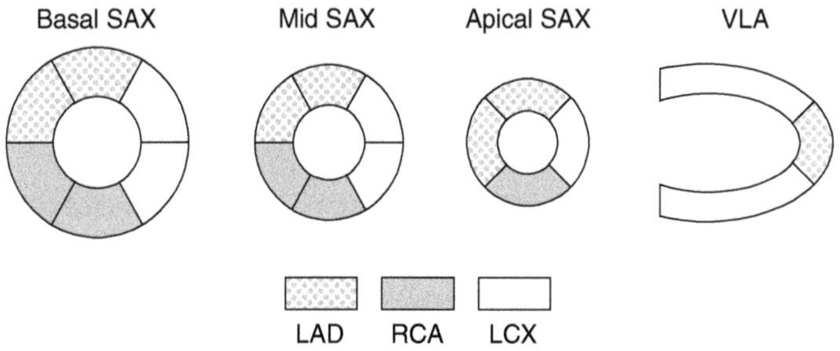

■ **Figure 9.5** Coronary artery supply. Left anterior descending (LAD) artery supplies anterior and apical walls. Left circumflex (LCX) artery supplies lateral walls. Right coronary (RCA) artery supplies inferior walls.

- Generally, specific coronary artery territories correspond to certain wall segments, taking into consideration normal anatomic variants and overlap
  - Left anterior descending artery supplies anterior and apical walls
  - Left circumflex artery supplies lateral walls
  - Right coronary artery supplies inferior walls
- Defect size (percentage of left ventricle)
  - Small (5% to 10%)
  - Medium (15% to 20%)
  - Large (> 20%)
- Defect severity
  - Mild—decreased counts without wall thinning
  - Moderate—decreased counts with wall thinning
  - Severe—decreased counts with wall thinning that approaches background
- Defect type
  - Reversible—defect present only on stress images
  - Persistent—fixed defect that is unchanged from rest to stress
  - Mixed—partial reversibility such as infarct with peri-infarct ischemia
- Transient ischemic dilation of left ventricle during stress
  - Marker of severe left main, proximal left anterior descending, or multivessel ischemia
  - Secondary to subendocardial ischemia and loss of subendocardial counts and/or persistent poststress dilation of left ventricle
- Presence of rest and stress left ventricular cavity enlargement
- Quantitative analysis (usually done with commercially available software)
  - Input from rest and stress projection, short-axis, and gated short-axis images generate automated quantitative values

- Allows comparison to gender matched and radiopharmaceutical matched normal patient database
- Quantitative perfusion SPECT
  - o LV myocardial uptake
    - ▪ Radial plots (Figure 9.6)
      - Counts are linearly graphed according to LV location
      - Resultant curve compared with normal patient database reference curve
      - Considered abnormal when patient's curve falls 2.5 standard deviations below reference curve
      - Area of deviation correlates with extent and severity of perfusion defect
  - o Semiquantitative analysis

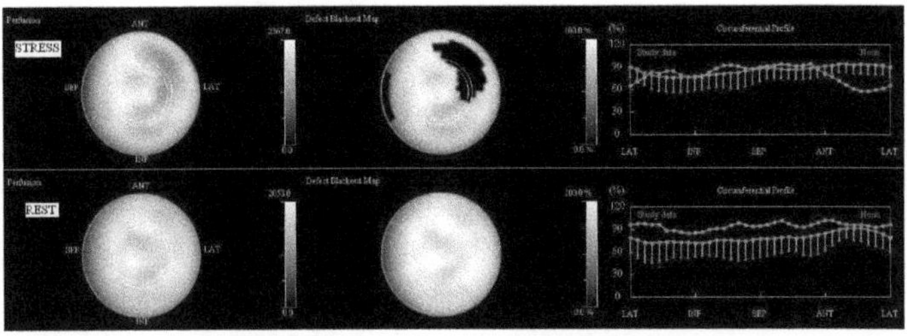

■ **Figure 9.6** Radial plots from same patient in figure 9.3B. Stress images are above rest images, with perfusion polar plots at left, defect blackout maps in middle and radial plots at right. Radial plots are representation of relative perfusion at level indicated by double white circle in defect blackout map (mid ventricular level in example). Single horizontal dotted line is relative perfusion from lateral (LAT) to inferior (INF) to septum (SEP) to anterior (ANT) to lateral (LAT) walls. Horizontal dotted line with individual vertical lines represents normal database with error bars indicating 2 1/2 standard deviations below the mean. In this example, radial plots indicate medium sized, moderate intensity reversible defect in anterolateral and lateral walls consistent with 90% ostial first diagonal stenosis confirmed by cardiac catheterization.

        - Count-based perfusion analysis: each Bull's Eye segment (of 17 or 20 segment model) given score 0 to 4
            - Normal tracer uptake = 0
            - Mild reduction of tracer uptake = 1
            - Moderate reduction of tracer uptake = 2
            - Severe reduction of tracer uptake = 3
            - Absent tracer uptake = 4
        - Summed stress score (SSS): addition of individual segment perfusion scores at stress
            - Mild intensity defect: 0 to 4
            - Moderate intensity defect: 5 to 8
            - Severe intensity defect: > 8
        - Summed rest score (SRS): addition of individual segment perfusion scores at rest (using same scoring system as for SSS)
        - Summed difference score (SDS): SSS–SRS, which corresponds to "reversibility" or ischemia
            - Mild reversibility: 0 to 2
            - Moderate reversibility: 3 to 7
            - Severe reversibility: > 7
        - Percent myocardium involved: divide summed score by worst segmental score possible (68 for 17 segment model) and multiplied by 100
            - Normal or minimally abnormal (< 5 %)
            - Mildly abnormal (5% to 9%)
            - Moderately abnormal (10% to 14%)
            - Severely abnormal (> 15%)
- Quantitative gated SPECT
    - Global LV function (ejection fraction [EF], end systolic volume [ESV], end diastolic volume [EDV]) and regional LV function
        - Location of myocardial borders calculated by software

      - Time–volume curves generated to identify end-diastolic and end-systolic volumes based on minimum of eight frames
      - Describe regional wall motion abnormalities by location and severity—hypokinesis, akinesis, dyskinesis
      - Small hearts can cause overestimation of left ventricular ejection fraction (partial-volume effect)
      - Hypertrophied hearts can lead to underestimation of EF due to calibration of software to normal patients
      - Eight-frame gating leads to overestimation of true end-systolic volume, thereby underestimating EF compared with 16-frame gating (due to smoothing effect of time–volume curves)
    - Right ventricular size and function
      - More difficult to visualize because of lower counts and partial volume effect, unless hypertrophied

D. Assessment of ventricular function
- Planar equilibrium radionuclide angiocardiography
  - Tc-99m labeled red blood cells
    - In vitro labeling most efficient (over in vivo modified and in vivo methods)
    - Tin used as reducing agent
    - Labeling efficiency adversely affected by heparin, digoxin, hydralazine, quinidine, penicillin, prazosin, propranolol, and others
  - Gated acquisition frame rate of at least 16 frames per cycle recommended
  - Anterior, LAO (best-septal) and lateral views acquired
  - Background correction performed, with lung counts (from region 0.5 to 1 cm outside end-diastolic border from approximately 2 o'clock to 5 o'clock) being subtracted from final systolic and diastolic counts

- Ejection fraction calculated from background corrected cycle as (end-diastolic counts–end-systolic counts)/end diastolic counts
- First-pass radionuclide angiography
  - Tc-99m diethylamine triamine pentaacetic acid preferred
    - Renally excreted
    - Limits dose to patient allowing for repeated studies
  - For right ventricular assessment, rest, and stress
  - For left ventricular assessment, rest, and stress
  - Background correction performed—counts from preinjection region of lung are subtracted from final systolic and diastolic counts
  - Ejection fraction calculated from background corrected cycle as (end-diastolic counts–end-systolic counts)/end diastolic counts
  - Also used to assess and measure left-to-right shunts
    - Assess counts over region of lung to detect early recirculation of tracer through shunt
    - Qp:Qs calculated by curve stripping
- SPECT equilibrium radionuclide angiocardiography
  - Tc-99m-labeled red blood cells as in planar equilibrium radionuclide angiocardiography studies except rest-only studies because of longer duration of image acquisition
  - Similar equipment, acquisition, gating and processing as in standard myocardial perfusion SPECT imaging

E. Clinical utility of myocardial perfusion imaging: diagnosis and prognosis

- Diagnosis
  - Perfusion imaging data are combined with pretest probability for disease and result of exercise stress ECG portion of test using Bayes' theorem (as described in exercise stress testing section) to determine overall predictive value of result

- Exercise SPECT sensitivity averages about 83% for thallium and 90% for Tc-99m; specificity averages about 80% for thallium and 93% for Tc-99m
- Diminished sensitivity seen with failure to reach target heart rate, antianginal medications, single vessel disease, left circumflex disease, branch vessel or distal stenosis, 50% to 70% stenoses
  - Quantitative assessment enhances both sensitivity and specificity

- Prognosis
  - The major goal is to identify high-risk patients with left main or severe multivessel disease at high risk for sudden cardiac death or infarction
  - Normal perfusion scan at peak exercise is associated with excellent outcome (combined mortality and nonfatal infarction rate of < 1% per year)
  - Prognosis worsens incrementally with number and extent of segments involved, severity, and reversibility
  - Major prognostic markers predicting future cardiac events
  - Large defect size involving > 20% of LV
    - Multiple reversible defects in multiple segments
    - Resting ejection fraction < 40%
    - Poststress ejection fraction < 45%
    - End-systolic volume > 70 ml
    - Transient ischemic dilation
    - Increased lung uptake with Tl-201
      - Strong linear relationship with pulmonary capillary wedge pressure
      - No clear data showing significance with Tc-99m agents

F. PET

- Equipment
  - Dedicated, multicrystal ring detector system

  - Crystals (bismuth germinate, lutetium oxyorthosilicate, or gadolinium oxyorthosilicate)
- Image acquisition
  - Positron emission leads to collision with nearby orbital electrons producing two 511 keV photons traveling 180° apart
  - Coincidence detection: detectors sense these two photons coincidentally identifying their axis or origin
  - Electronic collimation: eliminates need for physical collimators, as only coincidence detections are considered, increasing count statistics significantly, which improves temporal resolution
- Attenuation correction
  - Attenuation effects more significant than in SPECT due to photon attenuation along entire path between 180° coincidence detectors
  - However, attenuation correction easier to implement with PET than with SPECT because of the known distance between 180° coincidence detectors
  - Germanium-68 transmission
  - Combined PET/CT
- Perfusion radiopharmaceuticals
  - Rubidium-82 (Rb-82)
    - Potassium analog
    - Generator produced from electron capture of strontium-82 (Sr-82)
    - Decays by positron emission to Krypton-82 (Kr-82)
    - Half-life 75 seconds
    - Stress imaging limited to pharmacologic protocol due to short half-life
  - Nitrogen-13 (N-13)
    - Cyclotron produced
    - Decays by positron emission to carbon-13 (C-13)

- Half-life 10 minutes
- First pass myocardial extraction 95%
- Oxygen-15 (0-15)
  - Theoretical advantages for determining coronary blood flow
  - Very difficult to use, not used clinically and not Food and Drug Administration approved
- Metabolism radiopharmaceuticals
  - Fluorine-18 (F-18) 2-deoxyglucose (FDG)
    - Analog of glucose
    - Cyclotron produced
    - Decays by positron emission to oxygen-18 (O-18)
    - Half-life 110 minutes
    - In fasting state, myocardium preferentially metabolizes fatty acids
    - Image quality improved when myocardial glucose uptake enhanced with labs using various techniques
      - Oral glucose loading
      - Intravenous glucose loading with insulin protocols or euglycemic hyperinsulinemic clamp
    - FDG uptake occurs in both normal or ischemic myocardial segments, but not in scar
    - Used for assessment of viability with Rb-82 or N-13 perfusion
      - Matched defect (absence of both Rb-82 or N-13 perfusion and FDG metabolism) indicates scar
      - Mismatched defect (absence of Rb-82 or N-13 perfusion and presence of FDG metabolism) indicates viable myocardium
        - Revascularization likely to improve function

IX. Pharmacologic stress testing

A. Situations in which pharmacologic stress testing preferred over exercise stress testing

- Inability to perform adequate exercise

- LBBB—vasodilator stress testing with imaging preferred cause an inability to assess adequately ST segment changes and false-positive exercise stress septal defects in absence of significant epicardial artery disease
- Paced ventricular rhythm—inability to assess ST segment changes and severe inability to achieve target heart rate

B. Vasodilator stress agents
- A2A adenosine receptor agonists resulting in coronary arteriolar vasodilation
- Myocardial tracer uptake relative to regional coronary blood flow
- In presence of significant epicardial stenosis, relative coronary blood flow differences occur
- Hemodynamics—results in minimal increase in heart rate and decrease in blood pressure
- Combined vasodilator walking protocols
    - Decreases vasodilator induced bradycardia and hypotension
    - Promotes redistribution of blood flow away from liver, resulting in better imaging quality of heart compared with vasodilator stress alone
    - Reduces side effects
    - Generally use stage 0 of modified Bruce protocol (1.7 mph with no incline)
- Adenosine
    - Mechanism—nonspecific coronary arteriolar vasodilator resulting in 3.5- to 4-fold increase in myocardial blood flow
    - Adenosine receptors affected: A1, A2A, A2B, and A3
        - A1, A2B, and A3 receptor agonism responsible for undesirable side effects
            - A1: heart block
            - A2B and A3: bronchoconstriction

- Adenosine protocol—continuous infusion 140 μg/kg/min over 4 to 6 minutes, with injection of myocardial tracer at halfway point
- Adenosine side effects
  - Flushing (44%), chest pain (40%) (not specific for CAD), dyspnea (28%) headache (18%), throat/neck/jaw discomfort (13%), gastrointestinal discomfort (13%), lightheadedness/dizziness (12%), first- or second-degree AV block (3%), ST segment depression (3%), and hypotension (2%)
  - Caused by short half-life (< 10 seconds), side effects resolve in seconds on cessation of infusion, rarely requiring reversal with aminophylline (125–250 mg IV)
- Dipyridamole
  - Mechanism—indirect coronary arteriolar vasodilator via inhibition of intracellular reuptake and deamination of adenosine, causing native adenosine accumulation
- Dipyridamole protocol—continuous infusion 0.142 mg/kg/min over 4 minutes, steady, medium-intensity hand grip at 6 minutes for total 2 minutes, injection of myocardial tracer at 7 minutes, reversal with aminophylline at 10 minutes
- Dipyridamole side effects
  - Chest pain (20%), headache (12%), dizziness (12%), ST segment changes (8%), extrasystoles (5%), hypotension (5%), nausea (5%), flushing (3%), tachycardia (3%), and dyspnea (3%)
  - Effects can last longer than with adenosine (15–25 minutes) and often need reversal with aminophylline (125–250 mg IV)
- Regadenoson
  - Mechanism—A2A specific adenosine receptor agonist-inducing coronary arteriolar vasodilation

- Regadenoson protocol—administer 0.4 mg as rapid intravenous dose over 10 seconds, followed by a 5-ml saline flush, and then administer myocardial tracer 10–20 seconds after saline flush
- Regadenoson side effects
  - Dyspnea (28%), headache (26%), flushing (16%), chest discomfort (13%), angina pectoris or ST segment depression (12%), dizziness (8%), nausea (6%), abdominal discomfort (5%), dysgeusia (5%), and feeling hot (5%)
  - Aminophylline may be given (125–250 mg) to attenuate severe or persistent side effects
- Significant ST segment depression ≥ 0.1 mV (1 mm) during adenosine protocol
  - Occurs less commonly than during exercise
  - When present, may be indicative of significant CAD via steal phenomenon
  - Portend worse prognosis
  - Usually associated with abnormal myocardial perfusion imaging
  - When present with normal myocardial perfusion imaging, has been reported to denote an increased annual risk cardiac death or myocardial infarction
- Contraindications/precautions
  - Known or suspected bronchoconstrictive or bronchospastic lung disease, especially with ongoing wheezing (can cause bronchospasm via A3 adenosine receptor)
  - Sick sinus syndrome or more than first degree heart block without pacemaker (can cause AV block via A1 adenosine receptor)
  - Systolic blood pressure < 90 mm Hg
  - Adenosine and regadenoson protocol: dipyridamole, theophylline, or caffeine within last 12 hours

    - Dipyridamole protocol: theophylline or caffeine within last 12 hours
        - Oral dipyridamole is not contraindication to dipyridamole infusion
- Indications for termination of vasodilator (adenosine or dipyridamole) infusion
    - Severe hypotension (< 80 mm Hg)
    - Symptomatic second- or third-degree heart block
    - Wheezing
    - Severe chest pain with associated ST segment depression ≥ 0.2 mV (2 mm)

C. Dobutamine

- Mechanism—direct β_1 and β_2 agonist with dose-related increase in heart rate, blood pressure, and myocardial contractility with plasma half-life of 2 minutes
- Protocol—continuous infusion starting at 5 to 10 μg/kg/min and then increased at 3-minute intervals to 20, 30, and 40 mg/kg/min
    - Addition of atropine to maximum of 2 mg may be used if heart rate does not increase sufficiently
    - Contraindications to atropine include narrow-angle glaucoma or obstructive uropathy
- Contraindications to dobutamine protocol
    - Patients on β-blockers, which may limit the heart rate response
    - Myocardial infarction within 1 week or unstable angina
    - Hemodynamically significant left ventricular outflow tract obstruction or critical aortic stenosis
    - Atrial tachyarrhythmias with rapid ventricular response or ventricular tachycardia
    - Uncontrolled hypertension
    - Aortic dissection
    - Abdominal aortic aneurysm

  - Although some small series using stress echocardiography have reported no adverse events, currently not recommended, particularly for large aneurysms
- Reasons to stop dobutamine infusion—similar reasons to those for exercise stress test, but also stopped once target heart rate achieved
- Side-effects
  - Chest pain (31%), palpitations (29%), headache (14%), flushing (14%), dyspnea (14%), significant supraventricular or ventricular tachycardia (8% to 10%), hypotension can rarely occur
  - Severe side effects may require intravenous β-blocker

10 ■ Echocardiography

Barbara Berko, MD
Alyson Owen, MD
Donna Zwas, MD

Echocardiography is the most widely used diagnostic test within the field of cardiology. Continued improvements in image quality and the development of new technologies have enhanced the ability of the echocardiographer to diagnose and delineate the extent of cardiovascular pathology. Echo has the advantage of being noninvasive, portable, and very low risk, which can rapidly provide information about cardiac structure and function in the clinical setting for diagnosis and to guide therapy.

Uses and Indications

The American Society of Echocardiography has developed guidelines for the appropriate use of echocardiography. The following is a brief summary of appropriate indications.

General Evaluation of Cardiac Structure and Function

Echo is used to evaluate symptoms and abnormal findings when a cardiac etiology is suspected (e.g., shortness of breath, syncope, dizziness, cerebrovascular events, abnormal ECG, increased brain natriuretic peptide [BNP], suspected pulmonary hypertension).

Assessment of Arrhythmias

Echo can determine the presence or absence of structural heart disease in patients with paroxysmal or sustained supraventricular or ventricular arrhythmias—chamber sizes, ventricular function, hemodynamics, and valvular function can be defined and the underlying substrate for arrhythmias assessed. Transesophageal echo can be used to determine whether thrombus is present in the left atrial (LA) appendage to determine the safety of cardioversion or ablation in atrial fibrillation (AF) or flutter.

Ischemic Heart Disease

Echo provides an assessment of left ventricular (LV) function and segmental wall motion in the initial evaluation of acute myocardial infarction (MI) and identifies complications of infarction, such as pericarditis, LV thrombus, acute mitral regurgitation (MR), ventricular septal rupture or ruptured papillary muscle, right ventricular (RV) infarction, heart failure, or shock. It is used to assess LV function in the recovery phase to guide therapy, such as the need for prophylactic internal cardiac defibrillator (ICD). It can be used in the assessment of acute chest pain when labs and ECG are nondiagnostic and echo is obtained during episodes of chest pain. Stress echo can be used to identify the presence and extent of ischemia when exertional symptoms suggest underlying ischemic heart disease.

Heart Failure

Echo is used to determine the underlying cause of congestive heart failure (CHF), whether it is due to systolic or diastolic dysfunction, and to help guide and evaluate therapy. It is used to diagnose underlying cardiomyopathies (hypertrophic, restrictive, infiltrative, genetic, etc.), to screen relatives in familial cardiomyopathies, and to re-evaluate a change in clinical status or to guide therapy. Echo is used to evaluate for dyssynchrony and determine the appropriateness for cardiac resynchronization therapy or to optimize pacing devices. It is also used to obtain baseline and serial studies to follow patients receiving cardiotoxic chemotherapeutic agents such as Adriamycin.

Valvular Disease

Echo is the single most useful tool in the diagnosis of suspected valvular heart disease and the assessment of severity and hemodynamic consequences of valve disease. It is used to evaluate murmurs when underlying valvular or other structural heart disease is suspected, and in the initial assessment of mitral prolapse, native valve stenosis or regurgitation, and to establish a baseline after prosthetic valve replacement or to evaluate suspected prosthetic dysfunction. Re-evaluation with echo is appropriate yearly for asymptomatic patients with severe valvular regurgitation or stenosis or when a change in clinical status occurs. Transesophageal echo is used in MR to determine whether valve repair is feasible.

In suspected endocarditis, echo is used for initial diagnosis when blood cultures are positive or a new murmur is heard and for re-evaluation in diagnosed endocarditis when persistent fever or bacteremia are present and hemodynamic instability or clinical deterioration occurs or when there is either aortic involvement or a virulent organism. Transesophageal echo can also be used in the assessment of endocarditis and is particularly useful when prosthetic valve endocarditis is suspected or in the presence of potential infection of intracardiac devices.

Pericardial Disease

Echo is used to evaluate and diagnose suspected pericardial effusions, to assess for pericardial tamponade, to guide drainage of effusions, and to assess for constrictive pericarditis or the presence of pericardial masses.

Critical Care

In the intensive care unit setting, echocardiography can be very helpful in the assessment of hypotension, respiratory failure, or hemodynamic instability. In the presence of suspected pulmonary embolism, echo can assess the hemodynamic impact on the right ventricle to help guide treatment such as the use of thrombolytics.

Aortic Disease

Transthoracic echo is used to screen patients with Marfan's syndrome, or other connective tissue disorders, for involvement of the aortic root or ascending aorta. Transesophageal echo can be very useful in the diagnosis of suspected aortic dissection or aneurysm.

Congenital Heart Disease

Echo can be used in the adult with known or suspected congenital heart disease for diagnosis or follow-up.

Other Indications

Echo can be used to evaluate for possible source of embolism (cerebrovascular or peripheral) when a cardiac source such as patent foramen ovale (PFO), intracardiac thrombus or tumor, or complex atherosclerotic aortic plaque is suspected. Transesophageal echo can be used to guide invasive procedures such as PFO/ASD (atrial septal defect) closures, radiofrequency ablations, or mitral valvuloplasty.

Echocardiography—Modalities

Echocardiography is the use of reflected sound waves, reflected off both cardiac structures and off moving red blood cells, providing information about the structure and function of the heart. It is one of the most widely used techniques in cardiology, having as its advantages its noninvasive nature and lack of any harm to tissue or side effects.

M-Mode Echocardiography

It was one of the earliest modalities developed. It displays one slice of the heart as it moves over time and is used today for measurements and for accurate timing of events in the cardiac cycle (such as looking for diastolic collapse of the right ventricle in pericardial tamponade).

Two-Dimensional Echocardiography

This displays two-dimensional views of cardiac anatomy over time. The most commonly used is transthoracic echocardiography (using transducers from 2.5–5.0 MHz), for which pictures are taken by applying the ultrasound transducer directly to the chest wall with an ultrasound gel interface. Additional modalities include transesophageal echocardiography, in which an ultrasound probe (5.0–7.0 MHz), similar in appearance to an endoscopy probe, is placed in the esophagus under conscious sedation, allowing views of the heart and aorta unobstructed by chest wall and lungs. Also available are intracardiac ultrasound (7.5–10.0 MHz), used primarily in guiding placement of intracardiac devices such as ASD/PFO closure devices and in electrophysiologic procedures, and intracoronary ultrasound (20.0–30.0 MHz), used for evaluation of coronary plaque and flow within the coronary arteries.

Doppler Echocardiography

This is based on principles of sound waves explored by Christian Doppler in the 19th century. Sound waves reflected off moving red blood cells within the heart provide information on blood flow velocity and direction.

Spectral Doppler

This displays quantitative information about blood flow, both velocity and direction of flow, in the heart and vasculature. The pulse-wave Doppler displays information from a specific location defined by the sample volume but cannot display high velocities. The continuous-wave Doppler can evaluate high velocities but does not provided localizing information.

Color Flow Doppler

This is a special form of pulse wave Doppler that displays velocity and directional information in a color-coded format that allows for interrogating larger areas. Color Doppler is the mainstay for evaluation of valvular regurgitation in particular.

Tissue Doppler

This uses the same concepts as spectral and color flow Doppler (CFD), but it uses sound waves reflected off tissue rather than red blood cells, providing information about the velocity of tissue movement. It is used predominantly to evaluate systolic and especially diastolic function of the ventricles. Strain and strain rate evaluations use information derived from tissue Doppler (TD) and are used most frequently in the evaluation of cardiac dyssynchrony.

Three-Dimensional Echocardiography

This uses a series of two-dimensional views to reconstruct a three-dimensional image of the heart. Until recently, it was used mostly in research, but its current ability to do reconstructions in real time is increasing its use in clinical cardiology.

Transesophageal Echocardiography

This is the examination of structure and performance using an ultrasound probe mounted on a device similar to a gastroscope, which is inserted into the esophagus and stomach. Because of the proximity of the esophagus to the heart, a high-resolution probe can be used, leading to pictures with exquisite anatomic detail.

Indications

A transesophageal echocardiogram (TEE) should be performed when specific questions are not adequately addressed by the initial TTE examination or in cases in which TEE is clearly superior to TTE. The major clinical indications for TEE include the evaluation of native valve disease, prosthetic heart valve function and dysfunction, cardiac masses, hemodynamic instability, congenital heart disease, and evaluation of the left atrium in patients in AF. TEE is used to detect aortic dissection and endocarditis and to evaluate for cardiac sources of embolus. TEE also has a significant role as an adjunct to percutaneous cardiac procedures and cardiac surgical procedures.

Patient Safety

Despite the advantages of TEE and the low complication rate associated with the procedure, it is incumbent on the echocardiographer to assess whether the value of the question to be answered outweighs the risk to the patient. The major risks to the patient include bleeding, aspiration, and perforation, and these should be explained to the patient as part of the process of informed consent. A careful history should be obtained from the patient regarding any history of dysphagia or change in ability to tolerate oral intake and any esophageal surgery. Absolute contraindications include unrepaired tracheoesophageal fistula, perforated hollow viscus, poor airway control, severe respiratory depression, cervical instability, and the uncooperative unsedated patient. Esophageal diverticula, varices (greater than grade 2), recent surgery, active bleeding, malignancy, prior radiation, severe esophagitis, and scleroderma are also considered major contraindications to TEE. A history of aspiration should also factor into the risk profile of the patient, and special care should be taken after the procedure to prevent aspiration pneumonia. In nonurgent settings, TEE should be performed when the patient is not overanticoagulated, significantly thrombocytopenic, hypoxic, hypotensive, and severely hypertensive or has any evidence of metabolic disarray. The risks of all invasive procedures and of sedation increase with advanced age or confusion, and the procedure should be carefully discussed with the referring physician when requested for the very older population. Patients at increased risk of complications from sedation such as the morbidly obese, patients with sleep apnea, or the agitated patient should be performed with the assistance of an anesthesiologist. Patients with a history of narcotic or benzodiazepine abuse who will be difficult to sedate with routine quantities of sedating agents or patients who do not tolerate probe placement with routine sedation should also be anesthetized with the assistance of the anesthesia service.

Cardiac Chamber Quantification and LV Function

The assessment of chamber size and LV function is one of the most common reasons for obtaining an echocardiogram. Technical advances have provided significant improvements in image quality and endocardial definition, permitting more reliable measurements in a majority of patients. Guidelines for standardization of chamber quantification have been developed by the American Society of Echocardiography, and methods for obtaining quantitative measurements as well as normal and abnormal reference values for these parameters have been recommended.

LV Chamber Size

LV Dimensions

The left ventricle has been geometrically modeled as a prolate ellipse. Minor axis dimensions of the LV internal cavity and septal and posterior wall thicknesses can be measured from two-dimensional or two-dimensional–guided M-mode images. Although the upper limit of normal for LV end-diastolic dimension is generally considered to be 5.5 cm, differences in chamber dimensions have been recognized based on gender and body size. Left ventricular diastolic dimensions above 5.3 cm are considered abnormal in women, whereas 5.9 cm is the upper limit of normal in men. Measurements can be normalized for body size based on either body surface area or height, with 3.2 cm/m^2 in women or 3.3 cm/m^2 in men being considered the upper limits of normal. There is controversy about which is the best index, but measurements indexed for body surface area are traditionally used.

LV Volume and Geometry

To obtain LV volumes, the biplane Simpson's method of discs is recommended. The ventricular endocardium is traced (planimetered) in two views (apical four and two chamber) and then divided into a stack of elliptical discs of equal height from which ventricular volume can be calculated at end diastole and end systole. Normal end-diastolic volumes differ in men and women, but when indexed for body surface area, the upper limit of normal is 75 cc/m^2, regardless of gender. End-diastolic volume has important clinical and prognostic significance, independent of LV function, with poor clinical prognosis associated with very dilated ventricles in most disease processes.

Normal LV geometry is modeled as a prolate ellipse. As the ventricle dilates, it may become more spherical, and this change in geometry has also been associated with worse clinical outcomes.

LV Mass and Relative Wall Thickness

LV mass can be calculated from measurements of LV internal dimensions and wall thickness (see Table 10.1). One can also use two-dimensional measurement of myocardial area and LV length to calculate myocardial volume and LV mass. The ASE-recommended (American Society for Echocardiography) formula has been validated in autopsy studies.

LV mass is traditionally indexed to body surface area, although there is controversy as to the best index. Even when indexed, the LV mass differs between males and females.

Increased LV mass is a major risk factor for cardiovascular morbidity and mortality, and the geometry and pattern of hypertrophy provide additional prognostic information. Relative wall thickness (RWT) has been used to determine the pattern of hypertrophy and assess the adequacy of hypertrophy in response to increased wall stress. RWT is calculated as 2 × (PWT/LVID) and is directly proportional to systolic pressure in compensated ventricles. In ventricles that can no longer adequately normalize wall stress, RWT is disproportionately low and may reflect the transition to a decompensated state leading to heart failure. Normal RWT is defined as ≤ 0.45.

Table 10.1

$$\text{LV mass} = 0.8\{1.04\,[(\text{LVIDd} + \text{PWTd} + \text{SWTd})^3\ (\text{LVIDd})^3]\} + 0.6\text{g}$$

Where LVIDd = LV internal diameter at end diastole;

PWTd = posterior wall thickness at end diastole;

SWTd = septal wall thickness at end diastole;

1.04 = specific gravity of myocardium.

Concentric remodeling, in which LV mass is normal but RWT is increased, is typically the initial response to pressure overload and is associated with adverse prognosis. Concentric hypertrophy, in which both LV mass and RWT are increased, develops in response to pressure overload such as in hypertension and aortic stenosis (AS), along with other influences, including obesity and metabolic factors. It carries a worse prognosis than concentric remodeling. Eccentric hypertrophy usually results from volume overload, such as in valvular regurgitation, and is manifested as an increase in LV mass with normal RWT. Although cardiovascular morbidity and mortality are significantly higher than in a normal population, the increased risk is less than with concentric hypertrophy. Thus, the pattern of LV hypertrophy influences prognosis, with concentric hypertrophy conferring the worst prognosis, eccentric hypertrophy an intermediate risk, and concentric remodeling the least incremental risk compared with normal. Left ventricular hypertrophy is an independent predictor of cardiovascular outcomes and is as powerful a predictor as ejection fraction.

Assessment of LV Systolic Function

The most commonly used parameter for assessment of overall LV systolic function is the LV ejection fraction (EF). It is determined by preload, afterload, and contractility. In virtually all cardiac disease states, EF has been shown to have prognostic significance and is an important determinant of therapeutic options.

Ejection fraction is defined as follows:

$$\frac{\text{(end-diastolic volume)} - \text{(end-systolic volume)}}{\text{(end-diastolic volume)}} \times 100$$

Echocardiographic two-dimensional–derived volumes (discussed previously) can be used to calculate ejection fraction. The severity of LV dysfunction is graded by ejection fraction as shown in Table 10.2.

Fractional shortening (FS), the percentage change in LV internal diameter from diastole to systole, can be obtained from M-mode

Table 10.2

Degree of LV Dysfunction	Ejection Fraction
Normal	≥ 55%
Mild	45% to 54%
Moderate	30% to 44%
Severe	< 30%

Source: Adapted from Lang RM, Bierig M, Devereux RB, et al. Recommendations for chamber quantification: a report from the American Society of Echocardiography's Guidelines and Standards Committee and the Chamber Quantification Writing Group. *J Am Soc Echocardiogr* 2005;18:1440–1463.

or two-dimensional–derived linear dimensions of the left ventricle (normal FS ≥ 27%). Because measurements are obtained at the base of the LV, this parameter is unreliable in the presence of segmental wall motion abnormalities, but can be a useful parameter in disease states with global abnormalities, such as hypertension or valvular regurgitation. Other indices of LV systolic function can be obtained with echocardiographic techniques, including the velocity of fiber shortening (Vcf), dP/dt (the rate of pressure development during isovolumic contraction), stroke volume, cardiac output, longitudinal (long axis) shortening, and mitral annular excursion (see the section on hemodynamics).

All ejection phase parameters are very dependent on loading conditions and may not reflect true myocardial contractility. Isovolumic indices (such as dP/dt) are not as load dependent. The relationship between ejection fraction or FS and end-systolic wall stress provides a better index of myocardial contractility when loading conditions are abnormal.

Assessment of Left Ventricle Segmental Wall Motion

Coronary artery disease leads to segmental ischemia and infarction, which is reflected in abnormalities of motion of the LV walls. An understanding of the relationship between the myocardial segments and coronary perfusion aids the clinician in the assessment of the presence, severity, and significance of coronary artery disease. Echocardiography provides a unique tool for the evaluation of segmental wall motion, as the endocardial surface of multiple walls can be directly visualized. When image quality is poor, the use of echo contrast agents can aid in providing better endocardial definition. The American Society of Echocardiography has adopted the 17 segment model for depiction of segmental wall motion (Figure 10.1). Wall motion is traditionally described as normal, hypokinetic, akinetic, dyskinetic, or aneurysmal. Although "normal" wall motion has been defined as a more than 30% increase in wall thickness, assessment is usually done qualitatively. The wall motion score is an index of cardiac dysfunction wherein each visualized segment is given a score: 1 = normal, 2 = hypokinetic, 3 = akinetic, 4 = dyskinetic, and 5 = aneurysmal. The score is the total of all scores divided by the number of segments. Care should be taken to assess wall thickening/endocardial motion rather than motion of the segment as a whole. In the setting of left bundle branch block or postoperative paradoxical motion, the septum may move away from the center of the ventricle, but as it thickens normally, this should not be considered a hypokinetic segment. Similarly, akinetic or hypokinetic segments may be dragged by neighboring hypercontractile segments, leading to the appearance of motion, but without thickening. In addition to wall motion, the myocardial texture can be useful, as infarcted tissue may appear thin with increased echogenicity to suggest fibrous scar. Aneurysm formation and pseudoaneurysm, a localized rupture walled off by pericardium, can also be detected.

Assessment of Left Atrial Diameter and Volume

LA size is predominantly determined by LV filling pressure and reflects wall stress, and LA dilation is associated with an increased incidence of cardiac events, including death. LA diameter can be obtained by linear measurements of the atrium in the anterior–posterior plane. This linear measurement may misrepresent true

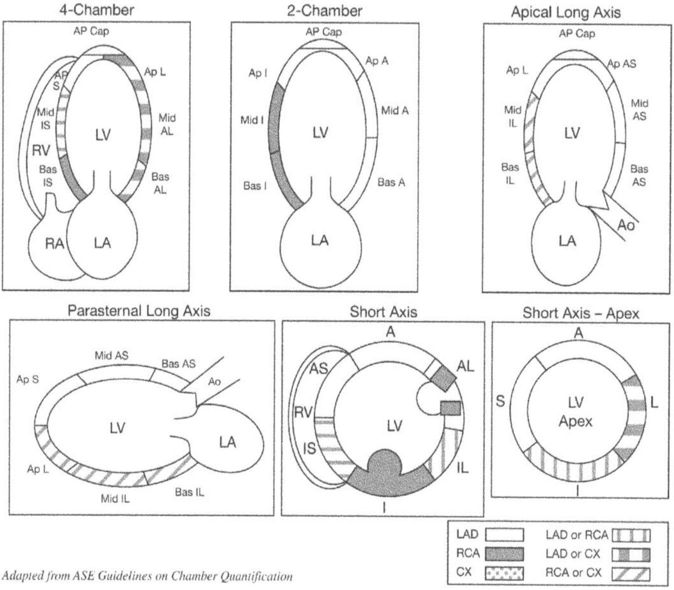

■ **Figure 10.1** 17-segment model demonstrating segmental analysis of the LV walls. Schematic representations of the standard echo views are shown with the wall segments identified. Superimposed on the segments is their typical coronary distribution. There is some individual variation in the coronary perfusion of LV wall segments. Right coronary artery(RCA); left anterior descending (LAD); left circumflex (Cx). Anterior(A); anteroseptal (AS); anterolateral(AL); apical (Ap); inferior(I); inferoseptal (IS); inferolateral(IL); septal (S); lateral (L); basal(Bas); left ventricle (LV); left atrium (LA); right ventricle (RV); right atrium (RA); aorta (Ao)

Source: Adapted from ASE Guidelines on Chamber Quantification.

LA size if atrial enlargement occurs in other planes. LA volume is a more reliable measure and correlates more closely with cardiovascular outcomes. Echocardiographic LA volume can be obtained by measuring the area of the LA in two views [apical 2- (Ap^2) and 4-chamber (Ap^4)] and the height of the atrium from the mitral annulus to the back wall. Using the shorter height from the two views, the following formula is used for calculating LA volume:

$$8/3\ \pi\ (\text{Area}_{\text{Ap4}} \times \text{Area}_{\text{Ap2}})/\text{height}$$

As for LV measurements, the LA volume can be indexed for body surface area to provide the most reliable clinical tool, and 22 ± 6 cc/m^2 is the normal range for both genders. An LA volume of greater than 40 ml/m^2 implies severe LA dilation.

Aortic Measurements

Aortic diameter is best measured from two-dimensional echo images and can be measured in different parts of the aorta. From standard images, measurement of the aortic root at the annulus of the aortic valve (AV), the sinuses of Valsalva, the sinotubular junction, and the proximal ascending aorta can be made. Aortic root diameter is dependent on body surface area and age, and nomograms have been developed for the normal range of aortic diameter for three age groups: less than 20 years old, 20 to 40 years, and older than 40 years. It is very important to index aortic root size for body surface area and compare it with these nomograms to determine accurately whether aortic dilation is present. The average normal aortic root diameter at the sinuses is 3.4 ± 0.3 cm (or 1.7 cm/m^2 indexed) in adult men and 3.0 ± 0.3 cm (1.8 cm/m^2) in women.

Aortic diameter is strongly predictive of the risk of aortic dissection or rupture and the severity and progression of aortic regurgitation (AR). Guidelines for elective surgical repair of thoracic aortic aneurysms have recommended repair for aortic roots measuring 5 cm or greater because of the high risk of dissection or rupture above this size.

Hemodynamics

Spectral Doppler echocardiography measures the velocity of blood flow within the heart and vasculature. By analyzing the Doppler shift, that is, the difference in the emitted and returning sound wave frequencies of ultrasound waves reflected off moving red blood cells, velocity of blood flow can be determined being expressed as meters per second or centimeters per second.

Determination of Pressure Gradient

The velocity of blood flow is determined by the pressure gradient (PG) down which the blood pool is moving. In the heart, this is determined by the PG between two cardiac chambers. Although the complete form of the Bernoulli equation, which allows us to convert from velocity to PG, includes a number of additional factors accounting for convective acceleration and viscous friction, the modified Bernoulli equation is sufficiently accurate to be used in clinical work. $PG = 4 \times (V2^2 - V1^2)$, with V1 being the velocity on the higher pressure side of the two chambers and V2 being on the lower pressure side. For example, when measuring an AV gradient, V1 is the LVOT velocity, and V2 is the velocity at the level of the AV. If V1 is low enough, less than approximately 2 m/sec, this factor can also be disregarded leaving us with $PG = 4(V2)^2$. The most frequent use of this formula is to assess the PG of stenotic lesions, such as AS and mitral stenosis (MS). A peak velocity may be used, leading to a value for peak gradient, or the complete spectral signal can be traced giving the velocity time integral, leading to a value for mean gradient (see Figure 10.2).

Estimation of Absolute Pressure

In many clinical situations, the actual peak pressure rather than the PG between two chambers is more clinically relevant. In order to go from PG to pressure, the pressure in the receiving chamber (either known or estimated) must be added to the PG. For example, the RV-RA gradient reveals the PG between the two chambers, but to obtain RV peak systolic pressure, an estimate of RA pressure must be added. The RA pressure is estimated from examination of the inferior vena cava (IVC) as to size and whether it collapses with inspiration, with an estimated pressure from 5 to 20 mm Hg being

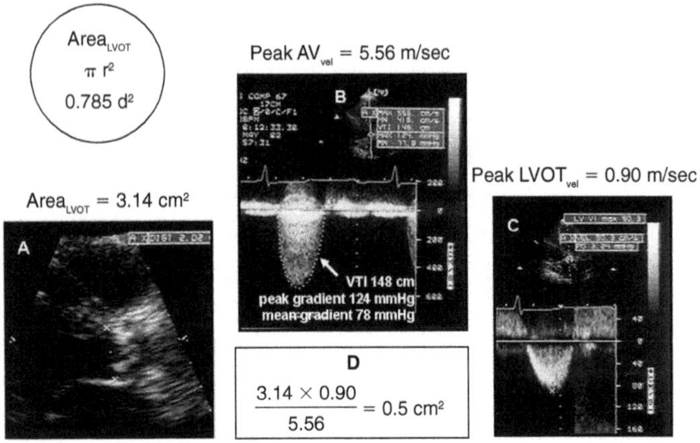

■ **Figure 10.2** Calculation of aortic valve area (AVA) in a patient with severe aortic stenosis. **(A)** Left ventricular outflow tract (LVOT) measurement. **(B)** Continuous wave spectral Doppler of aortic valve velocity, demonstrating measurement of velocity time interval (VTI) and peak velocity. **(C)** Pulse wave Doppler of LVOT velocity. **(D)** Calculation of AVA by continuity equation demonstrated.

assigned. This number is added to the RV-RA gradient, giving a value for RV systolic pressure, which in the absence of pulmonic stenosis, is the same as pulmonary artery systolic pressure, an important clinical piece of information (Figure 10.3).

Assessment of Volume of Flow

Estimation of volume of flow is useful, for example, to determine forward stroke volume (SV), regurgitant volume, or magnitude of intracardiac shunts. Volume is determined by multiplying the time velocity integral (TVI) of the spectral signal by the cross-sectional area at the same location from which the spectral signal is obtained. For this use, pulse wave (PW) Doppler must be used, as it allows the determination of the velocity at a specific point in space. When a structure is essentially circular, for example, the LV outflow tract

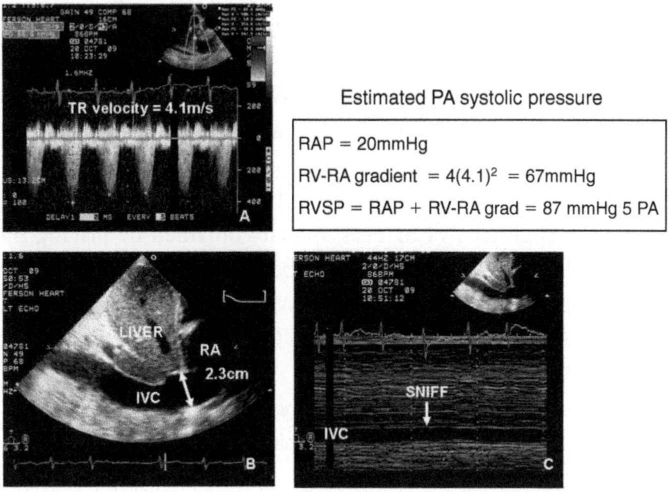

■ **Figure 10.3** Pulmonary Hypertension: Images from a patient with severe pulmonary hypertension, demonstrating the calculation of pulmonary artery (PA) pressure from tricuspid regurgitation (TR) jet. Panel **(A)** shows continuous wave Doppler of TR with measurement of the maximal TR velocity to obtain the right atrial (RA) to right ventricular (RV) gradient; **(B)** shows the dilated inferior vena cava (IVC) on subcostal view; **(C)** is an M-mode of the IVC during respiration, demonstrating a fixed, dilated IVC that fails to collapse during inspiration (sniff). RAP, right atrial pressure; RVSP, Right ventricular systolic pressure.

(LVOT), πr^2 may be used; therefore, SV = $LVOT_{Area} \times LVOT_{TVI}$ (Figure 10.2). This concept is also used in the continuity equation, from which, for example, AV area can be estimated (see Valvular Heart Disease), and in the evaluation of intracardiac shunts.

The Continuity Equation

This equation is based on the conservation of mass, which states that in a closed system the volume of flow at each individual point must be the same as at every other point. In the heart, the amount of blood crossing each area of the heart and vasculature must be the same; for example, the SV through the LVOT must be the same as the SV at the narrowest part of the AV. Aortic valve area may then be estimated using the continuity equation, $LVOT_{area} \times LVOT_{velocity} = AV_{area} \times AV_{velocity}$. The SV in the LVOT is estimated as $LVOT_{area} \times LVOT_{velocity}$. $LVOT_{area} = \Pi r^2$ or $3.14 \times (\frac{1}{2}\ LVOT_{diameter})^2$, and $LVOT_{velocity}$ is either TVI or peak velocity obtained by placing the PW sample volume in the LVOT just below the AV. The AV velocity is obtained by a continuous wave (CW) spectral signal of AV flow. Rearranging the equation, $AVA = LVOT_{area} \times LVOT_{velocity}/AV_{velocity}$ (Figure 10.2 and Table 10.3).

The proximal isovelocity surface area formula (PISA) is a special form of the continuity equation. As blood flows toward a limiting orifice, there is acceleration of flow in a series of concentric hemispheres, which can be visualized by CFD as a series of aliasing hemispheres of alternating red and blue. This information can be used to assess stenosis but is most frequently used to assess the severity of regurgitation, leading to an estimate of effective regurgitant orifice (ERO). In this case, the formula for a hemisphere ($2\pi r^2$) is used, with r being the distance between the limiting orifice and the first aliasing radius. This is multiplied by the aliasing velocity (the Nyquist limit of the CFD) to obtain the SV at that distance from the orifice. The continuity equation then becomes $6.28\ r^2 \times$ aliasing velocity (cm/sec) = ERO $\times$ peak velocity of the regurgitant spectral signal (cm/sec), or rearranging $6.28\ r^2 \times$ aliasing velocity (cm/sec)/peak velocity of the regurgitant spectral signal (cm/sec) (see Figure 10.4).

Assessment of Changes in PG Over the Cardiac Cycle

There are clinical situations in which the change in the PG over time provides very useful information (e.g., evaluation of the mitral inflow signal over diastole). The slope of the E wave deceleration, described in m/sec^2, describes the rate of change in velocity, which can be translated into the rate of change of pressure (i.e., the rate at which the two chambers are coming to equilibrium). For example, in MS, if the slope of the mitral inflow signal is steep, this

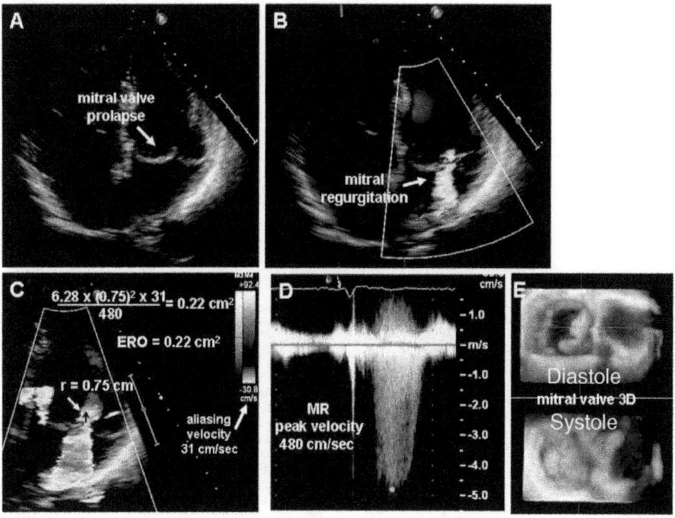

■ **Figure 10.4** Mitral valve prolapse and use of proximal isovelocity surface area formula (PISA) to estimate effective regurgitant orifice (ERO). **(A)** Apical four chamber view of patient with mitral valve prolapse (arrow). **(B)** Color flow Doppler signal of mitral regurgitation. **(C)** Color flow Doppler shown with baseline shifted in the direction of the regurgitant jet to obtain PISA aliasing radius (arrow). Calculation of ERO demonstrated. ERO of 0.22 cm^2 is consistent with moderate mitral regurgitation. **(D)** Continuous wave Doppler signal of (arrow) mitral regurgitation. (Peak velocity used in calculation of ERO.) **(E)** 3D reconstruction of prolapsing mitral valve in diastole (top) and systole (bottom).

means that the LV and the LA are coming to equilibrium rapidly (i.e., the severity of stenosis is mild). If the slope is flatter, the gradient between the LA and the LV is dissipating slowly (i.e., the stenosis is more severe) (see Figure 10.5). This information can be used quantitatively (e.g., in the pressure half-time [PHT], the speed at which the *pressure* declines from its peak in early diastole to half of its original value) and is used to estimate mitral valve (MV) area (Table 10.3). PHT measurements are also used in the evaluation of AR. Deceleration time (DT), for example, of the mitral inflow signal in the evaluation of LV diastolic function is the time interval from the peak velocity of the E wave to where the E-wave velocity reaches zero, with a shorter DT (< 150 msec) being associated with increased LV filling pressures.

Assessment of Tissue Velocity

In TD, the velocity of myocardium rather than the velocity of blood flow is measured. These measurements are typically carried out

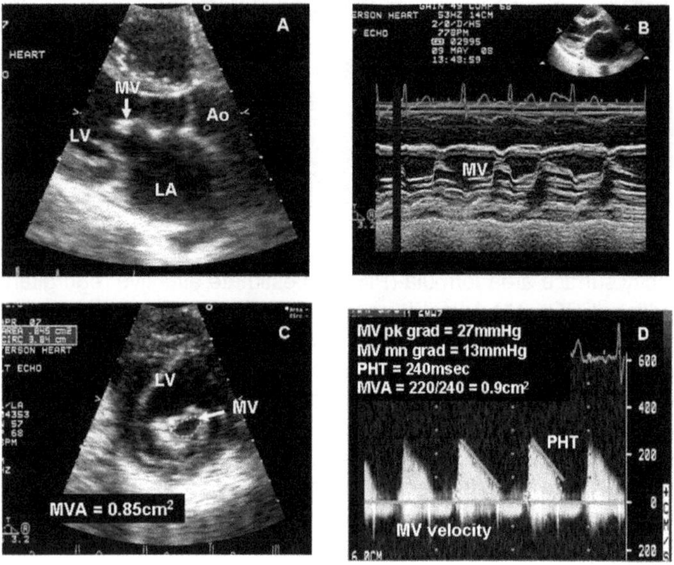

■ **Figure 10.5** Mitral Stenosis: Images from a patient with rheumatic mitral stenosis (MS). Panel **(A)** shows a 2D parasternal long axis view of the mitral leaflets with doming of the anterior leaflet; **(B)** is an M-mode of the mitral valve (MV) demonstrating restricted posterior leaflet which moves anteriorly to closure, mirroring the anterior leaflet motion; **(C)** is a 2D image of the short axis view of the MV with planimetry of the narrowest orifice to derive MV area (MVA); note the commissural fusion typical of rheumatic MS; **(D)** shows the CW Doppler of the mitral inflow velocity with pressure half-time (PHT) to calculate MVA. LA, left atrium; LV, left ventricle; Ao, aorta; pk grad, peak gradient; mn grad, mean gradient.

Table 10.3 Selected Echo Formulas

Application	Formula
LVOT area	$3.14 \times (\frac{1}{2}\ \text{LVOT diameter})^2$
Stroke volume (SV) (ml)	$SV = LVOT_{area} \times LVOT_{VTI}$
Cardiac output (CO) (L/min)	$CO = LVOT_{area} \times LVOT_{VTI} \times HR$
Aortic valve area (AVA) (cm^2)	$AVA = LVOT_{area} \times LVOT_{VTI} / AV_{VTI}$
Mitral valve area (MVA) by PHT (cm^2)	MVA = 220/PHT or 750/DT
Shunts (QP:QS)	$QP = RVOT_{area} \times RVOT_{VTI}$ $QS = LVOT_{area} \times LVOT_{VTI}$
Pulmonary artery systolic pressure (mm Hg)	PASP = RV/RA gradient + RA pressure*
Effective regurgitant orifice by PISA (cm^2)	ERO = 6.28 × first aliasing radius $(cm)^2$ × Nyquist limit (cm/sec)/ peak velocity of regurgitant signal (cm/sec)
Regurgitant volume (RV) (ml)	$RV = SV_{regurgitant\ valve} - SV_{competent\ valve}$ (e.g., SV_{LVOT} if no AR)
Regurgitant fraction (RF) (%)	$RF = RV / SV_{regurgitant\ valve}$

in the apical views and are a measure of longitudinal rather than radial myocardial function. Tissue Doppler measurements of the myocardium at the mitral annulus in diastole are used in particular to evaluate the diastolic function of the ventricles. Tissue velocity during early filling (E') can be obtained. Assessing the relationship between TD (E') and spectral signals of mitral inflow (E) provides information about LV filling pressures and provides prognostic information in patients with cardiomyopathy. The TD signal of the mitral annulus during systole can be used to assess LV longitudinal systolic function, which may be abnormal even when estimates of radial function, such as FS or ejection fraction, are preserved. Strain and strain rate imaging, which are derivatives of TD, can be used for evaluation of both systolic and diastolic function of the left ventricle and in particular have been used for the evaluation of ventricular dyssynchrony.

Echocardiography in Evaluation of Diastolic Function of the Left Ventricle

Although LV function refers most often to systolic function of the ventricle, evaluation of diastolic function is equally important, as the ventricle must be able to fill normally in order to empty normally. The inability to fill the ventricle adequately without elevation of LA pressure (i.e., a shift of the pressure–volume relationship upward and to the left) is termed diastolic dysfunction. Echocardiography is the widely used technique for evaluation of diastolic function, as it has many advantages over invasive evaluation (pressure-volume loops) and nuclear filling curves. From a clinical point of view, the important question is not "Is diastolic dysfunction present?" but rather "Is LV filling pressure elevated?" Diastole is a complex process involving both active (involving calcium uptake by the endoplasmic reticulum) and passive (compliance of the myocardium, which may be altered by hypertrophy, fibrosis, etc.) components. It is affected by many variables, including LV systolic function. The amount of deformation that the left ventricle experiences during systole is reflected in both a passive property, elastic recoil, and an active process, load-dependent inactivation; therefore, it can be said that when systolic dysfunction is present, diastolic dysfunction accompanies it.

There are four phases of diastole: (1) isovolumic relaxation (IVR), (2) early filling, (3) diastasis, and (4) atrial contraction (Figure 10.6). IVRT is the period of time between closure of the AV and opening of the mitral valve, during which ventricular pressure is falling but has not yet fallen below LA pressure. The duration of IVR can be measured by placing a PW sample volume between the mitral inflow and LVOT signals, whereby both closure of the AV and opening of the mitral valve can be seen and the time interval can be measured. Normal IVRT is 90 to 120 milliseconds. Early filling is

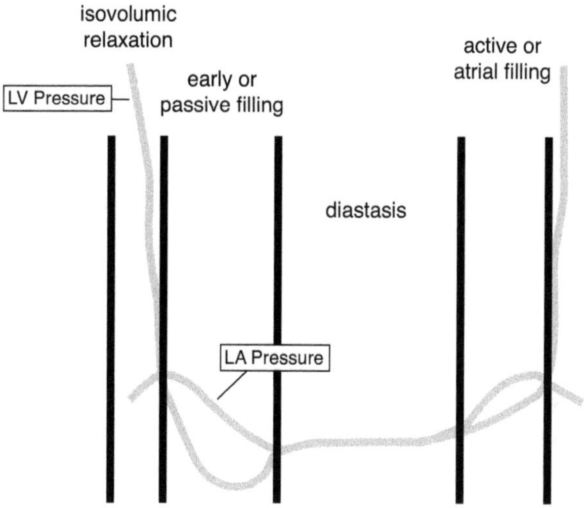

■ **Figure 10.6** Schematic of left ventricular (LV) and left atrial (LA) pressure curves, demonstrating the four phases of diastole.

driven by the PG between the LA and the LV in early diastole and is reflected in the velocity of the E wave. It is again important to distinguish between pressure (which is an absolute measurement) and PG (which is the relationship between the pressures in the two chambers). In other words, E-wave velocity could be high either because LA pressure is high or LV early diastolic pressure is low. The DT of the E wave (see Figure 10.7) is a marker of how rapidly LA and LV pressure comes to equilibrium. The DT will shorten if either the LA pressure falls rapidly or the LV pressure rises rapidly (e.g., because of decreased compliance of the LV). Normal value for mitral deceleration is 150 to 220 milliseconds. Diastasis is a period of time during which the LA and LV pressures have come to equilibrium and no significant net flow occurs. It is found at slower heart rates and is not generally seen if heart rate exceeds 60 beats

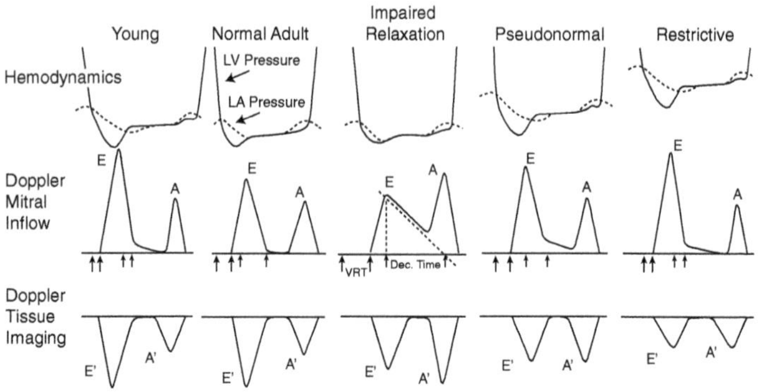

■ **Figure 10.7** Schematic of left ventricular (LV) and left atrial (LA) hemodynamics (top panel), pulse wave Doppler of mitral inflow (middle panel), and pulse wave tissue Doppler of the mitral annulus (bottom panel).

Source: Adapted from the Amer Soc of Echo Guidelines.

per minute. Atrial contraction occurs after the P wave on the ECG and is reflected by the A wave of the mitral inflow profile. A wave velocity is influenced by the compliance of the LV at end diastole, LA preload, and LA contractile state.

There has been a great deal of research into the mitral inflow patterns in normal and disease states and into the relationship between the E-wave velocity and the A-wave velocity (called the E/A ratio). The normal value for E/A ratio is between 1 and 2. This has led to the widely used schema seen in Figure 10.7. There is a "U"-shaped relationship, with the healthiest hearts (young adults or children) and the unhealthiest hearts (severe diastolic dysfunction with significant elevation of LV pressure) appearing exactly the same. To understand this, one must again return to the concept that the velocities recorded in the mitral inflow describe the PG between the LA and the LV and not the absolute pressure in either chamber. For example, the E-wave velocity is high in young, healthy individuals because early LV diastolic pressure is low (in fact being actually negative as the ventricle relaxes more quickly than it can fill), whereas in the group to the right of the figure (also called stage IV diastolic dysfunction or the restrictive pattern, characterized not only by an E/A ratio > 2, but also by a DT < 150 msec), E-wave velocity is high because LA pressure is high. Extensive research has demonstrated that the restrictive inflow pattern is associated with an LV filling pressure greater than 20 mm Hg; however, this is only valid in patients with decreased LV systolic function. In patients with normal LV systolic function and with supernormal LV systolic function (such as patients with hypertrophic cardiomyopathy), the mitral inflow parameters are inaccurate for the prediction of LV filling pressure.

Tissue Doppler has added a new dimension to the evaluation of diastolic function and LV filling pressures. To obtain TD, the sample volume of PW Doppler is placed not in the blood flow, but in the myocardium itself, and the velocity of tissue movement is recorded. Tissue velocity is much lower than most blood flows within the heart, measuring only from approximately 0 to 20 cm/sec (or 0.2 m/sec), and requires special software. A typical spectral Doppler profile is seen in Figure 10.7. With TD, that component of the E wave that is due to LA pressure can be separated from the component due to relaxation and elastic recoil of the myocardium. The velocity of the E wave (from the mitral inflow) is divided by the E' from TD (also known as Ea, Em). If E/E' > 15, LA pressure is estimated at > 15 mm Hg. If E/E' < 8, LA pressure is estimated as normal. If E/E' is between 8 and 15, no accurate estimation can be made. The positive predictive value of E/E' > 15 for LA pressure greater than 15 mm Hg is relatively low (64%); however, the negative predictive value (i.e., E/E' < 8 predicting that LA pressure is not elevated) is very good (97%). This relationship appears to hold for patients with normal as well as depressed LV systolic function, but with lower specificity and sensitivity. Subsequent research has identified subgroups for whom the relationship between E/E' and LV filling pressure is not good, such as healthy normal volunteers and patients with LBBB.

Additional factors that can be used to assess LV diastolic function and filling pressures are LA size (with larger atria being associated with the effects of increased LV filling pressure over time) and spectral Doppler of the pulmonary vein. Recent ASE guidelines provide an excellent review of this complex topic.

Ischemic Heart Disease

Echocardiography in Patients With MI

When a patient comes into the hospital with prolonged chest pain, the echocardiogram can easily and rapidly be performed at the bedside. The presence of an akinetic, hypokinetic, or dyskinetic myocardial segment in the distribution of a coronary artery can establish the presence of underlying coronary artery disease, although whether that is an acute finding cannot always be determined. If the segment is not only akinetic or dyskinetic, but also thin and hyperechoic, this suggests an old infarct. The extent and severity of the segmental wall motion abnormality can help in treatment plan and prognosis. The greater the number of abnormal segments the worse both early (30 day) and late prognosis. Additional prognostic information can be obtained from the mitral inflow profile, with a restrictive pattern being associated with a poorer prognosis. If the patient has an anterior infarct associated with overall reduced LV EF, then prophylactic anticoagulation to prevent the formation of apical thrombus should be considered. The presence of documented LV apical thrombus is also an indication for anticoagulation.

Echocardiography is key in the diagnosis of mechanical complications of acute MI. Significant MR caused by papillary muscle infarction or rupture, acute ventricular septal defect, myocardial rupture with formation of a pseudoaneurysm, and pericardial effusion and tamponade are all easily diagnosed with echocardiography. In the critically ill patient, in whom repositioning of the body may not be possible, TEE rather than TTE may be required.

Evaluation of LV EF at more than 40 days after MI is recommended to assess need for defibrillator placement. A LV EF < 35% when associated with NYHA class II or class III symptoms of CHF, or LV EF < 30% when such symptoms is absent, are indications for prophylactic defibrillator placement.

Echocardiography in Patients Who Have Episodic Chest Pain

When a patient presents with a chest pain syndrome that is not an acute coronary syndrome, a test that can establish the underlying presence of coronary artery disease is helpful. Stress testing is often used for this purpose. Stress echocardiography, unlike stress with nuclear perfusion imaging, requires that actual ischemia is present, with a resulting stress-induced wall motion abnormality in the myocardium served by a significantly stenotic coronary artery.

Stress Echocardiography

Stress echocardiography is used to screen patients for myocardial ischemia and to assess for myocardial viability (dobutamine echocardiography). In larger studies, the sensitivity for coronary disease ranges from 74% to 97%, and specificity ranges from 64% to 86%. A normal stress echo is associated with a very low risk of major cardiac events (< 1% per year) in the following 4 to 5 years.

Stress echocardiography for the evaluation of ischemic heart disease assesses the response of myocardial segments to the increased myocardial oxygen demand of exercise. At baseline, myocardial function may be normal even with severe obstructive disease. With exercise, blood flow in the normal coronary vasculature increases up to fivefold, leading to increased contractility of all segments. Left ventricular chamber size usually decreases as well. When a stenotic vessel precludes the increase in flow, the hypoperfused segment will become hypokinetic, akinetic, or even dyskinetic. Failure to augment is also consistent with ischemic, but less specific.

Routine Treadmill Stress Echocardiography

Routine treadmill stress echocardiography is performed by obtaining a baseline ECG and baseline two-dimensional images of the heart. The patient then exercises on the treadmill to maximal exertion (heart rate > 85% of maximal predicted heart rate) with ECG and blood pressure surveillance. The treadmill is abruptly stopped, and the patient is rushed to an imaging table, where images are obtained within 60 seconds of cessation of exercise. Wall motion is analyzed using the 17 segment model (see LV quantification). Images are compared side by side for evidence of normal augmentation of function. The presence of new segmental wall motion abnormalities suggests significant stenosis in the vessel perfusing that area.

Dobutamine Echocardiography

Dobutamine echocardiography is recommended for patients who are unable to exercise on the treadmill or for the assessment of viability in patients with severe resting segmental wall motion abnormalities. For this study, ECG monitoring is performed during the infusion of dobutamine. Protocols generally begin at 5 μg/kg/min for patients who have wall motion abnormalities and 10 μg/kg/min for patients who have normal resting wall motion. The dose is increased at 3-minute intervals to 10, 20, 30, and 40 μg/kg/min. If there is not an adequate increase in heart rate, atropine (0.5 to 1.0 mg) may be added beginning at 20 μg/kg/min. Images are obtained at baseline, low dose (5 μg/kg/min for patients with wall motion abnormalities and 10 μg/kg/min for patients with normal resting wall motion), and peak dose. Follow-up images are obtained during recovery (usually when heart rate is below 100 beats per minute). The interpretation of the response of normal segments to pharmacologic stress is similar to that of treadmill stress echocardiography. If there are abnormal segments, however, the low- and high-dose imaging allows for prediction of response to revascularization. Abnormal segments are evaluated as follows:

- Biphasic response: contractile improvement at low dose followed by deterioration at a higher dose. This is consistent with viable, ischemic myocardium and has a high predictive value for recovery of function after revascularization.

- Sustained improvement: improvement in function at a low dose that persists or further improves at higher doses. This is consistent with viable but nonischemic myocardium, for example, in a patient who underwent primary revascularization in the setting of MI.
- Worsening of function, without contractile reserve: This implies that myocardium is viable and ischemic and carries an intermediate likelihood of recovery of function.
- No change in function: This is seen in the setting of nonviable myocardium and predicts a low likelihood of recovery of function.

Patient Safety

The most frequent serious complications associated with dobutamine echocardiography are tachyarrhythmias, both supraventricular and ventricular. These may be associated with ischemia, but are usually mediated by β-adrenergic stimulation. Bradyarrhythmias (with very rare cases of asystole) have been reported and are thought to be a result of a vasodepressor response to LV mechanoreceptor stimulation. Dobutamine can lead to ischemia and may result in MI. Atropine toxicity is also a concern when this medication is used and should not be administered if that patient suffers from glaucoma or urinary retention. Dobutamine echocardiography should not be performed in patients with a history of paroxysmal atrial dysrhythmias (paroxysmal AF, paroxysmal supraventricular tachycardia), complex ventricular arrhythmias (sustained ventricular tachycardia or ventricular fibrillation), or moderate to severe hypertension.

Cardiomyopathies

Echocardiography is essential to the diagnosis and management of patients with suspected cardiomyopathies and is also useful for screening family members of patients with inherited cardiomyopathies. With its ability to assess LV morphology and obtain reliable chamber dimensions and wall thickness, as well as assess systolic and diastolic function and provide noninvasive hemodynamics, echo is uniquely capable of determining the type of cardiomyopathy and monitoring the progression of disease.

Hypertrophic Cardiomyopathy

Hypertrophic cardiomyopathy is an autosomal dominant disorder that is characterized by myocardial cellular disarray and has a wide spectrum of disease presentation. It is recognized when ventricular hypertrophy is present without another cause. The most common pattern of hypertrophy is asymmetric septal hypertrophy, with a septal to posterior wall thickness ratio of greater than 1.3 to 1; however, patterns of concentric hypertrophy and apical hypertrophy can also be seen. Abnormalities of diastolic function caused by the stiff myocardium are typical and can be assessed with Doppler and TD techniques. Hemodynamic consequences of elevated LV filling pressures, such as atrial dilation, are readily detected by echocardiography. Left ventricle systolic function is typically hyperdynamic and can result in cavity obliteration.

Systolic anterior motion (SAM) of the mitral valve is also a finding in hypertrophic cardiomyopathy. The presence of significant septal hypertrophy and SAM of the mitral valve is associated with ventricular outflow tract obstruction. The anterior mitral leaflet is pulled into the LVOT during systole, often contacting the ventricular septum and causing LVOT obstruction, as well as creating MR due to abnormal coaptation of mitral leaflets. Pulse Doppler along the ventricular septum into the LVOT can detect obstructive physiology if it is present. As systole progresses, there is an increasing gradient in the LVOT that produces a dagger-shaped profile (Figure 10.8). With any decrease in preload, such as with a Valsalva maneuver, which decreases LV size, the gradient will increase and can be unmasked if not present at rest.

Prognosis is related to the severity of LV hypertrophy, with severe septal hypertrophy (septal thickness > 2.5 cm) on echo being a marker of poor prognosis with a high risk of sudden death, largely

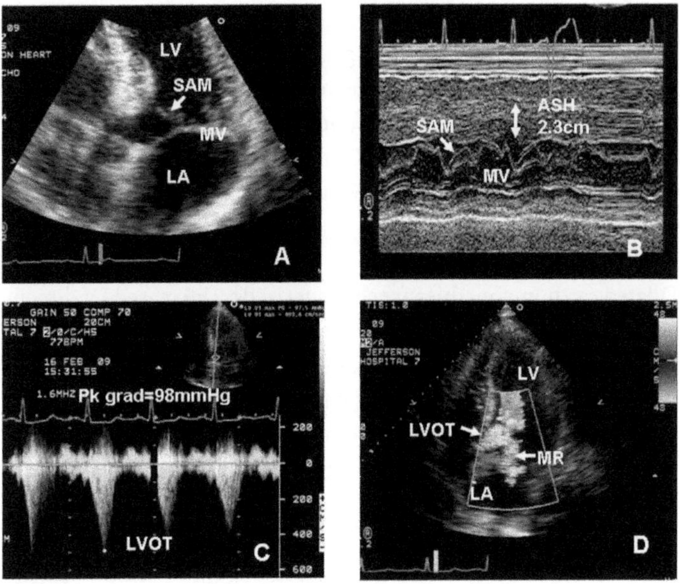

■ **Figure 10.8** A patient with hypertrophic cardiomyopathy (HOCM) with significant obstruction of the left ventricular outflow tract (LVOT). Panel **(A)** is a five-chamber view demonstrating systolic anterior motion (SAM) of the anterior mitral valve (MV) leaflet producing LVOT obstruction as it hits the thick, hypertrophied septum. **(B)** is an M-mode of the left ventricle (LV) at the level of the mitral valve showing asymmetric septal hypertrophy (ASH) and SAM. **(C)** is the CW Doppler profile of the LV outflow tract showing a typical late-peaking, "dagger" shaped velocity profile with a very high peak gradient (Pk grad); **(D)** is a color doppler image in this patient showing very turbulent high velocity flow in the LV outflow tract below the aortic valve and posteriorly directed mitral regurgitation (MR) jet resulting from malcoaptation of the mitral leaflets during systolic anterior motion.

because of ventricular arrhythmias. Other high-risk indicators include a family history of sudden death, young age at diagnosis, specific genetic mutations, nonsustained ventricular tachycardia, an abnormal blood pressure response to exercise, and significant

LVOT obstruction. Additionally, echo is used to monitor the effects of medical therapy by assessing the decrease in LVOT gradient, the decrease in SAM, and the decrease in MR, as well as monitoring improvements in diastolic function parameters. Echo can also be used to guide septal ethanol ablation and in the assessment of patients undergoing surgical myectomy.

Dilated Cardiomyopathy

Dilated cardiomyopathies are characterized by increased LV dimensions and volume, along with decreased systolic function. Eccentric hypertrophy is typically present. As the ventricle dilates, it becomes more spherical. This geometric change and increased LV dilation have been associated with a poor prognosis independent of LV ejection fraction. With dilation, the mitral annulus is stretched, resulting in abnormal coaptation of the mitral leaflets and producing MR. Left atrial enlargement is often present, resulting from significant MR or elevated filling pressures. The mitral inflow velocity profile and TD can be used to assess diastolic function and LV filling pressures. A restrictive mitral filling pattern, manifested by a rapid DT, is associated with poor prognosis in idiopathic dilated cardiomyopathy. A smaller radius to wall thickness ratio and lower wall stress are predictive of better outcomes. Assessment of RV size and function by echocardiography has also been found to have independent prognostic information, with worse outcomes predicted by RV dysfunction.

Hemodynamic parameters such as SV, cardiac output, estimated pulmonary artery pressures (see hemodynamic section), and diastolic filling parameters can be assessed from echo and Doppler information and can be followed to guide medical therapy and assess its impact on ventricular hemodynamics. Recently, echo has been used to evaluate patients for dyssynchrony and help determine whether they are likely to benefit from cardiac resynchronization therapy with biventricular pacing. The reliability of echo parameters in predicting response has been questioned in some studies.

Restrictive Cardiomyopathy

Restrictive cardiomyopathies are characterized by abnormalities of diastolic function with impaired filling and increased myocardial stiffness, and clinically, right heart failure caused by pulmonary hypertension usually predominates. Systolic LV dysfunction may develop in advanced stages. Restrictive cardiomyopathies include idiopathic disease, hypereosinophilic syndromes, and infiltrative cardiomyopathies such as amyloidosis and sarcoid. Although these may demonstrate distinctive morphology on echocardiography, normal systolic function is present in early stages, and abnormal diastolic function with evidence of impaired relaxation and elevated filling pressure can be identified from Doppler assessment of the mitral and tricuspid inflow patterns, pulmonary vein flow, hepatic vein flow, and TD. As the disease progresses, ventricular compliance decreases, and diastolic filling pressures rise. Atrial dilation is common as a result of the high filling pressures. Ultimately, a restrictive filling pattern becomes manifest with increased early mitral filling velocity (E), reduced e' on TD, short IVR time (< 60 msec), systolic blunting on the pulmonary vein flow pattern, and rapid mitral DT (< 150 msec).

Differentiation of restrictive cardiomyopathy from constrictive pericarditis can be difficult, and invasive hemodynamics can be similar in both disorders. Doppler techniques have been very helpful in making this differential diagnosis. Respiratory variation in ventricular filling is not seen in restrictive cardiomyopathies. Additionally, TD can be very useful, as diastolic function parameters will be very abnormal in restriction, with a reduced e' and systolic blunting, whereas intrinsic myocardial function is typically normal in constrictive pericarditis and e' will be normal and the systolic wave preserved.

Infiltrative Disorders

Amyloidosis is the classic example of restrictive cardiomyopathy. Amyloid fibrils are deposited in the interstitial tissue and produce a distinctive "sparkling" or granular appearance to the myocardium on echocardiography (Figure 10.9). The ventricular walls are significantly thickened, and the ventricular cavity is often small. Infiltration of the interatrial septum and valve leaflets is typical, and both atria are dilated. Doppler findings of abnormal diastolic function are present, and in advanced stages, classic restrictive physiology is demonstrated. Although the myocardium is thickened, QRS voltage on the electrocardiogram is often decreased, unlike other types of hypertrophy, and this characteristic pattern can be helpful in making the diagnosis of cardiac amyloid. The severity of increased myocardial wall thickness on echo, involvement of the right ventricle, and the presence of a restrictive diastolic filling pattern have all been associated with a poor prognosis.

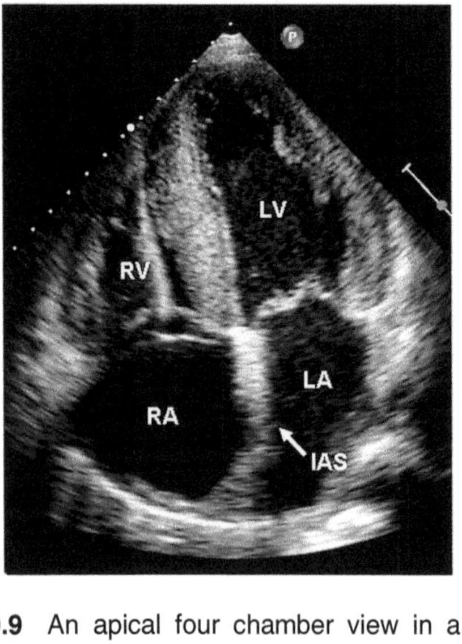

■ **Figure 10.9** An apical four chamber view in a patient with amyloid cardiomyopathy. Note the significantly thickened myocardium, of both left and right ventricles, with a characteristic "sparkling" appearance. Thickening of other cardiac structures is also seen, particularly of the interatrial septum, which is reasonably specific for amyloid involvement. LV, left ventricle; RV, right ventricle; LA, left atrium; RA, right atrium; IAS, interatrial septum.

Hemochromatosis, an iron-storage disease that can be primary or secondary, can involve the heart with iron deposits within the myocardium. Initially, this results in increased ventricular wall thickness and diastolic dysfunction, which can present as a restrictive cardiomyopathy. In the early stages, this can be reversible with phlebotomy, but if iron deposition increases, systolic dysfunction develops.

Sarcoidosis can also affect the heart, with granulomas found most often in the interventricular septum, papillary muscles, and ventricular free walls. Diastolic function abnormalities have been found on Doppler studies of patients with sarcoidosis, and systolic dysfunction has been found in a small percentage of patients; however, echo findings are not diagnostic for sarcoid. Segmental wall motion abnormalities can be seen; in particular, posterobasal aneurysms can be found in cardiac sarcoid. Clinically, conduction abnormalities and ventricular arrhythmias are the most common findings.

Endomyocardial Disease

Hypereosinophilic syndromes can present with hemodynamic findings of restrictive cardiomyopathy. These include endomyocardial fibrosis, which is endemic in Africa, South America, and India, and results from parasitic infection of the myocardium leading to a cytotoxic eosinophilic myocarditis, and Loeffler's endocarditis, which is part of the idiopathic hypereosinophilic syndrome. Both diseases are characterized by extensive endocardial fibrosis, which predominantly affects the apex leading to apical obliteration. Fibrosis can extend to the atrioventricular valves, causing valvular regurgitation. Both left and right ventricles can be involved, and mural thrombi are commonly found in the fibrotic apex. This pattern of apical obliteration seen on echocardiography is diagnostic.

Arrhythmic RV Dysplasia

Arrhythmic RV dysplasia is a genetic myocardial disease that affects the right ventricle with fibrofatty infiltration of the myocardial tissue. It presents predominantly with ventricular arrhythmias, and a variety of morphologic abnormalities of the right ventricle can be seen. Most often there is RV dilation, particularly of the RV outflow tract, and systolic RV dysfunction on echocardiography. There is no distinct pattern that is diagnostic, and prominent RV trabeculations and segmental wall motion abnormalities can also be seen. The EKG may demonstrate characteristic "epsilon" waves. Once suspected, imaging with MRI is the best diagnostic test, as the fatty infiltration can be identified and is a diagnostic feature.

Unclassified and Other Cardiomyopathies

A number of other cardiomyopathies present with distinctive echocardiographic findings, which can be diagnostic and are not classified with the major diagnostic categories.

Stress-Induced (Takotsubo) Cardiomyopathy

There has been increasing recognition of a distinct cardiomyopathy that appears to occur in situations of severe emotional or physical stress. Patients present with chest pain and a picture typical of acute MI, often with diffuse T-wave inversions on EKG and small troponin elevations; however, coronary artery angiography is normal. The echocardiographic picture is characteristic and demonstrates "apical ballooning." Wall motion abnormalities are typically extensive and involve the distal two thirds of the left ventricle, with akinesis to dyskinesis of the mid to distal segments of the anteroseptal, apical, anterior, inferior, inferolateral, and lateral walls. The extent and distribution of wall motion abnormalities go beyond any single coronary arterial territory. These abnormalities typically normalize, often resolving completely within several weeks of the acute presentation (Figure 10.10).

Left Ventricular Noncompaction

Left ventricular noncompaction is an inherited disorder in which the normal compaction of myocardial fibers becomes arrested during embryologic development. The epicardium forms a thin, compacted layer, whereas the endocardium is spongy, thick, and

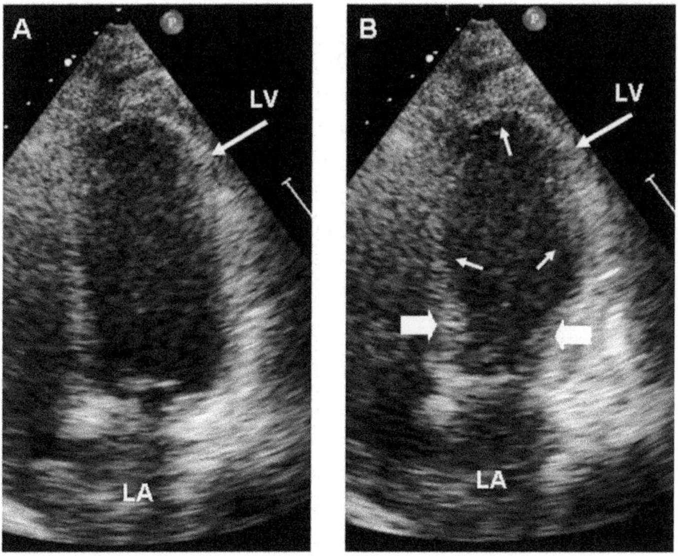

■ **Figure 10.10** Apical four chamber images of patient with Takotsubo cardiomyopathy. **(A)** Still frame of left ventricle at end diastole showing normal ventricular size and shape. **(B)** Still frame of left ventricle at end systole, demonstrating hyperdynamic contraction of basal segments with outward ballooning of distal two thirds of left ventricle. LV, left ventricle; LA, left atrium. Red arrows point to inward motion of basal segments. White arrows demonstrate outward movement, dyskinesis, of apical segments.

not compacted. This can be seen on echocardiography as very prominent trabeculations forming deep sinusoids invaginating the endocardial surface. These deep trabeculations preferentially involve the apex and inferior and lateral walls. They can be difficult to differentiate from increased trabeculation, which can occur in the setting of LV hypertrophy. The ratio of noncompacted to compacted myocardium must be greater than 2:1 in order to make a diagnosis of noncompaction. Echo contrast can be extremely useful in helping to differentiate noncompaction from normal trabeculation. Eventually severe systolic dysfunction and clinical heart failure develop.

Chagas Disease

Chagas disease is a disease found in tropical climates, in particular in South America and sub-Saharan Africa, and is caused by infection with *Trypnosoma cruzi.* In the acute phase, there is a myocarditis. In its chronic phase, the disease presents as a dilated cardiomyopathy with myocardial thinning and apical aneurysm formation, which can be found on echocardiographic imaging. Thrombus formation and thromboembolism are common.

Valvular Heart Disease

Aortic Stenosis (AS)

The underlying etiology of aortic stenosis can be readily determined with echocardiography. Aortic stenosis is now most often seen in older persons as a result of degenerative changes and valvular calcification resulting in restricted leaflet motion. Aortic sclerosis is often seen in the older population as a consequence of cholesterol deposition and appears as irregular calcification of the leaflets without hemodynamic stenosis. It has been associated with mitral annular calcification and aortic atheroma, all of which are markers of generalized atherosclerosis. Rheumatic AS is relatively rare in the United States and is characterized by fusion of the commissures with scarring and calcification. It is typically accompanied by mitral valve involvement. Congenitally bicuspid AVs can become stenotic over time, with progressive thickening and calcification of the two leaflets. Echocardiographic features characteristic of bicuspid AV include an eccentric closure line, doming of the valve, and aortic prolapse. Although classically there are only two sinuses, it is more common to have three sinuses with a raphe that can mimic a commissure but is underdeveloped and nonfunctional. Bicuspid valves are associated with ascending aortic aneurysms, and aortic root dimensions must be monitored. This is felt to be related to a connective tissue disorder similar to the abnormalities seen in Marfan's syndrome and may require aortic root repair as the diameter reaches 4.5 to 5.0 cm.

Assessment of AS Severity

Quantification of the severity of AS can be readily obtained using echo and Doppler techniques and has been shown to correlate well with more invasive techniques. Doppler-derived aortic gradients and valve area are used in decisions regarding the appropriateness of surgical intervention, and cardiac catheterization is reserved for preoperative coronary angiography or if the echo data and clinical scenario are discrepant. If imaging quality permits, AV area can be determined by planimetry of the valve orifice in the short axis view. Often this is not feasible, particularly if the valve is heavily calcified. Peak and mean gradients across the AV can be obtained by continuous wave Doppler in multiple views to determine the maximal transvalvular gradients. Doppler measures instantaneous gradients, whereas catheter-derived gradients are typically peak to peak, accounting for lower invasive peak gradients. Mean Doppler transvalvular gradients, obtained from the TVI, correlate well with mean catheterization gradients. Using pulse-wave Doppler, the level of obstruction can be determined to differentiate subvalvular, valvular, and supravalvular stenosis by detecting the location of an increase in velocity. AV area can be determined using the continuity equation (Figure 10.2). The greatest source of error in the continuity equation is the measurement of the LVOT diameter. A dimensionless index, the ratio of the LVOT over the AV peak velocities or TVIs, avoids this potential source of error (see Table 10.4).

In the setting of significant LV dysfunction with low cardiac output, transvalvular aortic gradients may be low, despite a small valve area. When this occurs, dobutamine stress echo can be used to differentiate LV dysfunction due to severe AS from LV dysfunction of other etiologies and mild or moderate AS. With low-dose dobutamine, the increase in cardiac output will result in an increase in gradients with no change in AV area in the setting of severe AS (which has a fixed valve orifice), whereas there will be little increase in gradient and an increase in calculated valve area (by $> 0.2\ cm^2$) in those patients with primary LV dysfunction and

Table 10.4 Grading of Aortic Stenosis Severity

	Peak Gradient (mm Hg) and Velocity	Mean Gradient (mm Hg)	Valve Area (cm^2)	Indexed Valve Area (cm^2/m^2)	Dimensionless Index
Normal	< 8		> 2 cm^2		0.9–1.0
Mild	< 36 (< 3 m/s)	< 20	> 1.5	> 0.85	> 0.50
Moderate	36–64 (3–4 m/s)	20–40	1.0–1.5	0.60–0.85	0.25–0.50
Severe	> 64 (> 4 m/s)	> 40	< 1.0	< 0.60	< 0.25

Source: Adapted from Baumgartner H, Hung J, Bermejo J, et al. Echocardiographic assessment of valve stenosis: EAE/ASE recommendations for clinical practice. *J Am Soc Echocardiogr* 2009;22:1–23.

mild or moderate AS in whom the valve area was inappropriately small because of the low cardiac output.

Hemodynamic Consequences

The left ventricle responds to the systolic pressure overload created by significant AS with concentric hypertrophy, resulting in increased wall thickness in an attempt to normalize systolic wall stress. The degree of hypertrophy can be determined with echocardiography by measurement of RWT and LV mass (see chamber quantification). With increasing hypertrophy, the myocardium becomes stiffer with decreased compliance and increased diastolic pressure, and diastolic dysfunction develops. The LV becomes more dependent on atrial contraction for adequate filling, and AF is poorly tolerated, often resulting in a drop in cardiac output. Coronary blood flow per unit mass is decreased in hypertrophied myocardium, and subendocardial ischemia can result without epicardial coronary disease, causing classic angina or, in some cases, infarction. When myocardial hypertrophy is inadequate, systolic wall stress increases, and this increase in afterload results in decreased ejection performance, and systolic dysfunction eventually develops.

Natural History, Prognosis, and Treatment

Patients who have AS often experience a long latent period in which they are asymptomatic and have a low morbidity. Several echocardiographic studies have demonstrated that the rate of progression of stenosis increases with increasing severity, such that once moderate AS is present the mean aortic gradient increases by 7 mm Hg per year and valve area decreases by 0.1 cm^2 per year. Thus, patients require close monitoring after significant AS is present and should be followed with yearly echocardiograms. Once severe AS is present, a high percentage of patients develop symptoms and cardiac events. The presence of angina, syncope, or heart failure portends a poor prognosis, with an average survival of only 2 to 3 years without surgical intervention. Symptomatic patients with severe AS, or those with systolic dysfunction, should undergo valve replacement. Surgery typically improves symptoms and survival, even in older patients ($>$ 80 years), and systolic dysfunction can be reversed if it is due to the excessive afterload associated with AS. ACC/AHA guidelines also suggest valve replacement in patients with moderate or severe AS who are undergoing coronary artery bypass graft (CABG) or other cardiac surgery.

Aortic Regurgitation (AR)

AR can be caused by intrinsic valvular disorders or dilation of the aortic root. Congenital bicuspid AVs, degenerative calcific disease, rheumatic heart disease, myxomatous disease, endocarditis, anorectic drugs, and trauma can all result in AR. Hypertension can result in aortic root dilation producing AR. Other problems causing aortic root dilation, most notably Marfan's syndrome and related connective tissue disorders, including bicuspid AV, can also produce AR. Acute AR can result from aortic dissection, trauma to the AV or aorta, and endocarditis. As with other valve lesions, echocardiography is central to the diagnosis, quantification, and clinical decision making in AR.

Quantification of AR can be determined from a variety of Doppler parameters. The results of various methods must be integrated together to derive a reliable assessment of AR severity. It is important that the regurgitant jet be assessed in multiple echo planes to assess its true severity. With CFD, the length, width, and area of the regurgitant jet can be obtained. The jet width measured just below the AV in the LVOT, as a percentage of the LVOT diameter, has proven to be more accurate than the jet length or area alone. Mild AR is present when the jet width ratio is less than 25% of the LVOT diameter, and severe AR is present when the ratio is greater than 65% (see Table 10.5). The narrowest area of the regurgitant jet at the AV level is the vena contracta, which can provide an estimate of the ERO area (EROA). A vena contracta width greater than 0.6 cm is a sensitive and specific indicator of severe AR. The PISA method can also be used to quantify AR, but is often difficult to perform. An EROA that is greater than 0.3 cm^2 suggests severe AR. From the ERO, regurgitant volume and regurgitant fraction can be derived.

In the presence of AR, LV diastolic pressure rises as the aortic pressure falls during diastole. The more severe the AR the more rapidly LV and aortic diastolic pressures will equilibrate. This

Table 10.5 Grading of Aortic Regurgitation

	Jet width / LVOT	Vena Contracta (cm)	PHT (msec)	EROA (cm^2)	RV (ml)	RF (%)
Mild	< 25%	< 0.3	> 500	< 0.10	< 30	< 30%
Moderate	25% to 64%	0.3–0.59	200–500	0.10–0.29	30–59	30–49
Severe	≥ 65%	≥ 0.6	< 200	≥ 0.30	≥ 60	≥ 50

Adapted from Zoghbi WA, Enriquez-Sarano M, Foster E, et al. Recommendations for evaluation of the severity of native valvular regurgitation with two-dimensional and Doppler echocardiography. *J Am Soc Echocardiol* 2003;16:777–802.

can be assessed by measuring the slope of the AR Doppler velocity profile and obtaining a PHT (time for the PG across the valve to decrease by half). A PHT above 500 msec is considered mild AR, and a PHT less than 200 msec is considered severe AR. Pressure half-time is influenced by intrinsic LV diastolic pressures and abnormal compliance and must be interpreted in relation to these factors. In addition to the PHT, diastolic flow reversal in the descending aorta is helpful in quantifying AR. The velocity and duration of flow reversal increase with increasing AR severity, and holodiastolic flow reversal in the descending aorta is a sign of at least moderate to severe AR. If present in the abdominal aorta, severe AR is present.

Hemodynamic consequences of chronic AR are a result of the increased volume load on the ventricle. The ventricle dilates in order to maintain a normal forward cardiac output, and eccentric hypertrophy develops. Diastolic compliance increases in order to normalize LV filling pressure. Increased LV volume produces an increase in systolic wall stress, triggering further hypertrophy in an effort to maintain normal ejection performance. After hypertrophy is no longer adequate to normalize LV wall stress, ejection fraction decreases. Initially, this reduction in ejection fraction is mostly due to afterload excess. Ejection fraction improves, and LV dilation reverses after valve replacement. Without surgical intervention, eventually intrinsic myocardial contractility becomes depressed and irreversible LV dysfunction develops.

Chronic volume overload is well tolerated, and patients with AR often remain asymptomatic for long periods of time. When preload reserve and hypertrophy are unable to normalize wall stress, symptoms often develop. As in AS, after symptoms of dyspnea, angina, and signs of heart failure develop, prognosis is poor without surgical intervention.

Acute AR is poorly tolerated, as the ventricle has not had time to become more compliant, and therefore, LV diastolic pressure rises rapidly with the acute volume overload. As a result, patients often develop acute pulmonary edema or cardiogenic shock, and emergency surgery is often required.

Natural History, Prognosis, and Management

Left ventricle systolic function and size correlate with clinical outcomes and prognosis in AR. Volume overload is very well tolerated for long periods because of the ventricle's ability to adapt. Just as with AS, the onset of symptoms carries with it a high mortality rate, greater than 10% per year. Unlike AS, LV systolic dysfunction can develop in asymptomatic patients with severe AR and predicts a rapid progression to symptoms, greater than 25% per year. In the asymptomatic patient, echocardiography provides key information regarding prognosis. Left ventricle size is directly related to prognosis. End-diastolic dimensions above 7.5 cm and end-systolic dimensions above 5.5 cm are predictive of a poor surgical outcome with persistent postoperative heart failure and high mortality. Close monitoring with serial echocardiography of patients with significant LV dilation caused by AR is recommended. Aortic valve replacement is indicated for asymptomatic patients when resting LV systolic dysfunction (EF $\leq$ 50%) is present or when EF is normal but severe LV dilation is present. Timely replacement of the AV will result in reversal of LV dysfunction and dilation.

Mitral Stenosis (MS)

Rheumatic heart disease is the major cause of MS. Rarely, other etiologies are present, including congenitally abnormal mitral valves and degenerative mitral annular calcification or LA myxoma. In rheumatic MS, the leaflets can become thickened and calcified, and commissural fusion is present. The chordae tendineae can also fuse and thicken. Typically, the posterior leaflet is restricted with doming of the anterior leaflet seen on echocardiography. An echo scoring index has been developed to determine the suitability for percutaneous mitral valvotomy, which is based on the degree of thickness calcification and mobility of mitral leaflets and the degree of subvalvular involvement.

Quantification of MS

Peak and mean PGs across the mitral valve are derived from the transmitral flow velocity using the modified Bernoulli equation and correlate well with catheter-derived gradients. A mean mitral gradient less than 5 mm Hg is consistent with mild stenosis, and a mean gradient above 10 mm Hg suggests severe MS. A normal mitral valve area (MVA) is 4.0 to 5.0 cm^2, and symptoms do not typically develop until the valve area is less than 1.5 cm^2. MS is considered mild when the valve area is > 1.5 cm^2 and severe when the MV area is < 1.0 cm^2 (Table 10.6).

If echo image quality is adequate, MVA can be determined by direct planimetry of the smallest mitral orifice in the parasternal short axis view. This is the most accurate assessment of MVA when it is obtainable. Mitral valve area can also be determined from the Doppler velocity profile using the PHT, the time for the PG to decrease to half of its peak gradient. The more severe the MS, the longer it will take for the pressure to decrease. Mitral valve area can be calculated using this formula: MVA = 220/PHT, where 220 is an empirically derived constant. This method is not reliable in the presence of other valvular lesions or when LV or LA compliance is abnormal (see Figure 10.5).

Table 10.6 Grading of Mitral Stenosis

	Mean Gradient (mm Hg)	PA Pressure (mm Hg)	Valve Area (cm^2)
Normal	< 2	< 30	> 4.0
Mild	< 5	< 30	> 1.5
Moderate	5–10	30–50	1.0–1.5
Severe	>10	> 50	< 1.0

Source: Adapted from Baumgartner H, Hung J, Bermejo J, et al. Echocardiographic assessment of valve stenosis: EAE/ASE recommendations for clinical practice. *J Am Soc Echocardiogr* 2009;22:1–23.

The continuity equation can also be used to determine MVA, using the same principles as for calculation of AV area. Flow volume (MVA × velocity time integral$_{mv}$) across the mitral orifice should be the same as flow across the AV, which can be calculated from the AV area and velocity. The PISA method using flow convergence can also be used, but must be corrected for the angle of the mitral leaflets, as the annulus is funnel shaped and not hemispheric.

Hemodynamic Consequences

As MS becomes hemodynamically significant, pressure increases in the left atrium, and diastolic filling of the left ventricle is slowed. The left atrium dilates in response to this increase in pressure, and pulmonary venous pressure rises. This may result in significant pulmonary arterial hypertension and subsequent RV dilation and dysfunction over time. Echocardiography can determine the LA size as well as estimate pulmonary artery pressure in the presence of tricuspid regurgitation (TR), and right heart size and function can be evaluated.

Natural History, Prognosis, and Management

Rheumatic MS has a long latent period, often decades, during which there is very gradual progression and no symptoms, except in undeveloped areas of the world in which progression can occur much more rapidly. Survival is greater than 80% over 10 years in asymptomatic or minimally symptomatic patients. When symptoms of pulmonary congestion become more significant, the 10-year survival decreases to 10% to 15%. The prognosis after severe pulmonary hypertension develops is very poor. Surgical intervention, or percutaneous balloon valvotomy in those with suitable valve morphology by echo, should be considered in patients with symptoms or pulmonary hypertension. Echocardiographic and Doppler assessment in MS are sufficient to make decisions regarding intervention without the need for cardiac catheterization. Catheterization is reserved for assessment of coronary anatomy prior to surgery if needed and for cases in which the Doppler data and clinical assessment are discrepant.

In addition to pulmonary congestion, high LA pressure and LA dilation predispose to the development of AF. Because of the need for a prolonged diastolic filling period to overcome the obstruction to mitral inflow, tachycardia and rapid AF are poorly tolerated and can result in a significant decline in cardiac output and rise in LA pressure. In this setting, β-blockers are particularly useful to control rate. Anticoagulation with warfarin is indicated in AF because of the risk of atrial thrombus formation and subsequent systemic embolization. Transesophageal echocardiography plays a major role in the evaluation of patients with AF prior to electrical cardioversion to detect LA and LA appendage thrombus.

Mitral Regurgitation (MR)

Mitral regurgitation can result from abnormalities of any of the structural components of the mitral apparatus, including the leaflets, chordae tendineae, papillary muscles, or mitral annulus. The most common causes include mitral valve prolapse, rheumatic heart disease, endocarditis, and collagen vascular disease. Degenerative calcific disease of the mitral annulus is common in association with atherosclerotic disease and renal disease. Dilation of the mitral annulus as a result of LV dilation is also a common cause of MR. Coronary artery disease can result in ischemia or infarction that involves the papillary muscles. With papillary muscle dysfunction, the mitral leaflet becomes tethered and produces malcoaptation of the leaflets resulting in MR. Chordae tendineae can rupture under mechanical strain resulting from infarction, endocarditis, mitral prolapse, or trauma and often results in hemodynamically significant acute MR. Echocardiography is critical in providing a morphologic assessment of the mitral apparatus to define the etiology of MR, as well as assessing its severity and hemodynamic consequences.

Quantification of MR is derived from a number of different Doppler indices, as with AR. Color flow Doppler can readily provide a visual assessment of severity using the jet area and length in multiple planes. The size of the regurgitant jet as a proportion of the LA area can give an indication of severity; however, eccentric jets may hug the atrial wall, and their severity is often underestimated by this method. The narrowest area of the regurgitant jet as it crosses the valve, the vena contracta, provides a more reliable estimate of MR severity; a vena contracta greater than or equal to 0.7 cm indicates severe MR (Table 10.7). The PISA method (see the hemodynamics section) can give a quantitative assessment of EROA from which regurgitant volume and regurgitant fraction can be derived. An EROA of 0.20 cm^2 or less indicates mild MR, and an EROA ≥ 0.4 cm^2 is consistent with severe MR (see Figure 10.4 and Table 10.7).

In addition to these parameters, severe MR often increases the early filling (E) velocity of the mitral inflow profile because of the significant increase in volume. The pulmonary veins can also be interrogated, and systolic flow reversal in the veins indicates at least moderate to severe MR. The density of the spectral Doppler jet from continuous wave Doppler also correlates with severity, becoming more intense with severe regurgitation.

Hemodynamic consequences of chronic MR initially include LA dilation. Atrial compliance increases in order to accommodate the large volume overload and prevent increases in pulmonary

Table 10.7 Grading of Mitral Regurgitation

	Jet Area (cm^2) Area/ LA (%)	Vena Contracta (cm)	EROA (cm^2)	RV (ml)	RF (%)
Mild	< 4 cm^2/ < 20%	< 0.3	< 0.2	< 30	< 30%
Moderate	4–10 cm^2	0.3–0.69	0.2–0.39	30–59	30% to 49%
Severe	> 10 cm^2/ > 40%	≥ 0.7	≥ 0.4	≥ 60	> 50%

Source: Adapted from Zoghbi WA, Enriquez-Sarano M, Foster E, et al. Recommendations for evaluation of the severity of native valvular regurgitation with two-dimensional and Doppler echocardiography. *J Am Soc Echocardiol* 2003;16:777–802.

venous pressure. With severe MR, the volume overload triggers eccentric hypertrophy over time, and the LV dilates and becomes more compliant to maintain adequate forward cardiac output. Ejection performance is maintained for long periods of time as a result of these compensatory mechanisms, and the decrease in ventricular afterload as a large percentage of the total cardiac output is ejected backward into the lower pressure left atrium. Chronic volume overload is therefore well tolerated for long periods, but eventually myocardial dysfunction develops. Reduced myocardial contractility can be masked by the reduced afterload faced by the LV. Once ejection parameters reach the low normal range, impaired contractility is already present and becomes irreversible when ejection performance declines further. LA pressure then rises, causing pulmonary congestion. After this occurs, EF may decrease significantly after MV surgery, unmasking the true myocardial contractility when afterload suddenly increases.

Acute MR is poorly tolerated, and with significant regurgitation, LA pressure rises rapidly, with a steep rise in pulmonary venous pressure. Ejection fraction is typically supernormal in the acute setting, despite the presence of pulmonary edema.

Natural History, Prognosis, and Treatment

Because of the compensatory mechanisms described previously here, patients with severe MR can remain asymptomatic for many years while progressive LA and LV dilation take place. With LA dilation, patients with severe MR often develop AF, which should be managed with rate control and anticoagulation. When symptoms develop, they are usually those of CHF, dyspnea, orthopnea, and paroxysmal nocturnal dyspnea. With worsening pulmonary hypertension, right-sided heart failure then develops. Once symptoms develop, prognosis is poor, with only a 30% 5-year survival without surgery. Mitral valve repair (for myxomatous valves) or replacement is indicated even for mild symptoms. Ideally, surgical intervention should take place before myocardial dysfunction is irreversible. Because of the abnormal loading conditions with MR, this can be difficult to detect, and irreversible dysfunction may be present before ejection fraction is significantly abnormal or symptoms develop. As with AR, LV size is a major predictor of clinical outcomes, along with ejection fraction. Poor surgical outcomes can be anticipated after the EF is less than 50% and/or LV end-diastolic dimension by echo is greater than 75 mm or end-systolic dimension > 52 mm. Echo measurements are therefore crucial for the timing of mitral valve surgery in order to preserve LV function. Mitral valve surgery is recommended even in asymptomatic patients with severe MR when EF drops below 60% or severe LV dilatation is present, particularly when end-systolic dimension reaches 40 mm or more or when AF develops.

Mitral valve repair, rather than replacement, is feasible in patients with MR caused by prolapse (particularly of the posterior leaflet) or chordal rupture and has been shown to have superior long-term results to valve replacement. When repair is felt to be possible with a high likelihood of success, it is reasonable to consider surgery in any patient with severe MR, even if EF and end-systolic dimension are relatively normal. Recent studies have shown that these patients have a better long-term prognosis than those who wait for the conventional indications. Transesophageal echocardiogram has been used to determine the likelihood of successful repair and to guide the surgical approach.

Mitral Valve Prolapse

Mitral valve prolapse is the most common cause of MR in the United States and results from myxomatous degeneration of the mitral leaflets, which become redundant, producing billowing of one or both of the mitral leaflets into the atrium during systole. It is seen in 1% to 2.5% of the population and presents with a wide spectrum of disease. Mitral prolapse can be familial and is often associated with connective tissue disorders, such as Marfan's syndrome. On echocardiography, one or both of the mitral leaflets must be displaced > 2 mm beyond the plane of the mitral annulus during systole to make a diagnosis of prolapse. Because the mitral annulus is saddle shaped, rather than planar, it is recommended that one use the parasternal long axis or the apical 2 chamber for diagnosis. Thickened mitral leaflets greater than 5 mm predict a higher incidence of complications of prolapse.

Mitral regurgitation results from malcoaptation of leaflets, and the regurgitant jet is typically eccentric and is usually directed away from the prolapsing leaflet. With prolapse, the severity of MR is dynamic and varies with changes in volume or preload. When volume decreases, the elongated leaflets prolapse earlier, and MR is more severe.

Significant MR is more common in males with prolapse. Complications of prolapse can include progressive MR, chordal rupture, an increased risk of endocarditis, and rarely embolic events or arrhythmias. With chordal rupture, the leaflet can become flail, with complete lack of coaptation. On echo this can be identified when the leaflet tip falls back into the atrium, usually producing severe acute MR.

When MR is severe, it behaves similarly to MR from other etiologies. Transesophageal echocardiography is particularly useful in evaluating severe MR caused by prolapse to determine the feasibility of MV repair when intervention is indicated. Posterior leaflet prolapse is usually amenable to successful repair, whereas anterior leaflet prolapse is surgically more challenging and has a significantly higher failure rate, necessitating valve replacement.

Prosthetic Valves

Prosthetic valves pose a challenging problem for imaging with ultrasound because of the acoustic shadowing from the prosthetic material, which can interfere with imaging and detection of abnormal flow. There are a large variety of prosthetic valves that can be bioprosthetic or mechanical, and each valve type has a distinctive echocardiographic appearance. All prosthetic valves are stenotic to some degree, with normal prosthetic AV mean gradients typically being less than or equal to 20 mm Hg, and normal mean gradients for mitral valve prosthetic valves typically being $\leq$ 5 mm Hg. A large degree of variability exists, however, based on prosthesis and patient characteristics, and it is therefore important to obtain a baseline echo Doppler study after valve replacement to define normal valve function for each individual. A small degree of regurgitation is often seen with prosthetic valves, and each valve type may have a particular pattern of regurgitation associated with normal function. Significant paravalvular regurgitation, at the edges of the prosthetic valve, is always pathologic when detected by Doppler and can be a sign of valve dehiscence from the sewing ring. Prosthetic valve dysfunction can result from structural deterioration, particularly of bioprosthetic valves, thrombus or pannus formation leading to valve stenosis, valve dehiscence, or endocarditis. Transesophageal echocardiogram is often required to obtain adequate imaging in the assessment of prosthetic valve function and the detection of prosthetic endocarditis.

Endocarditis

The diagnosis of infectious endocarditis is largely based on clinical criteria, such as the finding of a new murmur in a patient with fever and bacteremia, embolic vascular phenomena, or immunologic phenomena such as Osler's nodes, Roth spots, and so forth. Echocardiography has played a major role in making a definitive diagnosis, and the most recent Duke criteria for diagnosis of endocarditis incorporate echo findings as major diagnostic criteria, on par with positive blood cultures. Typical vegetations found on echo appear as tissue-density masses with independent chaotic motion and are usually adherent to the upstream surface of the valve leaflet (atrial surface for atrioventricular valves and the ventricular surface for the semilunar valves). Vegetations are found on transthoracic echo in approximately 60% to 75% of cases and on transesophageal echo in over 95% of patients with endocarditis. In addition to the finding of vegetations, echocardiography provides an assessment of the hemodynamic consequences and complications of endocarditis. The presence and severity of valvular regurgitation can be determined, and complications such as perforation, abscess, and fistula formation can be diagnosed. An abscess may appear as inhomogeneity of tissue density in the annulus or myocardium surrounding the infected valve and may develop an echo-free space because of liquefaction of the infected contents of the abscess. Fistulas can be identified from abnormal Doppler jets in the region of the infected valve. Transesophageal echo may be required for better visualization of these complications. It is often necessary for diagnosis in the presence of prosthetic valves and intracardiac devices, such as pacemakers and ICDs, because of acoustic shadowing from the foreign material. In these settings, it is reasonable to proceed directly to TEE when endocarditis is suspected. Transesophageal echocardiogram should also be considered when the clinical index of suspicion is high, but the transthoracic echo is nondiagnostic.

Echocardiography in the Evaluation of Right Heart Disease

The right heart is well seen by transthoracic echocardiography because it is an anterior structure. Right heart pathologies such as RV infarction, tricuspid and pulmonic valve disease, and congenital abnormalities such as Epstein's anomaly are well seen by TTE. In fact, the sensitivity of TTE for some pathologies, such as tricuspid valve endocarditis, is as high, if not higher, than TEE.

Evaluation of Pulmonary Hypertension

Pulmonary hypertension is a clinical entity that is seen as a consequence of both left heart disease and pulmonary pathology, as well as occurring without an underlying etiology as primary pulmonary hypertension. Estimation of pulmonary artery pressure can be performed by TTE in the majority of patients. Pulmonary artery systolic pressure can be determined from TR velocity (see Hemodynamics). The TR velocity is converted to PG in mm Hg between the RV and the RA using the modified Bernoulli equation ($PG = 4V^2$). To this number is added an estimate of RA pressure according to the size and inspiratory collapse of the IVC. The normal IVC is < 2 cm in diameter approximately 1 cm into the IVC from the RA-IVC junction and collapses by at least 50% with inspiration or sniff (IVC flat = low RA pressure [0 to 5 mm Hg]; IVC < 2.0 cm and with normal inspiratory collapse = 5 mm Hg; IVC > 2.0 cm with normal inspiratory collapse = 10 mmHg; IVC < 2.0 cm but without inspiratory collapse = 15 mm Hg; and IVC > 2.0 cm and without inspiratory collapse = 20 mm Hg). For example, if TR velocity is 2.5 m/sec and IVC is normal in size and collapses—$4(2.5)^2 = 25$ mm Hg + 5 mm Hg (estimated RA pressure), PA systolic pressure is estimated at 30 mm Hg. PA diastolic pressure can be estimated from the spectral Doppler signal of pulmonic regurgitation (PR). The end-diastolic velocity of PR describes the PG between the PA and the RV at end diastole. The end diastolic pressure in the RV is the same as RA pressure; therefore, PA diastolic pressure can be estimated by the equation – PA diastolic pressure = 4(PR end-diastolic velocity)^2 + RA pressure. PA mean pressure is estimated by the PG of the PR signal at the beginning of diastole, without an additional factor added (empirically derived data) (see Figure 10.3).

Evaluation of Patient with Pulmonary Embolism

When a patient has had a large pulmonary embolism, this may put acute pressure strain on the right ventricle. The RV handles pressure poorly and may undergo acute dilation as well as decreased RV systolic function as a result of the acute increase in afterload. The size and function of the RV are some of the most important factors in deciding whether either thrombolytic therapy or surgical embolectomy is necessary. A classic pattern of RV systolic dysfunction in acute pulmonary embolism has been described. Known as McConnell's sign, there is akinesis of the free wall of the right ventricle, with sparing of the apical segment. This phenomenon has a 77% sensitivity and a 94% specificity for the diagnosis of acute pulmonary embolism.

Echocardiography in the Patient Who Has Atrial Fibrillation (AF)

Atrial fibrillation is a rhythm characterized by disorganized electrical and mechanical activity and is usually accompanied on presentation by rapid ventricular response rate. Atrial fibrillation is important not only for its hemodynamic effects with its associated symptoms, most commonly palpitations and shortness of breath, but also for its association with thromboembolism. With ineffective mechanical activity, blood stasis in the atria occurs, which may lead to frank thrombus formation. More than 95% of atrial thrombi occur in the LA appendage, a crescent-shaped outpouching of the atrial wall. This thrombus may dislodge, leading to peripheral embolization, the stroke being the most serious manifestation. The vast majority of patients with AF have underlying structural heart disease, an enlarged left atrium being the most common, but a small percentage do not, often called "lone AF." The rate of embolization is approximately 5% per year, including a low-risk population that has a stroke rate of < 1% per year, increasing with advancing age and comorbidities to > 10% per year.

Evaluation for the Presence of Structural Heart Disease

LA Size

Information about LA size is crucial, not only as an underlying cause of AF, but also as it predicts the likelihood of restoring and maintaining sinus rhythm. Classically, a LA anteroposterior dimension of > 5 cm predicts a high likelihood of recurrent AF and is associated with increased stroke risk.

LV Systolic Function

Decreased LV systolic function is an important precursor of AF and increased thromboembolic risk. Associated heart failure is one of the most important factors in most systems, which attempt to quantify thromboembolic risk. It is also necessary to know LV systolic function to choose antiarrhythmic therapy, as the majority of antiarrhythmic medications are contraindicated in patients with LV systolic dysfunction, with the notable exception of amiodarone.

TEE and Cardioversion

Conventional therapy for patients with AF in whom restoration of sinus rhythm is considered beneficial is to anticoagulate them for 4 weeks before cardioversion (CV) to allow for resolution of any thrombi which may have formed. This approach reduced the risk of CV associated embolism from 5% to less than 1%. The LA appendage, the most common site of thrombus formation, is well seen on TEE. If a patient has no LA appendage thrombus visualized on TEE, he or she can undergo immediate cardioversion, assuming full anticoagulation at the time of CV. Transesophageal echocardiogram studies have shown that there is an additional period of atrial stunning after CV during which de novo thrombi may form. This necessitates the continuation of anticoagulation for a minimum of 4 weeks after CV. The ACUTE trial, comparing conventional strategy with TEE-guided CV, demonstrated that TEE-guided CV was noninferior, also reducing CV-related stroke to less than 1%, provided that full anticoagulation is present at the time of CV and for at least 4 weeks thereafter.

Pericardial Disease

Echocardiography has become the critical tool for the evaluation of pericardial disease. Pericardial effusions can be visualized and assessed for their size and their hemodynamic significance. The size of the echo-free space surrounding the heart can be determined, as well as whether it is circumferential or loculated. An effusion is considered small if it is < 1.0 cm, large if it is ≥ 2 cm, and moderate if it is between these measurements.

Cardiac tamponade results when the pressure within a pericardial effusion exceeds the intracardiac pressure, compromising cardiac filling. Tamponade is a clinical diagnosis that is characterized by a decrease in cardiac output resulting from pericardial effusion. Echocardiographic findings reflect the increase in intrapericardial pressure, which is determined by the volume of fluid, the rate of accumulation, and the compliance of the pericardium, such that tamponade physiology can develop from a small effusion that accumulates rapidly in a stiff pericardium. Because right atrial pressure usually has the lowest intracavitary pressure, the earliest signs of increased intrapericardial pressure are collapse or inversion of the right atrial wall, followed by early diastolic collapse of the right ventricle. As pericardial pressure rises, the degree and duration of collapse increase.

M mode through the RV can be particularly useful in detecting RV diastolic collapse. As right-sided pressure rises, the IVC may dilate and fail to collapse with inspiration. Left atrial and LV collapse can be seen when right-sided pressures are high or the effusion is loculated. In tamponade, the total intracardiac volume is relatively fixed because of compression from the pericardial effusion, and there is increased ventricular interdependence. During inspiration, venous return to the right heart increases, the septum shifts, and LV filling decreases. This results in the physical finding of pulsus paradoxus and in marked respiratory variation of the inflow velocities across the mitral and tricuspid valves, with an increase in tricuspid inflow and decrease in mitral inflow with inspiration (see Figure 10.11). Reciprocal changes occur in the inflow velocities during expiration. These changes can be readily detected from assessment of Doppler inflow velocities using a respirometer and are an important adjunct in making the diagnosis of tamponade. When hemodynamic compromise is present, pericardiocentesis can be lifesaving.

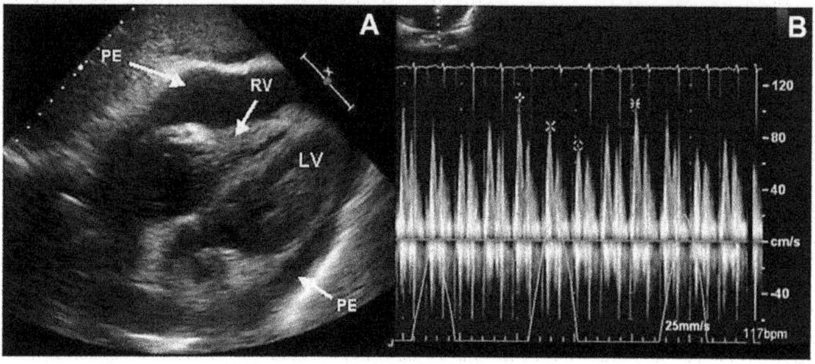

■ **Figure 10.11** Large pericardial effusion with pericardial tamponade. **(A)** Subcostal view showing large pericardial effusion (PE) compressing the right ventricle (RV). (Left ventricle LV). **(B)** Pulse wave spectral Doppler of mitral inflow demonstrating significant respiratory variation consistent with pericardial tamponade.

Echo guidance for pericardiocentesis has proven to be very helpful in locating the optimal site for percutaneous drainage and directing the placement of the pericardiocentesis needle. The position of the needle can be confirmed by injecting agitated saline to outline the pericardial space. Subsequent monitoring of the adequacy of drainage and reaccumulation of pericardial fluid is done with follow-up echo studies.

Constrictive pericarditis develops when the pericardium becomes thickened, adherent, or calcified. Constriction can be very difficult to diagnose, and patients often present with signs of right heart failure. Although echo is not very sensitive for detection of thickened pericardium in the absence of fluid, the hemodynamic effects of constriction can be detected with echo techniques. Abnormal septal motion, a "septal bounce," can be seen, along with respiratory variation of ventricular size and dilation of the IVC. As in tamponade, total intracardiac volume is restricted, and ventricular interdependence is exaggerated. Respiratory variation of mitral and tricuspid inflow velocities can be seen on Doppler, similar to those seen in tamponade. Constriction can often be difficult to differentiate from restrictive physiology seen in cardiomyopathies. The respiratory variation of inflow velocities seen in constriction is typically absent in restriction. Additionally, TD can be very useful, as diastolic function is usually normal in constriction and the E' velocity on TD is normal. In restriction, diastolic dysfunction is paramount, and tissue E' is significantly reduced.

Aortic Diseases

The major diseases of the aorta include aortic aneurysm and aortic dissection. With a combination of transthoracic echo and TEE, most of the aorta can be visualized, although the distal ascending aorta is generally not well seen with either technique. The aortic root and proximal ascending aorta are visualized on transthoracic, and careful measurement of the size of the root, the aortic sinuses, and the proximal ascending aorta are crucial, particularly in the assessment of patients with Marfan's disease or other connective tissue disorders in which ascending aortic aneurysms occur. Aortic root dilation is also often seen with bicuspid AVs, and ascending aneurysms are thought to be similar to those in Marfan's disease. Outcomes with surgical repair of ascending aneurysms in this setting have been shown to be superior if done electively when the aortic diameter reaches 4.5 to 5.0 cm.

Hypertension and atherosclerosis are common causes of aortic aneurysms, but the majority of these develop in the descending thoracic aorta, where surgery is generally recommended when the aortic diameter reaches 6.0 cm. The aortic arch and descending thoracic aorta are best visualized with TEE but can often be seen from a suprasternal notch view on transthoracic imaging. Involvement of the arch is important to determine before surgical repair of aneurysms, as involvement of the arch may require total circulatory arrest.

Aortic dissection is diagnosed by finding an intimal flap on echocardiography. Transesophageal echo is the procedure of choice for the rapid diagnosis of dissection. The true and false lumens can be distinguished echocardiographically, and Doppler can detect flow within the false lumen. Thrombus within the false lumen can also be identified, and intramural hematoma can be differentiated from dissection. The extent of the dissection can be determined to guide the surgical approach. Additionally, involvement of the AV, the presence of AR, the presence of pericardial effusion or tamponade, and involvement of the arch vessels can be assessed with TEE.

Aortic atherosclerosis can range from intimal thickening or calcification to focal rupture of plaque, or in its most severe form, mobile atheroma may be seen in the aortic lumen. The size of atheroma, the presence of ulceration, and the detection of mobile components are all analyzed when imaging the aorta on TEE. This can be very important as a potential source of embolism.

Cardiac Source of Embolus

Although transthoracic echo can detect LV mural thrombus, cardiac masses such as myxoma or vegetations, and structural heart disease that may predispose to systemic embolization, the yield is low. Transesophageal echocardiogram is far superior, partly because of better visualization of areas such as LA appendage, aorta, and atrial septum, which are poorly seen on TTE. In several studies looking at the yield of echo in identifying a potential cardiac source of embolism, the yield from TTE ranges from 15% to 30%, whereas TEE provides a yield of 55% to 65%. The majority (approximately 75%) of cardiac emboli travel to the brain resulting in stroke, whereas 25% are peripheral. When embolic stroke is clearly present, the yield with TEE is significantly higher.

Left atrial thrombi are relatively common, particularly in the setting of AF. Because most are found in the atrial appendage, TEE is needed to detect them, although treatment is rarely altered as AF is often present, necessitating anticoagulation. Spontaneous echo contrast can also be seen in the atria and represents a low flow state that has been associated with an increased risk of thromboembolism.

Aortic atheromas have clearly been identified as a potential source of embolism, especially when mobile debris is found in the ascending aorta or arch (debris in the descending aorta can cause peripheral embolization). The finding of complex, particularly mobile, plaque may prompt treatment with full anticoagulation with warfarin rather than aspirin, although the data to support this are limited.

Patent Foramen Ovale (PFO) with right to left shunting or atrial septal aneurysm is the other major potential source of embolism, particularly in patients under the age of 55 years. Because PFO is present in approximately 25% of the population, the finding of PFO on TEE does not necessarily identify this as a source of embolization; however, studies have shown that in the presence of atrial septal aneurysm there is a much stronger association with stroke. A small PFO may not be easily detected, even with TEE, and agitated saline is therefore injected to provide contrast. A Valsalva maneuver may be necessary to increase right atrial pressure and reveal right to left shunting. When PFO and atrial aneurysm are diagnosed without another source of embolism, the treatment with antiplatelet agents or warfarin is indicated. Surgical closure or percutaneous closure devices can be used to close a defect to prevent recurrent embolic events. Transesophageal echocardiogram plays a key role in guiding these catheterization procedures and establishing proper sizing and placement of the device. Percutaneous closure devices are now also being used for closure of actual atrial septal defects when appropriate, with or without embolic events.

11 ▪ Cardiac Computed Tomography and Magnetic Resonance Imaging

Alexander Rubin, MD
Ethan J. Halpern, MD
Christopher G. Roth, MD

Computed tomography (CT) and magnetic resonance (MR) can provide either cross-sectional or volumetric images in the heart. As compared with echocardiography, both CT and MR require less technical operator expertise to acquire the images and are therefore less subject to variability based on differences among the technologists who acquire the images. Nonetheless, imaging of the heart with either CT or MR does require an understanding of the underlying cardiac anatomy as well as the intricacies of imaging technology. In order to be useful, the CT/MR examination must be tailored to answer the specific clinical question that is posed. This chapter briefly reviews technical issues involved with CT/MR imaging and discusses clinical applications of these techniques. As might be expected, the clinical indications for CT/MR imaging of the heart are evolving with the rapidly advancing technology. CT has a superior resolution for evaluation of coronary anatomy, and MR has the advantage of imaging without exposure to ionizing radiation.

Cardiac CT

Technical Considerations

There are two major types of modern CT scanners: electron-beam computed tomography (EBCT) and multislice/multidetector computed tomography (MDCT). EBCT has no moving parts, and its main advantage is a very fast scanning time (< 50 msec), which is important for imaging a moving heart. EBCT has been very useful for cardiac calcium scoring. MDCT is superior to EBCT for evaluating coronary anatomy with CT angiography. Currently, MDCT most commonly uses 64 slice scanners with a temporal resolution of 165 to 210 msec that can image the coronary tree in 6 to 9 seconds; however, newer MDCT scanners may provide improved temporal resolution or more rapid coverage of the heart in fewer heartbeats with 256 or 320 slices. Cardiac CT requires injection of an iodinated contrast material. Consequently, all patients should be screened for a history of prior allergic reactions to X-ray contrast material or history of anaphylaxis to other drugs. Iodinated contrast should be used judiciously, and premedication with steroids may be necessary depending on the severity of dye allergy. A prior anaphylactic reaction to iodinated contrast should raise a red flag—these patients should not be evaluated with an injection of iodinated contrast material unless this is absolutely necessary. Other patients with less severe allergic reactions may be premedicated with steroids. The protocol in our institution includes 32 mg of oral Medrol given once at 12 hours before the scan and repeated at 2 hours before the procedure.

Patients with abnormal renal function can be pretreated with hydration before administration of iodinated contrast material. We generally advocate hydration for any patient with an estimated glomerular filtration rate (GFR) < 60 ml/min. There may be additional benefit from administration of oral N-acetylcysteine 600 to 1,200 mg every 12 hours for a total of four doses and intravenous sodium bicarbonate 150 mEq in 1,000 ml of 0.45% of normal saline with an infusion rate of 3 ml/kg/hr for the first hour before the scan and then 1 ml/kg/hr for the next 6 hours.

Because of the limitation of temporal resolution, coronary CT image quality is limited in patients with tachycardia and/or irregular rhythms. Rapid, irregular cardiac rhythms, such as poorly controlled atrial fibrillation, often result in suboptimal coronary CT studies.

The optimal heart rate for most scanners is 50 to 60 beats per minute. In order to achieve this goal, many patients will require pretreatment with a β-blocker. Patients may be pretreated with oral metoprolol 50 to 100 mg 1 to 2 hours prior to the study. Alternatively, intravenous metoprolol may be administered at the time of the study to titrate to a target heart rate. In hypotensive patients (systolic blood pressure < 100) and patients with active asthma, β-blockers should be avoided. Calcium channel blockers may be more effective for control of heart rate in patients with atrial fibrillation. Calcium channel blockers may be used in place of β-blockers in patients with active asthma.

Sublingual nitroglycerin is routinely used 2 to 3 minutes prior to the scan to promote coronary vasodilation; however, hypotension-induced reflex tachycardia may have a negative impact on image quality.

Radiation dose with cardiac CT is a moving target. Early cardiac CT studies used radiation doses as high as 30 to 35 mSv. Recent advances, including ECG-gated tube current modulation and "step and shoot" axial imaging, have lowered doses to 3 to 5 mSv for the study. Nonetheless, the presence of ionizing radiation is an important issue with CT and is a major reason that CT is not used for evaluation of cardiac morphology in children with congenital heart disease.

Cardiac CT angiography was first introduced into clinical practice in the mid 1990s and since then has become a widely accepted cardiac imaging modality because of rapidly improving technology. Currently, cardiac computed tomography angiography (CTA) allows excellent imaging of native coronary vessels as well as coronary artery bypass grafts. In addition, it provides additional diagnostic information about cardiac morphology and function, making it possible to evaluate valvular disease, cardiac neoplasms, and pericardial disease.

Coronary Artery Disease, Native Vessels Considerations

Coronary artery atherosclerosis is a very common problem. The lifetime risk of developing coronary heart disease after the age of

40 years is 49% for men and 32% for women. The disease progresses from nonobstructive to more extensive with diffuse or focal narrowing of the vessels by atherosclerotic plaque.

A ruptured plaque with partial or complete occlusion of the coronary vessel is the culprit in acute coronary syndrome. No single study can currently predict which plaque will become unstable. It is known, however, that plaques with a large lipid core and thin fibrous cap are more likely to rupture. Cardiac CT may be helpful in defining plaque morphology—including size, contour, lipid content, and calcifications—to predict instability. Clinical trials are needed to determine whether it is possible to predict the likelihood of plaque rupture based on these radiologic characteristics.

A number of studies have compared 64-slice CT coronary angiography with conventional angiography, the latter used as the gold standard. In most studies, the sensitivity and specificity of CT angiography for detecting the presence of coronary artery disease were over 90% and close to 100%, respectively.

Both sensitivity and specificity of coronary CTA are reduced in patients with significant coronary artery calcifications caused by blooming artifact. In a cohort of patients referred for cardiac catheterization, the negative predictive value for coronary CTA was 98%. Based on these data, CT angiography is a reliable, noninvasive alternative to cardiac catheterization to exclude the presence of coronary artery disease.

A CT will be less cost-effective in high-risk patients who are likely to have coronary calcifications and stenosis. It is likely that CT will simply confirm the need for further testing in such patients.

Computed tomography angiography is not cost-effective for risk stratification of asymptomatic patients. There are no outcomes data to demonstrate a mortality benefit for interventional treatment of coronary lesions detected by CT in the asymptomatic patient. It is likely that the radiation risks outweigh the benefit of CT angiography in the asymptomatic population.

Clinical Indications for Coronary CTA, Native Vessels

Coronary CT angiography is commonly used for evaluation of persistent chest pain in the setting of a negative stress test. Perfusion stress tests can be falsely negative in the setting of triple vessel disease with balanced ischemia. A normal coronary CT angiogram excludes the possibility of coronary disease.

Coronary CT angiography may be used to follow up a positive or equivocal stress test result when the patient is considered to be low risk for coronary disease.

Coronary CT angiography is useful in the evaluation of patients with acute chest pain presenting to the emergency department, as part of a triple rule-out scan for coronary artery disease, pulmonary embolism, and acute aortic dissection. The triple rule-out scan is most cost-effective in low-risk patients who can be discharged on the basis of a normal coronary CT angiogram. Our experience suggests that CT will define a noncoronary cause of chest pain in approximately 11% of these patients.

Coronary CT angiography may be useful as a primary imaging modality for the workup of chest pain and suspected CAD.

Indications for CT angiography as well as study quality are rapidly evolving. At this point, the major limiting factor of the widespread use of CT angiography is a lack of major prospective randomized trials identifying the role of this modality in patient risk stratification and prognosis.

Coronary Artery Disease, After Coronary Artery Bypass Graft Surgery

Presently, coronary artery bypass graft (CABG) is the procedure of choice for left main disease and three vessel disease. Both venous and arterial grafts are used. The best patency rates (90% in 10 years) are achieved with the use of the left internal mammary artery (LIMA) to the left anterior descending (LAD) artery.

Because of their relatively large size, good visualization of venous grafts can be achieved using the 64-slice CT detector system. Patency of LIMA and radial artery conduits is also easily established by CTA; however, imaging of distal anastomoses can sometimes be challenging. A number of studies have shown promising results for the detection of graft disease by coronary CTA. Routine use of this modality for the evaluation of patients after CABG is not recommended. Coronary CTA is most useful in the postbypass patient with clinical symptoms in whom possible graft thrombosis is suspected.

Coronary CTA can be useful for patients with unknown bypass graft anatomy in whom conventional angiography would otherwise be challenging. Coronary CTA in the bypass patient should extend cranially to the level of the subclavian artery in order to visualize the origin of a LIMA graft.

Coronary Artery Disease, After Coronary Artery Stenting

High-density material used in stents creates blooming and beam hardening artifacts, making imaging of the stent lumen very difficult by the current 64-slice detector systems. Coronary CTA is generally adequate to document patency or occlusion of a stent. Limited data suggest that reliable imaging of internal stent lumen in large caliber stents (> 3.0 mm) is possible. Routine use of coronary CT angiography after stenting is not recommended. It is likely that blooming artifacts will be reduced with increased resolution of the new generation systems currently under investigation.

Coronary Artery Anomalies

Coronary artery anomalies are relatively uncommon, with a prevalence of about 1% in the general population. Coronary anomalies are classified into benign or malignant, with the latter predisposing patients to sudden cardiac death especially during exercise. In malignant coronary anomalies, the coronary artery runs between the trunk of the pulmonary artery and the aorta, making it vulnerable to compression. Coronary CTA is very reliable in identifying coronary anomalies and an excellent alternative to cardiac catheterization.

Coronary Artery Aneurysm

A coronary artery aneurysm is defined as abnormal coronary dilation that exceeds the diameter of the normal adjacent segment by 1.5 times. More than 50% of aneurysms are caused by atherosclerosis. Less common causes include congenital aneurysms, post-Kawasaki syndrome, Takayasu's arteritis, adult polycystic kidney disease, lupus erythematosus, and Ehlers-Danlos syndrome. Iatrogenic coronary pseudoaneurysms can be a complication of interventional coronary procedures.

The most common complication of coronary aneurysms is thrombosis with potential distant vessel embolization resulting in myocardial infarction. Based on this observation, many patients are empirically treated with antiplatelet therapy. CT angiography is an excellent modality for the diagnosis of coronary aneurysms.

Preoperative Imaging for Aortic Aneurysm Repair

CT is an excellent modality for imaging aortic aneurysms. CT demonstrates the extent and size of the aneurysm as well as the distribution of calcium within the aorta. Coronary CTA can be used to image the coronary arteries and the thoracic aorta in a single study. A normal coronary CTA study can eliminate the need for cardiac catheterization prior to aortic aneurysm repair.

Preoperative Imaging for Aortic Valve Surgery

CT is an excellent modality for imaging the aortic root and proximal ascending aorta. CT demonstrates the true size of the aortic valve annulus and the sinuses of Valsalva, as well as the distribution of calcium within the wall of the ascending aorta. CT of the chest is usually requested prior to aortic valve surgery to assess the location and extent of calcium within the ascending aorta. Coronary CTA can be used to image the coronary arteries and the aortic root in a single study. A normal coronary CTA study can eliminate the need for cardiac catheterization prior to aortic valve replacement.

Assessment of Cardiac Morphology

In addition to imaging the coronary arteries, gated cardiac CT allows for excellent imaging of the cardiac chambers, including their size, morphology, and function. Accurate estimation of left ventricular ejection fraction, as well as assessment of regional segmental wall motion abnormalities, provides additional pivotal information for clinicians. Evaluation of the right heart during CT angiography is possible but is often limited by heterogeneous mixing of contrast from the superior vena cava (SVC) with unopaticified blood from the inferior vena cava (IVC).

CT would never be used as a primary modality for assessment of cardiac function but can be used to provide this information when a CT scan is requested for other reasons (such as coronary artery disease). CT is often used as a preprocedure study in patients with atrial fibrillation for ablation procedures in the left atrium. CT angiography can be used to map the locations of the antra of the pulmonary veins and to exclude the presence of coronary disease simultaneously. Pathologies such as atrial enlargement, symmetric and asymmetric ventricular hypertrophy, and atrial and ventricular septal defects can also be adequately assessed with this modality; however, this information can be readily obtained by an echocardiogram without the additional risk of radiation exposure.

Assessment of Pericardial Disease

A cardiac CT provides detailed images of the pericardium and is very sensitive for the presence of calcification (which may not be detected with MRI). Increased pericardial thickness with or without calcifications can help in the diagnosis of constrictive pericarditis.

The diagnosis of constrictive pericarditis is based on a combination of clinical, hemodynamic, and radiologic findings. Some patients with constrictive pericardial disease can have a normal pericardial thickness without calcifications, whereas other patients with thickened and/or calcified pericardium may not have significant hemodynamic impairment of ventricular filling.

Cardiac Neoplasms

Primary neoplasms are rare, with an estimated incidence of 0.02%, with cardiac myxomas, lipomas, and papillary fibroelastomas being the most common. Cardiac CT can provide a detailed assessment of tumor size, location, myocardial invasion, as well as possible compression of intracardiac and extracardiac structures. Masses in the right heart, particularly in the right atrium, are more difficult to define due to heterogeneous contrast opacification. Cardiac MRI may be a preferred modality here as it provides the same information as CT without the risks associated with iodinated contrast and radiation exposure.

Specific Considerations Associated with Radiation Exposure

A typical 64-slice detector coronary angiography without dose-reduction techniques results in patient exposure to approximately 10 mSv. This is about the same dose as 200 chest X-rays or 3 years of normal environmental background radiation.

Based on extrapolation of data from atomic bomb survivors, a radiation exposure of 10 mSv may be associated with an increased frequency of death from malignancy in 1 of every 2,000 patients. This risk is thought to be significantly higher in younger patients and females. It is thus imperative to exercise appropriate clinical judgment and to weight the risk of radiation exposure against the risk of the disease that might be discovered by the CT scan.

Newer CT techniques such as "prospective tube current modulation" and "step and shoot" that reduce the radiation dose should be encouraged, especially for imaging of younger patients.

Calcium Scoring

Coronary calcium scoring should not be used for evaluation of the symptomatic patient. Coronary calcium scoring has been extensively evaluated for risk assessment of asymptomatic patients for future cardiovascular events. This technique is associated with a relatively low radiation exposure (about 1 mSv). Based on the extent of coronary calcification, an Agatston score is assigned to each patient: from 0 to 100 for minimal plaque, 100 to 400 for moderate plaque burden, and greater than 400 for extensive plaque burden. The risk of future cardiovascular events is extremely low, about 0.1% per year, for patients with a low score. The risk is significantly higher for a calcium score above 100, estimated to be above 2% per year.

The coronary calcium score is a strong predictor of incident coronary heart disease and provides predictive information beyond that provided by standard risk factors. It is most useful in patients who have an intermediate risk based on a Framingham score or other clinical data and when there is a need to decide upon more aggressive medical management. In these patients, the coronary calcium score can provide independent risk data above and beyond that which is obtained in the Framingham risk score.

Technical Issues in Cardiac MRI: Pulse Sequences and their Applications

Cine Gradient Echo Sequences

Gradient echo sequences are useful for creating "bright blood" cine images of cardiac function. A commonly used gradient echo sequence for evaluation of cardiac function is steady-state free precession. One of the major advantages of gradient echo sequences is rapid image acquisition. Images are acquired during a single breath hold, minimizing motion artifact. Blood pool and abnormal myocardium appear bright, whereas normal myocardium appears dark. Cine gradient echo sequences are useful to assess left and right ventricular function, detect regional wall motion abnormalities, and assess valvular function (stenotic or regurgitant jets appear as hypointense blushes against the normal bright blood pool) (see Figure 11.1).

Fast Spin-ECHO Sequences

Fast-spin echo sequences are useful for creating "black blood" images to evaluate cardiac morphology. Most commonly used black blood sequences are ECG-gated (fast) spin echo or double-inversion recovery sequences. Additional pulses may be used to "null" the signal from blood in fast spin echo sequences. The absence of signal from blood on the "black blood" images facilitates better

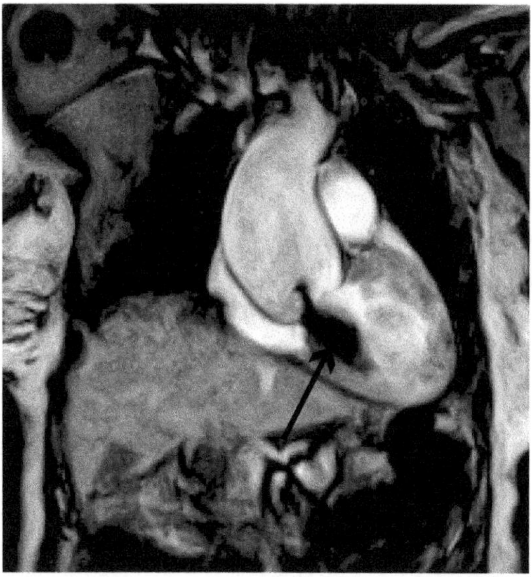

■ **Figure 11.1** The snapshot image from a cinegraphic gradient echo "bright blood" sequence oriented to the aortic outflow tract shows a dilated ascending aorta with a turbulent flow jet regurgitating into the left ventricular cavity (arrow) in a patient with aortic insufficiency.

appreciation of myocardial tissue, which appears bright, improves the surface definition of the myocardium, and aids in the definition of thrombus and mass lesions that may project into cardiac chambers. These techniques can be very sensitive to myocardial water content and can be used to detect edema from capillary leakage due to recent injury as opposed to old scar tissue. T1-weighted spin echo sequences are particularly important for detection of fat in the myocardium for the diagnosis of arrhythmogenic right ventricular dysplasia and for definition of the pericardium, which is surrounded by fat planes on both sides (see Figure 11.2).

Contrast-Enhanced Gradient Echo Sequences

Magnetization-prepared gradient echo sequences are used to "null" signal from viable myocardium. An inversion recovery pulse is generally used for this purpose. Gadolinium-diethylenetriamine pentaacetic acid (Gd-DTPA) is an intravenous MR contrast agent that accumulates in the extracellular space. Gd-DTPA accumulates in

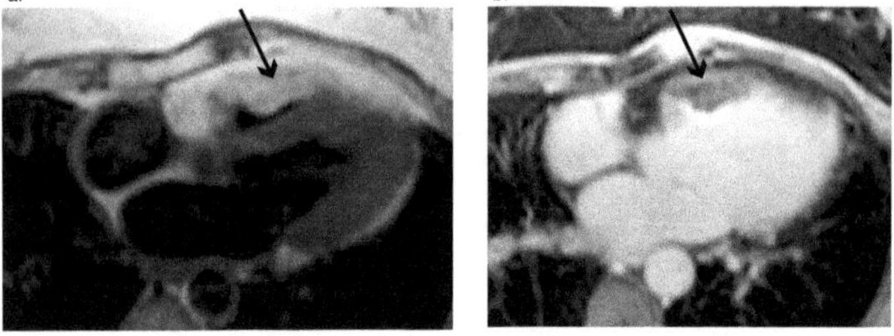

■ **Figure 11.2** The T1-weighted "black blood" image **(a)** eliminates signal from flowing blood in the cardiac chambers, optimizing discrimination of the abnormally thickened right ventricular wall (arrow) infiltrated with hyperintense fat in a patient with arrhythmogenic right ventricular dysplasia. The corresponding snapshot image from a fat-suppressed gradient-echo "bright blood" cinegraphic sequence **(b)** depicts hyperintense blood in the cardiac chambers contrasting against the signal-suppressed fat in the right ventricular free wall (arrow).

necrotic and scar tissue because of increased extracellular space and relatively slow washout. Areas of ischemic injury or scar are seen to enhance on delayed images after administration of Gd-DTPA. Echo planar gradient echo images may be used for very rapid acquisition of the entire heart to detect ischemia.

Cine Phase Contrast Sequences

Phase contrast sequences allow quantification of blood flow velocity and directionality. Phase contrast imaging can be used to calculate gradients across stenotic valves and regurgitant flow velocity.

Angiographic Sequences

Coronary MRA can be performed without a contrast agent, but most sequences employ Gd-DTPA as a contrast agent to enhance vascular conspicuity. A variety of angiographic sequences are used to evaluate coronary arteries for anomalies and stenosis.

Other Technical Considerations

The demands of cardiac MRI require a high-field MR system (at least 1.5 Tesla) with relatively strong gradient strength. ECG gating is required in order to eliminate cardiac motion artifact. Most cardiac sequences are triggered by the R wave (beware of the distorting effects of the magnetic field on the ECG waveform artifactually elevating the T wave). Cardiac arrhythmias often degrade image quality by the absence of predictable R waves to trigger image acquisition. A dedicated cardiac coil optimizes signal to noise, allowing for improved image quality, better spatial resolution, and potentially decreased image acquisition time. Consider oxygen by nasal cannula to improve breath-holding capability and minimize breathing motion artifact. Remember (relative) the contraindications to MRI: pacemaker, defibrillator, other implanted devices, and recent coronary stenting ($<$ 6 weeks). Postprocessing saves time and magnifies the utility of MR by yielding accurate assessment of chamber volumes, ejection fractions, and wall motion.

Gd-DTPA

This is the most commonly used MR contrast agent. In May 2007, the Food and Drug Administration introduced a new boxed warning for Gd-DTPA. The patients who are most at risk are those with kidney malfunction, patients just before or after liver transplantation, or patients with chronic liver disease. These patients are at risk to develop nephrogenic systemic fibrosis or nephrogenic fibrosing dermopathy. The risk of nephrogenic systemic fibrosis should be considered before administration of Gd-DTPA for any patient with an estimated GFR of < 60 ml/min, although the few cases observed to date have occurred in patients with severe renal failure with a GFR < 30 ml/min.

Imaging Planes

Imaging planes can be prescribed in any orientation desired. Conventional planes coincide with nuclear cardiographic planes and include the four-chamber (horizontal long axis) view, the two-chamber (vertical long axis) view, the short-axis view, and the left ventricular outflow (three-chamber) view. Cardiac imaging planes are referred to as "double oblique," oriented at arbitrary angles to the MR scanner and requiring two orthogonal planes to be accurately prescribed. Modern imaging systems allow real-time (interactive) image assessment, permitting the operator to continuously adjust the imaging plane to yield the desired image orientation.

Ischemic Heart Disease

Stress Testing

Stress MRI provides superior image quality to nuclear stress or stress echo with no exposure to radiation. Standard exercise treadmill stress testing is not commonly used with MRI because of logistical constraints. Pharmacologic testing is carried out with the standard adenosine or dobutamine infusion protocols or a combination of both. The magnetic gradients used in MRI will interfere with the normal ECG signal, most commonly producing "pseudo-R waves," which reflect T waves magnified by the magnetohydrodynamic effect (of moving blood protons in a magnetic field generating their own magnetic field).

Adenosine—Dynamic First-Pass Perfusion Imaging

This is used to identify perfusion defects immediately after contrast injection and is performed with short axis views of the heart. Ischemic areas appear dark in contrast to normal myocardium, which appears bright because of the relative hyperemia from adenosine-induced vasodilation. Clinical studies show comparable sensitivity and specificity to an adenosine nuclear stress test, approximately 85%.

Dobutamine—Wall Motion Cine Imaging

This is used for detection of wall motion abnormalities and has been found to have superior sensitivity and specificity, 86% versus 74% and 86% versus 70%, respectively, to conventional stress echo due to improved endocardial border definition.

Adenosine and Dobutamine Combined Protocol

This protocol provides advantages of both techniques by first looking for perfusion defects with adenosine and then using dobutamine in the second part of the study to identify wall motion abnormalities. This protocol has a highly specific protocol with a 3-year event-free survival of 99.2% for patients with a normal study.

Coronary Magnetic Resonance Angiography

Most sequences employ a contrast agent, most commonly Gd-DTPA. Coronary magnetic resonance angiography does not require ionizing radiation exposure (unlike cardiac CT angiography). This type is technically challenging because of motion artifact caused by respiratory motion and cardiac contraction, exacerbated by long acquisition times (up to 10 minutes) necessary to achieve adequate spatial resolution. Based on small studies, cardiac magnetic resonance angiography is highly sensitive and specific for the detection of proximal vessel disease only. Routine use for diagnosis of coronary artery disease currently not recommended. Currently, it is most commonly used for evaluation of congenital coronary artery anomalies. Strategies to minimize motion artifact and improve resolution of smaller vessels are still under development.

Infarct Detection and Sizing: Late Enhancement Imaging

Late enhancement imaging obtained 15 to 20 minutes after contrast injection is used for the detection and sizing of infarcts. Infarcted myocardium appears hyperenhanced and is clearly demarcated from normal myocardium. This is one of the best currently available ways to assess for the presence of acute or chronic myocardial infarction (MI), with 99% sensitivity for acute and 94% sensitivity for chronic MI. A highly accurate and reproducible test that provides the exact anatomic location and size of the MI as well as define the infarct related artery. It can be used for the detection of RV infarct, however, with lower sensitivity.

Myocardial Viability

After ischemic injury, areas adjacent to the infarct may remain viable but lose their contractile function. It is important to identify the presence of viable, yet stunted tissue because revascularization may improve contractility, patient functional status, and long-term prognosis. A number of modalities, including thallium-nuclear scans, low-dose dobutamine echocardiography, and positron emission tomography (PET), have been used to assess myocardial viability. Late-enhancement cardiac MRI is one of the best available techniques for defining myocardial viability. In the dysfunctional area of the heart, scar tissue appears hyperenhanced as compared with viable, but dysfunctional adjacent myocardium. MRI precisely delineates the extent of salvageable myocardium. MRI has a very high correlation with PET scan for detecting scar tissue and viability. The detection of viable myocardium by cardiac MRI has clinical significance. Areas found to have viable myocardium by MRI were found to have significant functional recovery after bypass surgery.

Cardiomyopathy and Myocardial Disease

Ischemic Versus Nonischemic Cardiomyopathy

Cardiac MRI (CMR) can help distinguish ischemic cardiomyopathy (ICM) from nonischemic cardiomyopathy (NICM). During myocardial infarction, the subendocardium is the most vulnerable area to ischemic injury. Late enhancement of the subendocardial layer on CMR is invariably present in patients with ICM, but can occasionally be found in patients with NICM. The absence of late enhancement is highly suggestive of a nonischemic origin of disease.

Hypertrophic Cardiomyopathy

MRI is the best available study to quantify left ventricular mass. It can also help to define regional wall thickness as well as regional contraction abnormalities. This makes it particularly suited to evaluate hypertrophic cardiomyopathy (HCM). Some patients with HCM have late enhancement on cardiac MRI with involvement of RV septum and anterior and posterior right ventricular junctions. There is evidence to suggest that a higher degree of late enhancement is associated with more progressive disease and can potentially correlate with a worse prognosis. Cardiac MRI can help to define precisely the location and severity of obstruction, as well as the gradient across the aortic valve. This makes it particularly helpful in the diagnosis and follow-up of patients with HCM. Despite the fact that MR is the most sensitive and specific study for the evaluation of HCM, most of the same findings can be obtained by transthoracic echocardiography, which is more readily available and cost-effective.

Right Ventricular Size and Function

Right ventricular size and function are difficult to assess by echocardiography. MRI can provide quantitative assessment of RV volume and ejection fraction.

Arrhythmogenic Right Ventricular Cardiomyopathy

Arrhythmogenic right ventricular cardiomyopathy (ARVD) is a rare cardiomyopathy that often affects young individuals and presents with intractable ventricular tachycardias, right heart failure, or sudden cardiac death. The diagnosis is extremely difficult and requires a combination of clinical, ECG, and imaging findings. Presently, no single study is sensitive enough to make the diagnosis. Earlier studies found that replacement of the myocardial RV wall with fatty tissue was present in some patients with ARVD. When present, it is extremely helpful in making the diagnosis; however, its absence does not exclude ARVD. Fat is bright on T1-weighted images; however, it is sometimes difficult to distinguish myocardial fat, which is pathologic, from epicardial fat, which is a normal finding. This is further complicated by the fact that not all patients with ARVD have myocardial fat infiltration. The size, shape, and function of the RV on CMR are additional findings that can aid in making the diagnosis.

Cardiac Sarcoidosis

Sarcoidosis is a systemic inflammatory process, which can involve any organ of the body, most commonly the lungs, lymph nodes, and skin. Subclinical cardiac involvement is relatively common and is found in about 25% of affected patients at the time of autopsy. In patients with clinically significant cardiac sarcoidosis, the most common manifestations are congestive heart failure, heart block, malignant ventricular arrhythmias, and sudden cardiac death. Cardiac biopsy can help to establish the diagnosis; however, because of patchy myocardial involvement, the biopsy can often be falsely negative. Cardiac MRI has proven to be extremely helpful in the diagnosis of cardiac sarcoidosis. The late gadolinium enhancement images can help identify patchy areas of myocardial inflammation and scarring caused by sarcoidosis with a sensitivity of close to 100%. The left ventricular free wall and intraventricular septum are the two most commonly involved areas in this disease process. MRI findings are not entirely specific for cardiac sarcoidosis, as other inflammatory processes involving the heart can have a similar radiologic appearance.

Acute Myocarditis

Acute myocarditis is an inflammatory process that is most commonly caused by a viral infection. Patchy late enhancement of the left ventricular wall is the most common contrast-enhanced MR finding, usually suggesting an acute inflammatory process. In addition to its diagnostic value, late enhancement is extremely helpful in guiding and increasing the diagnostic yield of endomyocardial biopsy. Contrast-enhanced MR can also be helpful in patient follow-up because the myocardial enhancement disappears with resolution of the disease.

Cardiac Neoplasms

Contrast-enhanced MR is the best study for evaluating cardiac neoplasms and differentiating between thrombus and solid tissue with the use of intravenous gadolinium. MR can precisely define tumor location, size, and its relationship to adjacent structures such as blood vessels and the mediastinum. Superior tissue contrast properties of MRI improve diagnostic accuracy by distinguishing different tissue types. Fat (lipoma, lipomatous hypertrophy of the interatrial septum, etc.) is confirmed using fat-suppression techniques. Fibrous tissue (fibroma, etc.) is usually uniformly dark. Melanin (melanoma metastasis) is usually T1 hyperintense. Myxoid tissue (left atrial myxoma) is relatively T2 hyperintense. Contrast-enhanced MR can identify tumor-specific characteristics, such as solid, cystic, or vascular areas. It is also useful for planning of biopsy and surgical resection.

Ventricular Thrombi

The detection of left ventricular (LV) thrombi can be challenging by transthoracic (TTE) or transesophageal echocardiography (TEE). MR has a much higher sensitivity than TTE or TEE and should be considered as a gold standard for the diagnosis. Thrombi appear hypointense against the bright blood pool on gradient echo ("bright blood" images) and exhibit an absence of enhancement. This is particularly clinically relevant when managing patients with large anterior wall myocardial infarctions in determining the need for anticoagulation.

12 ■ Noncardiac Surgery for the Patient with Cardiovascular Disease

Howard Weitz, MD

Risk Assessment Prior to Noncardiac Surgery

The American College of Cardiology-American Heart Association guideline for preoperative evaluation of patients who are to undergo noncardiac surgery emphasizes that preoperative tests are indicated only if the results will affect perioperative care. A theme of the American College of Cardiology-American Heart Association guideline is that cardiac intervention is rarely necessary to lower risk of surgery. The guideline uses a strategy that requires assessment of active cardiac conditions, clinical predictors, functional status, and surgery specific risk.

Active cardiac conditions (Table 12.1) when present indicate major perioperative risk. Active cardiac conditions are unstable coronary syndrome (unstable angina, acute myocardial infarction [MI] within prior 7 days), recent MI (MI occurring more than 7 days but less than 1 month before the evaluation), and decompensated heart failure. Patients with active cardiac conditions in whom noncardiac surgery is planned should be evaluated and treated before noncardiac surgery with the goal of resolving the active cardiac condition prior to surgery. Clinical risk factors (Table 12.2) if present may contribute to the risk of perioperative cardiac complications. Clinical risk factors include a history of ischemic heart disease, a history of compensated or prior heart failure, and a history of cerebrovascular disease, diabetes mellitus, and renal insufficiency (serum creatinine $\geq$ 2.0 mg/dl). Functional capacity if poor has been shown to be an indicator of perioperative risk. If a patient is unable to reach or exceed an aerobic demand of 4 metabolic equivalents (METs), even if a noncardiac cause is the

Table 12.1 Active Cardiac Conditions

- Unstable coronary syndromes (unstable angina, recent MI [MI more than 7 days but less than 1 month before evaluation])
- Decompensated heart failure
- Significant arrhythmias
- Severe valvular disease

Source: Adapted from: Fleisher LA, Beckman JA, Brown KA, Calkins H, Chaikof E, Fleischmann KE, Freeman WK, Froehlich JB, Kasper EK, Kersten JR, Riegel B, Robb JF. ACC / AHA 2007 guidelines on perioperative cardiovascular evaluation and care for noncardiac surgery: a report of the American College of Cardiology / American Heart Association Task force on Practice guidelines (Writing Committee to Revise the 2002 Guidelines on Perioperative Cardiovascular Evaluation for Noncardiac Surgery). J Am Coll Cardiol 2007;50:e159–242.

reason for their inability, their risk for perioperative cardiac complication may be increased. An example of 4 METs aerobic demand is climbing one flight of stairs. Surgery-specific risk (Table 12.3) is determined by the type of surgery and its associated hemodynamic stress. After the patient's active cardiac conditions, clinical risk factors, functional capacity, and surgery specific risks are identified,

Table 12.2 Clinical Risk Factors

- History of ischemic heart disease
- History of compensated or prior heart failure
- History of cerebrovascular disease
- Diabetes mellitus
- Renal insufficiency (serum creatinine $\geq$ 2.0)

Source: Adapted from: Fleisher LA, Beckman JA, Brown KA, Calkins H, Chaikof E, Fleischmann KE, Freeman WK, Froehlich JB, Kasper EK, Kersten JR, Riegel B, Robb JF. ACC / AHA 2007 guidelines on perioperative cardiovascular evaluation and care for noncardiac surgery: a report of the American College of Cardiology / American Heart Association Task force on Practice guidelines (Writing Committee to Revise the 2002 Guidelines on Perioperative Cardiovascular Evaluation for Noncardiac Surgery). J Am Coll Cardiol 2007;50:e159–242.

Table 12.3 Surgery-Specific Risk

- High (reported cardiac risk, often > 5%)
  - Emergency major operations, particularly in older patients
  - Aortic and major vascular surgery
  - Peripheral vascular surgery
  - Anticipated prolonged surgical procedures associated with large fluid shifts or blood loss
- Intermediate (reported cardiac risk, 1% to 5%)
  - Carotid endarterectomy
  - Head and neck surgery
  - Intraperitoneal and intrathoracic surgery
  - Orthopedic surgery
  - Prostate surgery
- Low (reported cardiac risk, < 1%) (patients who are to undergo these procedures do not generally require further perioperative cardiac testing)
  - Endoscopic procedures
  - Superficial procedures
  - Cataract surgery
  - Breast surgery
  - Ambulatory surgery

Source: Adapted from: Fleisher LA, Beckman JA, Brown KA, Calkins H, Chaikof E, Fleischmann KE, Freeman WK, Froehlich JB, Kasper EK, Kersten JR, Riegel B, Robb JF. ACC / AHA 2007 guidelines on perioperative cardiovascular evaluation and care for noncardiac surgery: a report of the American College of Cardiology / American Heart Association Task force on Practice guidelines (Writing Committee to Revise the 2002 Guidelines on Perioperative Cardiovascular Evaluation for Noncardiac Surgery). J Am Coll Cardiol 2007;50:e159–242.

the ACC/AHA 2007 Perioperative Guideline recommends a five-step algorithm to guide decision making regarding further cardiac testing, proceeding to surgery, or both (Figure 12.1). Key points include the following: If the surgery is an emergency, the patient

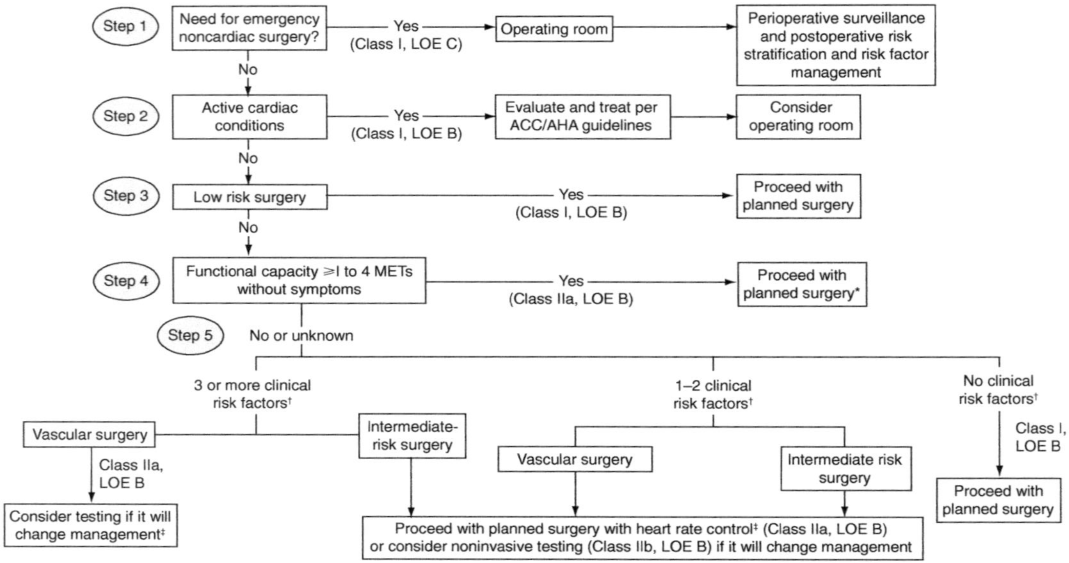

*Noninvasive testing may be considered before surgery in specific patients with risk factors if it will change management.
†Clinical risk factors include ischemic heart disease, compensated or prior heart failure, diabetes mellitus, renal insufficiency, and cerebrovascular disease.
‡Consider perioperative beta-blockade for populations in which this has been shown to reduce cardiac morbidity/mortality.
LOE = level of evidence; MET = metabolic equivalent

■ **Figure 12.1** American College of Cardiology / American Heart Assn Risk Stratification Algorithm

Reprinted with permission. *Circulation*, 2007; 116; 1971–19996. ©2007 American Heart Association, Inc.

should proceed to surgery without delay for further preoperative testing. Noninvasive cardiac testing, if clinically indicated, should only be performed if the results will change patient management.

Recommendations for Noninvasive Stress Testing Before Noncardiac Surgery

This is considered for the following patients if the results of stress testing will change perioperative management. Patients may be considered if they have three or more clinical risk factors and poor functional capacity (less than 4 METs) who require vascular surgery. Stress testing may be considered for patients with one or two clinical risk factors and poor functional capacity (less than 4 METs) who require intermediate risk noncardiac surgery. Stress testing may be considered for patients with at least one or two clinical risk factors and good functional capacity (greater than or equal to 4 METs) who are undergoing vascular surgery. Preoperative stress testing is not considered useful for the following patients: patients with no clinical risk factors undergoing intermediate risk noncardiac surgery and patients undergoing low-risk noncardiac surgery. When stress testing is indicated, pharmacologic modalities should be used for the patient who is unable to exercise as well as for the patient with left bundle branch block (exercise-based stress tests can be associated with false positive suggestion of anterior wall myocardial ischemia in the patient with left bundle branch block).

Anesthesia Considerations

Physiologic Response to Anesthesia and Surgery

Catecholamine production increases in response to the stress of surgery. This may increase myocardial oxygen demand, leading to myocardial ischemia in the patient with coronary artery disease. Hypoventilation as well as perioperative atelectasis may decrease myocardial oxygen delivery. Anemia decreases myocardial oxygen delivery. Perioperative volume depletion or hypotension may result in coronary artery hypoperfusion.

Cardiovascular Effects of Anesthetic Agents

Inhalation Agents

Inhalational agents may cause hypotension and/or dose-dependent myocardial depression. This may result in clinically significant intraoperative hypotension in the patient who is concurrently receiving vasodilators (e.g., nitrates and hydralazine) or who is volume depleted. The depressant effects of inhalational agents may be accentuated in the patient with left ventricular systolic dysfunction.

Intravenous Agents

Opioids (e.g., sufentanil and fentanyl) are commonly used in anesthesia to blunt the sympathetic response to intubation and surgical manipulation. This serves to decrease myocardial oxygen demand by preventing increases in heart rate. Propofol, commonly used in outpatient surgery because of its short duration of action, may result in hypotension, especially after bolus administration.

Spinal Anesthesia

Spinal anesthesia is relatively contraindicated in patients with critical aortic stenosis or severe left ventricular dysfunction. These patients are unable to increase their cardiac output ("fixed cardiac output") in response to vasodilation, and subsequent hypotension may accompany this technique.

Regional Versus General Anesthesia

There is no difference between the effects of regional and general anesthesia on cardiovascular morbidity or mortality. Regional anesthesia produces less respiratory and myocardial depression than general anesthesia and may be advantageous for the patient with left ventricular dysfunction, congestive heart failure, or pulmonary disease.

The Patient with Ischemic Heart Disease

Prevention of Perioperative Myocardial Ischemia and Myocardial Infarction

Coronary Artery Revascularization

Coronary artery bypass surgery before noncardiac surgery is indicated for the patient who otherwise meets criteria for coronary revascularization (significant left main coronary artery stenosis, stable angina, and triple vessel coronary artery disease, especially when left ventricular ejection fraction less than 50%, stable angina and two-vessel coronary artery disease with significant proximal left anterior descending [LAD] coronary artery stenosis and either left ventricular ejection fraction less than 50% or demonstrable ischemia on noninvasive testing, high-risk unstable angina or recent NSTEMI, acute ST elevation myocardial infarction [STEMI]). Coronary artery angioplasty before noncardiac surgery is indicated for a patient who meets indications for angioplasty, even if noncardiac surgery was not planned. There is no evidence that prophylactic angioplasty before noncardiac surgery in patients with asymptomatic ischemia or stable angina decreases the incidence of perioperative cardiac complications. Medical therapy decreases perioperative myocardial ischemia and myocardial infarction.

β-*Blockers*

Data supporting the use of beta blockers in the perioperative period are sparse, with most recommendations based on clinical consensus and small clinical trials. According to the American College of Cardiology-American Heart Association 2006 focused guideline update on perioperative β-blocker use, β-blockers should be used in the perioperative period for patients who take them chronically or those who have an indication for β-blockers (e.g., angina) but were not otherwise receiving them. They should also be considered for patients undergoing vascular surgery in whom preoperative testing identifies the presence of coronary artery disease, patients with multiple cardiac risk factors (ischemic heart disease, compensated or past heart failure, diabetes mellitus, renal insufficiency, cerebrovascular disease) who undergo vascular surgery, and patients with coronary heart disease or those with multiple predictors of coronary risk who undergo intermediate or high-risk procedures. The role and indications for perioperative β-blocker use are controversial. The POISE trial showed that although perioperative β-blockers (in patients who were not already receiving them) decreased perioperative myocardial infarction, their use was associated with an increased incidence of stroke and mortality. The increased morbidity and mortality were often preceded by β-blocker–medicated hypotension. Based on POISE and its demonstrated risks, it has been our approach to continue β-blockers for those already receiving them and to initiate β-blockers well in advance of surgery (e.g., 2 to 4 weeks) for those in whom the preoperative evaluation identifies an indication for chronic beta blocker use. This advanced initiation of β-blockers facilitates identification of potential β-blocker–related complications (e.g., bradycardia, hypotension).

Statins

Evidence suggests that statins may decrease the risk of perioperative cardiac complication. Statins should be continued in the perioperative period for patients already receiving them. Preoperative initiation of statins is reasonable for patients undergoing vascular surgery or those with at least one clinical cardiac risk factor who are undergoing intermediate-risk procedures.

The Patient Who Has Chronic Coronary Artery Disease

For patients who have chronic coronary artery disease, it is important to continue chronic antianginal medications in the perioperative period. This may require substituting parenteral agents for oral medications for the patient who is unable to resume oral intake after surgery. For patients receiving chronic aspirin therapy for the treatment of coronary artery disease, aspirin should be continued in the perioperative period if possible and should only be discontinued if its perioperative use is associated with risk for major bleeding (e.g., prostatectomy) or if the surgical procedure is one where a small degree of bleeding may be associated with significant complication (e.g., intracranial surgery).

Perioperative MI

Most perioperative myocardial infarctions are non–ST-segment elevation MIs (NSTEMI) and occur during the first 48 hours after surgery. Perioperative myocardial infarction is typically not associated with chest pain. Typical clinical features include congestive heart failure (CHF), ventricular arrhythmia, hypotension, and confusion. In the patient with diabetes, unexplained hyperglycemia should lead to a consideration that perioperative MI may be the precipitant. Troponin is the most sensitive and specific biomarker of perioperative MI. The goals for treatment of the patient with a perioperative MI are the same as those for the treatment of MI in the nonsurgical setting. These include reperfusion of ischemic myocardium, antithrombotic therapy to prevent thrombosis of subtotal coronary stenoses, and adjunctive measures to decrease myocardial oxygen demand (e.g., β-blockers). Thrombolytic therapy will be contraindicated in the majority of patients who have undergone recent surgery. Recent surgery during the prior 2 weeks has been considered as a relative contraindication to its use. Urgent coronary angiography with coronary angioplasty should be considered for perioperative patients with evolving acute MI. Heparin and antiplatelet agents are of benefit during and after acute MI. They may increase bleeding in the perioperative period. The benefits versus risks of these agents must be considered before they are used in the perioperative period.

The Patient Who Has a Coronary Stent

Premature discontinuation of antiplatelet therapy places the patient at risk of acute stent thrombosis. Antiplatelet agents mandated by stent placement may increase the risk of perioperative bleeding. Neurosurgical procedures are of special concern given the impact that perioperative bleeding has in those cases. Elective procedures associated with a significant risk of perioperative bleeding should be deferred until patients have completed the minimum course of dual antiplatelet therapy (aspirin + thienopyridine) (12 months after implantation of a drug-eluting stent and 4 weeks after implantation of a bare metal stent). Patients who are to undergo coronary artery angioplasty and stent placement who are likely to undergo invasive or surgical procedures within the next 12 months should probably receive a bare metal stent rather than a drug-eluting stent. Surgery can proceed after completion of 4 weeks of dual antiplatelet therapy. This approach will minimize the risk of premature discontinuation of antiplatelet therapy.

Hypertension

The Patient Who Has Chronic Hypertension

Despite the extent of preoperative blood pressure control, perioperative hypertension or hypotension occurs in up to 25% of hypertensives who undergo surgery. Data are conflicting regarding the role of preoperative hypertension as a cause of postoperative cardiac complications. There is little evidence for an association between a systolic blood pressure of 180 mm Hg or less and perioperative cardiac complication. In patients with chronic hypertension, as long as the diastolic blood pressure is < 110 mm Hg, hypertension in and of itself is not an indication to cancel surgery.

Perioperative Hypertension

Risk factors for perioperative hypertension are history of hypertension (especially a diastolic blood pressure > 110 mm Hg as well as the surgical procedure itself [carotid surgery, abdominal aortic surgery, peripheral vascular procedures, intraperitoneal, intrathoracic surgery]). The importance of perioperative hypertension as a risk factor for cardiac complication is unclear. There is no evidence that systolic blood pressure < 180 mm Hg or diastolic blood pressure < 110 mm Hg is related to perioperative cardiac complication.

When Does Perioperative Hypertension Occur?

This tends to occur at four distinct time periods:

1. During endotracheal intubation and induction of anesthesia as a result of sympathetic stimulation.
2. Intraoperatively as a result of pain induced adrenergic stimulation resulting in vasoconstriction.
3. In the early postanesthesia period as a result of various factors: pain, intravascular volume overload, and hypothermia.
4. Twenty-four to 48 hours after surgery, as fluid is mobilized from the extravascular space. It is also during this time that hypertension may occur as a result of the withdrawal of chronic antihypertensive medications.

Treatment of Perioperative Hypertension

Rapid control of perioperative hypertension is rarely necessary. Too aggressive of an attempt at blood pressure control may result in hypotension, placing the patient at risk for myocardial ischemia and infarction. Indications for acute postoperative blood pressure control are severe hypertension, for example, BP > 180/110 mm Hg with evidence of end-organ involvement, that is, acute myocardial ischemia, stroke, and acute renal failure. Because many cases of perioperative hypertension are a result of withdrawal of chronic antihypertensive medications, reinstitution of antihypertensive therapy is often all that is needed. Consider the possible causes for the patient's hypertension in planning the approach to treatment (e.g., β-blocker therapy) when sympathetic stimulation is the cause, analgesia if pain is implicated, diuretic if volume overload is documented, and warming if the patient is hypothermic.

Perioperative Hypotension

Iatrogenic is probably most common cause (i.e., too aggressive of treatment of perioperative hypertension). Other causes include intravascular volume depletion and excessive vasodilation. This may be caused by anesthetic agents (e.g., isoflurane, desflurane, and sevoflurane). The patient particularly at risk is one who is receiving chronic vasodilator medications and presents to surgery with volume depletion (diuretic induced, preoperative fasting, etc.). Consider sepsis, pulmonary embolism, and myocardial infarction if unexplained hypotension occurs during the 72 hours after surgery. Hypotension caused by volume depletion or vasodilation is treated by volume expansion. When clinically significant vasodilation-induced hypotension does not respond to volume expansion, consider using a peripheral vasoconstrictor (phenylephrine). Hypotension caused by direct myocardial depression is treated with inotropes (dopamine, dobutamine, and milrinone).

Valvular Heart Disease—Perioperative Considerations

Mitral Stenosis

Perioperative intravascular volume status and heart rate are key factors that require attention. Left atrial pressure may increase putting the patient at risk for pulmonary edema as a result of volume overload or tachycardia (tachycardia decreases diastolic filling time thereby increasing left atrial filling pressure). The patient with chronic hemodynamically significant mitral stenosis often has atrial fibrillation. Atrial fibrillation with rapid ventricular response may be treated with β-blocker, calcium channel antagonist (diltiazem, verapamil). The patient with mitral stenosis and atrial fibrillation typically receives chronic warfarin anticoagulation. For the patient who undergoes a surgical procedure, the time during which the patient is not anticoagulated should be as brief as possible. Strategies to minimize time off anticoagulation include performing surgery while receiving anticoagulants (cataract surgery, dental procedures) and the use of heparin to maintain anticoagulation while warfarin is withdrawn.

Mitral Regurgitation

Left ventricular dysfunction is a risk factor for perioperative congestive heart failure for the patient with severe mitral regurgitation.

The patient with severe mitral regurgitation and normal left ventricular function should have a "greater than normal" (e.g., > 60%) left ventricular ejection fraction (LVEF) because the mitral regurgitation facilitates left ventricular unloading. If the LVEF is not greater than normal, we are particularly vigilant to avoid volume overload in an effort to prevent congestive heart failure.

Aortic Regurgitation

In noncardiac surgery, operative risk correlates more with the status of left ventricular function than with the degree of aortic regurgitation. Vasopressors that increase peripheral vascular resistance may increase the degree of regurgitation. Excessive bradycardia is associated with increased diastolic filling time, which raises the magnitude of regurgitant volume by lengthening the period during which regurgitation may occur. Patients typically tolerate vasodilation (spinal anesthesia) well with a subsequent increase in cardiac output.

Aortic Stenosis

Critical or severe aortic stenosis is a risk factor for perioperative cardiac mortality and morbidity. Most patients with asymptomatic severe aortic stenosis who require emergency surgery can do so at relatively low risk with monitoring of anesthesia and attention to fluid balance. Spinal anesthesia is relatively contraindicated for the patient with severe aortic stenosis because of the risk of peripheral vasodilation induced by the anesthesia in a patient with "fixed cardiac output" who cannot increase his cardiac output any further because of aortic stenosis.

Bacterial Endocarditis Prophylaxis (Table 12.4)

Bacterial antibiotic prophylaxis should be administered only to patients who have cardiac abnormalities associated with high risk of adverse outcome from endocarditis. Surgical procedures that warrant prophylaxis include (1) dental procedures that involve manipulation of gingival tissues or periapical regions of teeth or

Table 12.4 Cardiac Conditions Associated with the Highest Risk of Adverse Outcome from Endocarditis for Which Prophylaxis with Dental Procedures Is Recommended

- Prosthetic heart valve
- Previous infective endocarditis
- Congenital heart disease
  - Unrepaired cyanotic congenital heart disease, including palliative shunts and conduits
  - Completely repaired congenital heart defect with prosthetic material or device, whether placed by surgery or by catheter intervention, during the first 6 months after the procedure.
  - Repaired congenital heart disease with residual defects at the site or adjacent to the site of a prosthetic patch or prosthetic device (which inhibit endothelialization)

Source: Adapted from: Fleisher LA, Beckman JA, Brown KA, Calkins H, Chaikof E, Fleischmann KE, Freeman WK, Froehlich JB, Kasper EK, Kersten JR, Riegel B, Robb JF. ACC / AHA 2007 guidelines on perioperative cardiovascular evaluation and care for noncardiac surgery: a report of the American College of Cardiology / American Heart Association Task force on Practice guidelines (Writing Committee to Revise the 2002 Guidelines on Perioperative Cardiovascular Evaluation for Noncardiac Surgery). J Am Coll Cardiol 2007;50:e159–242.

perforation of oral mucosa, (2) invasive procedures of the respiratory tract that involve incision or biopsy of the respiratory mucosa (i.e., tonsillectomy and adenoidectomy), and (3) surgery involving infected skin, skin structures, or musculoskeletal tissue. Antibiotic prophylaxis is not routinely recommended for genitourinary or gastrointestinal tract procedures. Prophylactic antibiotic regimens should focus on the bacteria at the site most likely to result in bacteremia and endocarditis (e.g., dental procedures—*Streptococcus viridans*; gastrointestinal or genitourinary procedures—enterococci; infected skin, skin structures, or musculoskeletal tissue—staphylococci and β hemolytic strep). It is recommended that patients at high risk for endocarditis who have an established genitourinary or gastrointestinal tract infection have included in their antibiotic regimen an agent active against enterococci (e.g., penicillin, ampicillin, piperacillin, or vancomycin). It is recommended that enterococcal urinary tract infection or colonization be eradicated prior to elective cystoscopy or urinary tract manipulation in the patient at high risk for endocarditis.

Perioperative Antithrombotic Management for the Patient Who Has a Mechanical Heart Valve Who Requires Interruption of Warfarin in the Perioperative Period

According to guidelines of the American College of Cardiology-American Heart Association, risk factors for mechanical valve thrombosis include atrial fibrillation, previous thromboembolism, left ventricular dysfunction, hypercoagulable conditions, older-generation thrombogenic valves, mechanical tricuspid valve, and more than one mechanical valve. In patients at low risk of thrombosis (i.e., those with a bileaflet mechanical AVR with none of the previously mentioned risk factors), warfarin may be stopped 48 to 72 hours before the surgical procedure (so that the international normalized ratio [INR] falls to less than 1.5) and restarted within 24 hours after the procedure. Heparin is usually unnecessary. In patients at high risk of thrombosis, defined as those with any form of mechanical mitral valve or a mechanical aortic valve prosthesis with any of the previously mentioned risk factors, therapeutic doses of intravenous unfractionated heparin (UFH) should be started when the INR falls below 2.0, stopped 4 to 6 hours before the surgical procedure, restarted as soon as possible after surgery and continued until the INR is again therapeutic with warfarin therapy. In patients at high risk of thrombosis, therapeutic doses of subcutaneous UFH (15,000 U every 12 hours) or LMWH (100 U per kg every 12 hours) may be considered during the period of subtherapeutic INR. It is reasonable to give fresh frozen plasma to patients with mechanical heart valves who require interruption of warfarin therapy for emergency noncardiac surgery. Fresh frozen plasma is referable to high-dose vitamin K. If possible, antithrombotic therapy should not be stopped in the perioperative period for procedures in which bleeding is unlikely or inconsequential (e.g., surgery on the skin, dental cleaning, treatment of dental caries, cataract surgery, and glaucoma surgery).

Congestive Heart Failure

Risk for the Development of Perioperative Congestive Heart Failure

Decompensated heart failure is a major predictor of increased perioperative risk. Compensated heart failure is an intermediate predictor of risk.

When Does Perioperative Congestive Heart Failure Occur?

There are two periods in the perioperative period when the risk for acute congestive heart failure is greatest. The immediate postoperative period is a time when congestive heart failure may occur as a result of excessive intraoperative fluid administration, perioperative hypertension or hypertension, myocardial ischemia, sympathetic stimulation, cessation of positive pressure ventilation, or hypoxia. The second peak period for perioperative acute congestive heart failure is 24 to 48 hours after surgery as a result of reabsorption of interstitial fluid, effects of perioperative withdrawal of chronic oral congestive heart failure medications, or myocardial ischemia.

Approach to Patients Who Have Chronic Compensated Congestive Heart Failure Who Require Noncardiac Surgery

Identify, prevent, and treat destabilizing factors that may occur in the perioperative period (e.g., fluid overload, anemia, fever). Before surgery, plan the resumption of the patient's chronic heart failure medications substituting a parenteral regimen for the patient who will be unable to resume oral medications after surgery. Evaluate the patient for evidence of decompensated congestive heart failure before surgery. Consider cancellation of nonemergency surgery in order to treat congestive heart failure if the patient with chronic congestive heart failure has evidence of congestive heart failure decompensation before surgery or if the patient has had decompensated congestive heart failure during the prior 7 days.

Use of Chronic Congestive Heart Failure Medications in the Perioperative Period

During the preoperative examination, assess for an orthostatic change in blood pressure in patients who receive chronic diuretic or vasodilator therapy. If orthostatic blood pressure change is found, intravascular volume depletion may be present that should be assessed and corrected prior to surgery. Continue β-blockers in the perioperative period. If β-blockers are interrupted for a period in excess of 72 hours in the perioperative period, consider resuming them at 50% of their previous dose if the patient is still deemed to be a candidate for their use. The dose is then titrated cautiously to the preoperative dose no sooner than 2 weeks. Consider withholding or reducing the dose of angiotensin-converting enzyme inhibitor, the diuretic, or both the day of surgery to minimize the risk of perioperative electrolyte abnormality, renal insufficiency, and hypotension. For the patient receiving chronic angiotensin-converting enzyme inhibitors or angiotensin receptor blockers who is unable to resume oral medications immediately after surgery, consider intravenous enalaprilat (0.625 mg every 6 hours increasing to 1.25 mg every 6 hours) until oral medication intake resumes. Serum potassium should be checked preoperatively for patients who are receiving diuretics. For patients who receive chronic digoxin therapy, a digoxin level should be measured if there is a perioperative decline in renal function.

Management of Acute Congestive Heart Failure in the Perioperative Period

Treatment is directed at the primary cause of the acute episode of congestive heart failure (e.g., diuretics to treat perioperative volume overload, antihypertensives to treat hypertension that has provoked CHF, control of atrial fibrillation ventricular response if that is the etiology of decompensation or inotropes to treat perioperative decline in left ventricular function).

Hypertrophic Cardiomyopathy—Perioperative Considerations in Noncardiac Surgery

Patients with hypertrophic cardiomyopathy with left ventricular outflow obstruction are at risk for worsening of outflow obstruction in the perioperative period. Perioperative factors that may increase the left ventricular outflow tract gradient include excessive reduction in preload or afterload (result of volume depletion or vasodilator therapy) or catecholamine-induced increased myocardial contractility.

Arrhythmias and Conduction Disorders

Incidence and Clinical Significance of Perioperative Arrhythmias

Cardiac arrhythmias are common in the perioperative period and are usually benign and clinically insignificant. Perioperative ventricular premature contractions and related ventricular ectopy are markers of risk if they occur in the setting of ischemic or structural heart disease. If significant ventricular ectopy occurs in the perioperative period, an evaluation to rule out ischemic or structural heart disease, electrolyte disorder (e.g., hypokalemia and hypomagnesemia), or hypoxia should take place.

Perioperative Considerations for Patients Who Have Preoperative Cardiac Arrhythmias

Atrial Fibrillation

Consider preoperative initiation of β-blocker or amiodarone for the patient at high risk of developing perioperative atrial fibrillation. For patients with chronic atrial fibrillation and receiving oral anticoagulation, consider their thromboembolic risk when planning the management of their perioperative anticoagulant therapy. For patients undergoing surgery not associated with an increased risk of bleeding, surgery can often be performed while receiving anticoagulation (e.g., dental surgery and selected ophthalmologic procedures). For patients in whom perioperative bleeding is of concern, warfarin is withheld prior to surgery. Typically, patients at low risk of thromboembolism can discontinue warfarin 4 to 5 hours prior to surgery with resumption of warfarin as soon as possible after surgery. Patients at high risk for thromboembolism should have short-term therapy with heparin while they are not receiving oral anticoagulation.

Ventricular Arrhythmias

Ventricular arrhythmias (ventricular premature contractions, nonsustained ventricular tachycardia) usually do not require treatment in the perioperative period unless they are associated by acute myocardial ischemia and/or are associated with hemodynamic compromise. Perioperative ventricular premature contractions and nonsustained ventricular tachycardia are not associated with an increase in perioperative death. The occurrence of perioperative frequent ventricular premature contractions or nonsustained ventricular tachycardia should result in assessment of the patient for myocardial ischemia or infarction, electrolyte abnormality, drug toxicity, or hypoxia. Sustained ventricular tachycardia in the perioperative period should be treated in the same fashion as in the nonperioperative setting.

Identification and Treatment of Specific Perioperative Disorders of Cardiac Rate and Rhythm

Sinus Tachycardia

Sinus tachycardia is the most common cardiac arrhythmia and is almost always benign. The most common causes of perioperative sinus bradycardia are perioperative pain, hypovolemia, anemia, fever, hypoxia, and hypercarbia.

Atrial Flutter and Fibrillation

Perioperative atrial fibrillation or atrial flutter is treated in the same fashion as atrial fibrillation or atrial flutter that occurs as a result of noncardiac surgery. If perioperative atrial fibrillation results in hemodynamic instability, then the immediate goal is to restore sinus rhythm, usually by direct current (DC) cardioversion. If perioperative atrial fibrillation is well tolerated, the approach should be to control the ventricular rate (β-blockers or diltiazem) and consider adding heparin or warfarin anticoagulation if the atrial fibrillation persists for 24 to 48 hours or more. Atrial fibrillation, atrial flutter that starts in the perioperative period and is hemodynamically well tolerated, often reverts to sinus rhythm within 4 to 6 weeks after surgery. For the patient whose new onset perioperative atrial fibrillation persists more than 4 to 6 weeks after surgery, we often consider elective cardioversion to restore sinus rhythm.

Paroxysmal Supraventricular Tachycardia

Paroxysmal supraventricular tachycardia (PSVT) is characterized by a sudden onset of rapid regular rhythm, with rates between 150 and 250 beats per minute. If the patient is hemodynamically unstable, immediate synchronized DC cardioversion should be performed. If the QRS complex is wide and the rhythm has not definitely been proven to be supraventricular, the rhythm should be treated as ventricular tachycardia. If the rhythm is narrow complex and the patient is hemodynamically stable, vagal maneuvers or medical therapy (intravenous adenosine, calcium channel blockers, β-blockers) may be effective in restoring sinus rhythm.

Multifocal Atrial Tachycardia

Multifocal atrial tachycardia (MAT) is an automatic arrhythmia characterized by an atrial rate $>$ 100 beats per minute with organized, discrete, nonsinus P waves of at least three different morphologies. Multifocal atrial tachycardia is usually associated with severe pulmonary disease. When MAT occurs in the perioperative period, respiratory failure, pneumonia, and congestive heart failure are common causes. Perioperative treatment centers on the treatment of the precipitating medical cause.

Ventricular Premature Contractions and NSVT

Common causes of acute ventricular arrhythmias in the perioperative period include acute myocardial ischemia, hypoxia, hypokalemia, and hypomagnesemia. Right heart catheters inserted to facilitate hemodynamic monitoring may induce ventricular arrhythmias as a result of irritation or micro trauma of the left ventricular outflow tract. Treatment of perioperative ventricular ectopy focuses on identification of its cause and correction if possible.

Sustained Ventricular Tachycardia and Ventricular Fibrillation

Patients who develop perioperative sustained ventricular tachycardia or ventricular fibrillation should be treated according to the American Heart Association Advanced Cardiac Life Support (ACLS) protocol (see the ACLS guideline: http://circ.ahajournals.org/cgi/content/full/112/24_suppl/IV-67).

Significance of Perioperative Conduction Abnormalities

Sinus bradycardia and Mobitz I second-degree A-V block (characterized on electrocardiogram by progressive prolongation of PR interval until a P wave is not conducted to the ventricles) are common, usually clinically insignificant, and typically a result of increased vagal tone. Mobitz II second-degree A-V block (characterized on electrocardiogram by a fixed P-R interval with P-wave conduction to the ventricles blocked on a constant [e.g., 2:1, 3:1,

4:1] or variable basis). This is indicative of diffuse clinically significant conduction disease with risk of progression to complete heart block. A means of temporary cardiac pacing should be available in the perioperative period for the patient with Mobitz II A-V block in the event that it progresses to complete (third degree A-V block) heart block in the perioperative period. Chronic bifascicular block (i.e., right bundle branch block with either left anterior hemiblock or left posterior hemiblock, or left bundle branch block) rarely progresses to complete heart block in the perioperative period. Placement of a temporary cardiac pacemaker should be considered for the patient who is identified during preoperative to meet criteria for implantation of a permanent cardiac pacemaker, and surgery cannot be delayed to allow permanent pacemaker insertion.

Preoperative and Perioperative Management of the Patient with Pacemaker

For the patient with a cardiac pacemaker, the reason for pacemaker implant should be to know prior to noncardiac surgery, and the pacemaker should be interrogated prior to surgery to obtain and document pacemaker settings and battery reserve. The most significant potential pacemaker problem in the perioperative period is pacemaker inhibition resulting from electrocautery-induced electromagnetic interference (EMI). Some pacemakers respond to EMI pacing in an asynchronous (fixed-rate) mode. Some pacemakers may reprogram in response to EMI. The risk of EMI-induced pacemaker interference may be decreased by avoiding the application of electrocautery directly over the pacemaker pulse generator and by keeping the electrocautery current path as far away as possible from the pacemaker generator. Another approach to avoidance of perioperative alteration of pacemaker function by electrocautery induced EMI to temporally programming the pacemaker to an asynchronous fixed rate mode. Many pacemakers assume fixed rate mode pacing (insensitive to EMI) when a magnet is placed over them. This is a common approach to temporary asynchronous pacing in the perioperative period. Permanent pacemakers should be interrogated and the patient's chronic pacemaker setting restored after surgery.

Preoperative and Perioperative Management of the Patient with an Automatic Implantable Cardioverter-Defibrillator

Automatic implantable cardioverter-defibrillators (AICDs) are found in the patient who has survived sudden cardiac death or has ischemic or nonischemic cardiomyopathy and has had an AICD implanted for primary prevention of sudden cardiac death. EMI from electrocautery may be interpreted by the AICD as ventricular tachycardia or ventricular fibrillation resulting in AICD electrical discharge during surgery. Before surgery, if electrocautery is to be used, the AICD should be temporally programmed to avoid EMI-induced AICD discharge. It is essential to reprogram the pacemaker to the patient's baseline settings immediately after surgery.

Role of Perioperative Invasive Hemodynamic Monitoring

There is no evidence that routine perioperative pulmonary artery catheterization offers any advantage when compared to standard care. Individual situations in which invasive hemodynamic monitoring may facilitate management include the patient with severe left ventricular dysfunction or "fixed cardiac output" (e.g., critical or severe aortic stenosis) who requires surgery involved with significant fluid administration.

When should an electrocardiogram be performed prior to surgery for a patient who is not known to have cardiovascular disease? Guidelines from the American College of Physicians recommend that a preoperative ECG be performed to test for the presence of asymptomatic cardiac disease in men older than 40 years and women older than 50 years having major surgery. For patients undergoing minor surgery in whom the history and physician exam is normal, a routine ECG is unlikely to improve outcomes and can be omitted. Some abnormalities on ECGs (e.g., ST-T wave changes, left ventricular hypertrophy are of unknown prognostic value), whereas others (left bundle branch block) are not predictive of perioperative cardiac events.

13 ■ Bradyarrhythmias and Indications for Pacemaker Implantation

Behzad B. Pavri, MD

Anatomy and Physiology of the Cardiac Conduction System

The cardiac conduction system is comprised of the sinus node, the atrioventricular (AV) node, the bundle of His, bundle branches, and the Purkinje network. The sinus node is the dominant pacemaker of the normal heart, but the AV node, bundle of His, and the left bundle branch are capable of "backup" automaticity in case of sinus node failure or atrioventricular block.

The Sinoatrial Node

- The sinoatrial node (SAN) is a large, comma-shaped collection of specialized cells capable of spontaneous firing (automaticity). When viewed from the surface of the heart, the SAN is located along the posterolateral aspect of the right atrium in the sulcus terminalis. Its upper end lies at the juncture of the superior vena cava and trabeculated right atrial appendage. The lower end of the SAN extends toward the inferior vena cava.
- When viewed from inside the right atrium, the SAN is located along the crista terminalis.
- The SAN shows heavy innervation with parasympathetic (vagal) and sympathetic nerve fibers. Vagal effects result in slowing of SAN firing rate (such as during sleep—physiologic bradycardia), whereas sympathetic effects result in sinus rate acceleration (such as during exercise—physiologic sinus tachycardia).

- The site of impulse formation shifts within the SAN. Under sympathetic drive, faster rates originate from the superior portions of the SAN, whereas during parasympathetic states, slower rates originate from the lower portions of the SAN.
- Blood supply typically arises from the proximal right coronary artery (70%) or circumflex branch of the left coronary artery (30%).
- Normal SAN impulse generation is mainly driven by the pacemaker current, I_f ("funny" current).

The AV Node

- The compact portion of the AV node is located near the crux of the heart between the right and left atria, just above the membranous portion of the interventricular septum.
- The sinus impulse arrives at the AV node over the "fast" (anterior) and "slow" (posterior) approaches to the AV node. These approaches to the AV nodes are often referred to as the fast and slow "pathways" of the AV node, although they are not discrete bundles in the human heart. Rather, they represent preferential conduction due to longitudinal fiber orientation.
- The AV node exhibits "decremental conduction," delaying the sinus impulse on its way to the ventricles. This allows time for the thin-walled atria to complete systolic emptying while the ventricles are held in diastole. Decremental conduction also protects the ventricles from rapid rates during atrial arrhythmias such as atrial fibrillation and atrial flutter by acting as an electrical "filter."
- The AV node functions as the first "backup" pacemaker in case of SAN failure, typically providing heart rates of between 40 and 55 beats per minute.
- Blood supply to the AV node derives from the A-V nodal artery, which arises from the right coronary 90% of the time and from the circumflex branch of the left coronary artery 10% of the time.

The Bundle of His

- This arises from the lower end of the compact AV node and crosses the annulus fibrosus that electrically isolates atria from ventricles.
- The bundle of His is capable of rapid, "all-or-none" conduction and no decremental properties (when healthy).
- The bundle of His can serve as a "backup" pacemaker in case of SAN and AV node failure, providing heart rates of 30 to 40 beats per minute. Such "escape" rhythms are often unstable and can result in loss of consciousness.
- Blood supply is typically derived from the first septal perforator branch of the left anterior descending coronary artery but can occasionally arise from the posterior descending coronary artery.

Left Bundle Branch

- This is a fan-like structure that immediately splits into two or three broad fascicles.
- The left septal fascicle (when present) runs along the left side of the interventricular septum.
- The left anterior fascicle runs along the anterolateral wall of the left ventricle.
- The left posterior fascicle runs along the inferior base of the left ventricle.
- This allows rapid propagation of electrical impulse to all portions of the Purkinje network (discussed later here).
- The fascicles can also serve as "backup" pacemakers in case of SAN, AV node, and His bundle failure, providing heart rates of 30 to 40 beats per minute.
- The blood supply to the left anterior and septal fascicle is primarily derived from septal perforators from the left anterior descending artery.
- The blood supply to the posterior fascicle derives from both the left anterior descending and the posterior descending artery.

Right Bundle Branch

- This is a discrete nerve-like structure that travels down the right side of the interventricular septum before branching to innervate the Purkinje network near the right ventricular apex and free wall. A prominent branch to the right ventricular free wall near the terminus is called the moderator band.
- The right bundle branch is not capable of "backup" automaticity.
- Blood supply to the proximal right bundle branch can be from both the A-V nodal artery and septal branches of the left anterior descending artery (50%), the septal branch only (40%), or the A-V nodal artery alone (10%).

The Purkinje Network

- This is a diffuse, rapidly conducting reticulum of fibers that covers large area of the ventricular endocardial surface.
- The final pathway of impulse spreads from the specialized conduction system to the working ventricular myocardium.

Clinical Pearls

- A right bundle branch block (RBBB) is seen in conditions that cause chronic right ventricular overload such as atrial septal defects with left to right shunting, chronic pulmonary disease that results in pulmonary hypertension and valvular disorders such as pulmonary stenosis and mitral stenosis—both of which can cause pulmonary hypertension in their severe forms.
- RBBB can be seen in acute RV overload states such as pulmonary embolism.
- RBBB that occurs after coronary artery bypass surgery (CABG) appears to be of benign clinical significance.
- The finding of RBBB in an otherwise asymptomatic individual does not mandate further diagnostic evaluation.

- The left bundle branch block (LBBB) typically occurs in the setting of structural heart disease and is often related to chronic severe hypertension, coronary artery disease, valvular pathology, or a cardiomyopathy; therefore, the recognition of LBBB should prompt further investigation.
- The ECG pattern of bundle branch block does not necessarily imply that the bundle is incapable of conduction. More often, it simply reflects slower conduction in that bundle as compared with the other bundle.

Sino Atrial Node (SAN) Dysfunction

Sino atrial node (SAN) dysfunction may present in many ways:

- Sinus bradycardia
  - Heart rate less than 60
  - Increased vagal tone in healthy young adults and trained athletes may result in physiologic sinus bradycardia at rest. Labeling a bradycardia as abnormal requires careful correlation of symptoms with bradycardia.
- Sinus pause
  - Cessation of sinoatrial activity
  - Asymptomatic pauses can occur in athletes or during sleep
  - Typically, pauses greater than 3 seconds require clinical correlation and further evaluation
- Sinus exit block: The P wave represents atrial depolarization recorded from the body surface. Sino atrial node depolarization is not seen on the ECG because of the small amount of tissue that is depolarized.
  - Sinus exit Wenckebach or type 1 sinus exit block—progressively longer delay in sinoatrial conduction time, followed by failure of a sinus impulse to reach the atrium. This results in a pause on surface ECG (see Figure 13.1).
  - The clues to a type 1 exit block are as follows:
    - Grouped beating
    - Shortening of the P-P interval prior to a pause
    - Sinus pauses less than twice the shortest P-P interval

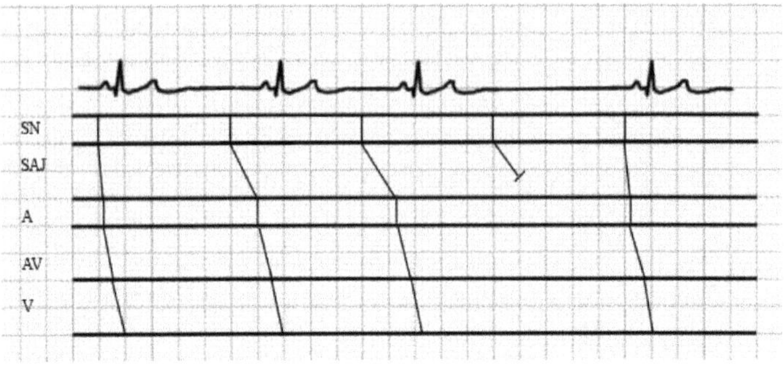

■ **Figure 13.1** Sinoatrial Wenckebach or Type 1 Sinus Exit Block. Note the decremental conduction that is seen between the sinus node and atria. Each progressive sinus impulse takes longer to conduct to the atria until finally one impulse fails to reach and depolarize the atria. The only evidence of this on the surface electrocardiogram is a pause that is preceded by shortening of the P-P interval. Shortening of the P-P interval is seen because the first increment in SAN-to-atrium conduction is the largest; each subsequent increment is smaller than the last. Failure of conduction is followed by improved conduction of the next sinus impulse, resulting in the longest PP being less than twice the shortest PP cycle length. This behavior explains the 'grouped beating' of P waves seen during Type 1 Sinus Exit Block. (SAN = Sinoatrial Node, SAJ = SinoAtrial Junction, A = Atria, AV = AV node, V = Ventricle)

- Type 2—an intermittent and abrupt failure of conduction from SAN to atria results in sinus pause that is an exact multiple of the p-p interval.

- Sick sinus syndrome
  - This is a broad term used to describe a constellation of findings, including failure of sinoatrial impulse generation, failure of escape pacemakers, and a predilection for atrial tachyarrhythmias.
  - Atrial tachyarrhythmias can be atrial tachycardia, atrial flutter, or atrial fibrillation (Figure 13.2).
  - Because of inappropriate suppression of sinus node and escape pacemakers, it is common to see prolonged sinus arrest and asystole after termination of the atrial

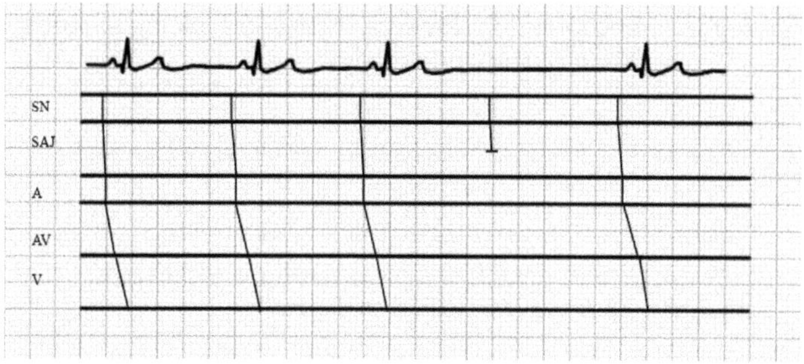

■ **Figure 13.2** There is intermittent failure of conduction from sinus node to atria. Note that the P-P interval prior to the pause is stable and that the pause is an exact multiple (two times) of the P-P interval.

tachyarrhythmia, often referred to as "tachybrady" or "sleepy sinus" syndrome.

- ECG manifestations of sick sinus syndrome are as follows:
  - Sinus bradycardia that is persistent, severe, and symptomatic
  - Sinus arrest without the emergence of a subsidiary pacemaker
  - Sinoatrial block
  - Atrial fibrillation
  - Alternating bradycardia and tachycardia
  - Chronotropic incompetence (inappropriate SAN response to exercise)
- Indications for pacing in sinus node dysfunction (American College of Cardiology [ACC]/American Heart Association [AHA]/Heart Rhythm Society [HRS] 2008 Guidelines)

Atrioventricular Block

General Considerations

AV nodal dysfunction or His-Purkinje dysfunction results in varying association (or dissociation) between atrial and ventricular activity. Block at the level of the AV node has a benign prognosis

Table 13.1 Recommendations for Permanent Pacing in Sinus Node Dysfunction (SND)

Class I

1. Indicated for symptomatic bradycardia, including frequent sinus pauses that produce symptoms
2. Indicated for symptomatic chronotropic incompetence
3. Indicated for symptomatic sinus bradycardia that results from required drug therapy for medical conditions

Class IIa

1. Reasonable for SND with heart rate less than 40 bpm when a clear association between significant symptoms consistent with bradycardia and the actual presence of bradycardia has not been documented
2. Reasonable for syncope of unexplained origin when clinically significant abnormalities of sinus node function are discovered or provoked in electrophysiological studies

Class IIb

1. Consider for minimally symptomatic patients with chronic heart rate less than 40 bpm while awake

Class III

1. Not indicated for asymptomatic patients
2. Not indicated for SND in patients for whom the symptoms suggestive of bradycardia have been clearly documented to occur in the absence of bradycardia
3. Not indicated for SND with symptomatic bradycardia due to nonessential drug therapy.

and usually does not require electronic pacing. Block below the AV node, within the His bundle, or in the bundle branches has a poor prognosis, and requires electronic pacing.

Types of AV block are discussed as follows:

- First-degree AV block or prolonged PR interval (Figure 13.3)
  - The normal PR interval (measured from the beginning of the P wave to the beginning of the QRS complex) is between 0.12 and 0.2 seconds.

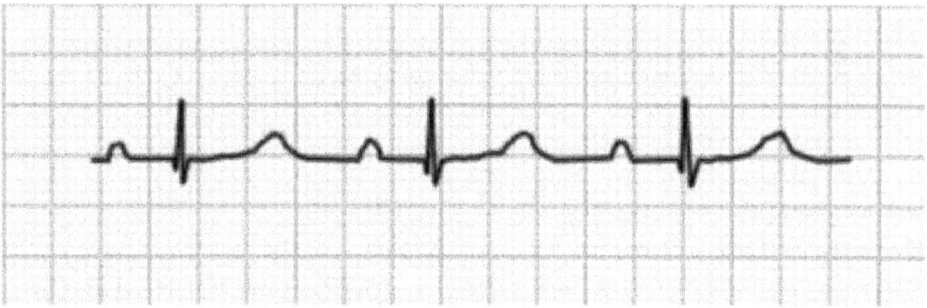

■ Figure 13.3 First degree AV block. Every PR interval is longer than 0.2 seconds and is stable.

- A prolongation of the PR interval to > 0.2 seconds is referred to as "first-degree AV block."
- In this setting, the term block is a misnomer, as none of the sinus impulses actually fail to conduct to the ventricles.

- Second-degree AV block: Some sinus P waves fail to conduct to the ventricles ("blocked" or "dropped" beats). An analysis of a second-degree AV block includes two steps: step 1, ECG pattern characterization, and step 2, localization of site of block.
  - Step 1: ECG patterns of a second-degree AV block
    - Second-degree Mobitz type 1 (Wenckebach): progressive PR interval prolongation, followed by failure of AV conduction (see Figure 13.4).
    - Second-degree Mobitz type 2: abrupt failure of P-wave conduction, not preceded by PR prolongation. Before the dropped beat, at least two consecutive PR intervals should be of equal duration (Figure 13.5).
  - Second-degree 2:1 AV block: alternate P waves fail to conduct; the PR interval associated with conducted P waves is constant (Figure 13.6a/b).
  - Step 2: Localization of site of AV block: Analysis of the PR interval and QRS complex width allows accurate localization of the site of block in the majority of patients:
    - A markedly prolonged PR interval with a normal (narrow) QRS complex localizes the site of block to be

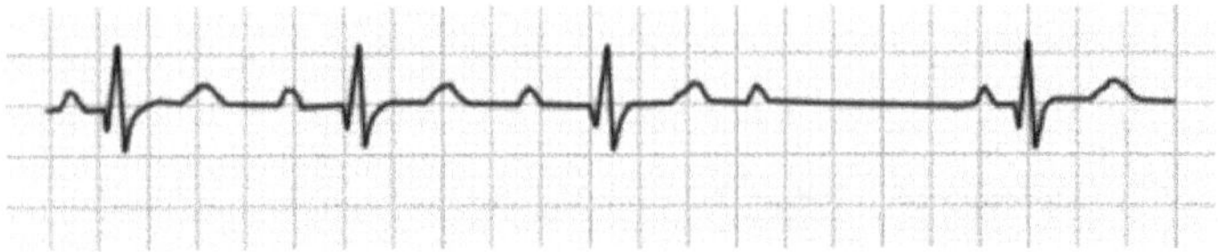

■ **Figure 13.4** Second Degree Mobitz Type 1 (Wenckebach). Progressive PR interval prolongation can be seen before a P wave fails to conduct. Notice the R-R interval shortens before the dropped beat. Shortening of the R-R interval is seen because the first increment in atrium-to-ventricle conduction time (PR interval) is the largest; each subsequent increment is smaller than the last. Failure of conduction is followed by improved conduction of the next sinus impulse, resulting in the longest RR being less than twice the shortest RR cycle length. This behavior explains the 'grouped beating' of QRS complexes seen during AV Wenckebach Mobitz Type 1 Block. The narrow QRS strongly suggests that the level of block is within the Atrioventricular node, and is thus likely to be a stable rhythm that is prognostically benign.

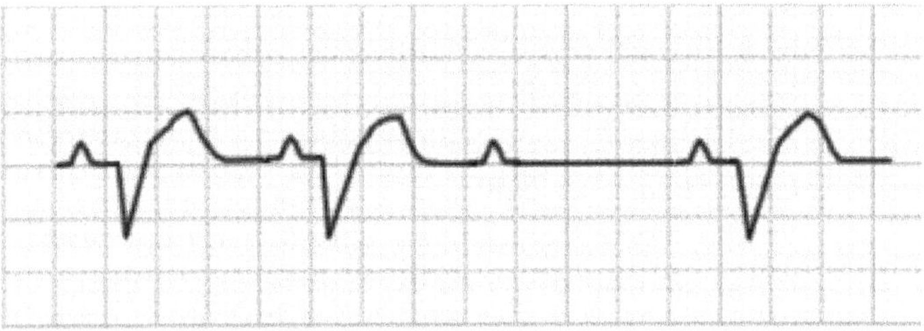

■ **Figure 13.5** Second Degree Mobitz Type 2 Block. A stable PR interval is seen prior to a non-conducted P wave. The non-conducted P is not premature and is expected to conduct to the ventricles. These features are diagnostic of Mobitz Type 2 behavior. Notice that the wide QRS complex suggests an intra-ventricular conduction delay. The presence of a bundle branch block, minimally increased PR interval, and Mobitz Type 2 behavior on the electrocardiogram very likely localizes the block to be below the AV node. Block below the AV node is always pathologic, is associated with a poor prognosis and commonly requires artificial pacing.

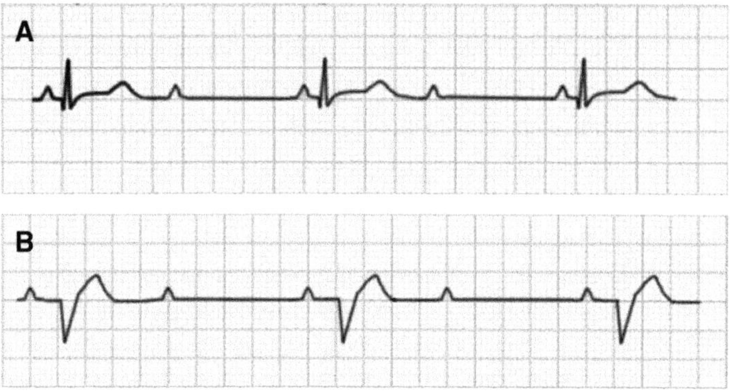

■ **Figure 13.6A/B** Second degree 2:1 AV block. The failure of every other P wave to conduct can be a result of Mobitz Type 1 or Mobitz Type 2 block. The inability to accurately discriminate the two entities results in the description of the conduction ratio—which in this case is 2 to 1 atrioventricular block. In the first example, the narrow QRS complex and mildly prolonged PR interval suggest that the anatomic level of block may be within the AV node. In the second example, the normal PR interval and the widened QRS complex suggest that the anatomic level of block may be below the AV node. This figure emphasizes the importance of describing rate as well as the conduction ratio. The sinus rate is approximately 70 bpm, but the ventricular rate is 35 bpm because only every other sinus beat is conducted. Block at this rate is almost always pathologic even though the anatomic location of this block may be within the AV node.

within the AV node. This is most commonly seen in Mobitz type I AV block (Wenckebach). Block within the AV node may be physiologic or pathologic. Physiologic AV Wenckebach may be observed during states of increased vagal tone, such as during sleep.

- A normal or minimally prolonged PR interval and a widened QRS complex (bundle branch block) localize the site of block to be below the bundle of His. This is most commonly seen in Mobitz type II AV block. The block below the AV node is always pathologic.

        - An AV block without preceding PR prolongation but with a normal or slightly prolonged PR interval and a normal (narrow) QRS complex suggests the site of block to be within the bundle of His. This is an uncommon finding, is often pathologic, and usually requires an electrophysiology (His bundle) study to confirm the correct diagnosis.
        - The surface ECG pattern will allow accurate localization of block in the majority of patients; however, invasive electrophysiology study with direct recording of His bundle electrograms may be required in some patients.
    - Third-degree block (complete heart block): defined as complete failure of conduction from atrium to ventricle. Making the diagnosis of complete AV block from a surface ECG requires three criteria:
        - More P waves than QRS complexes (atrial rate greater than ventricular rate)
        - No association between atrium and ventricle as demonstrated by varying P to R relationships with a regular ventricular rate
        - A ventricular rate that is slow enough (usually < 45 beats/min) so that it is clear that P waves fail to conduct even though they have ample opportunity to do so. This criterion is very important and often not appreciated.
        - The recognition of AV dissociation does not automatically imply the presence of complete AV block! The diagnosis of complete AV block requires that ample opportunity be present for P waves to conduct (see Figure 13.7).
- High-grade AV block

  High-grade AV block is recognized when
    - There is intermittent conduction between atria and ventricles
    - At least two consecutive P waves fail to conduct
    - All blocked P waves must have ample opportunity to conduct
    - The atrial rate is physiologic (typically < 135 beats/min) (Figure 13.8)

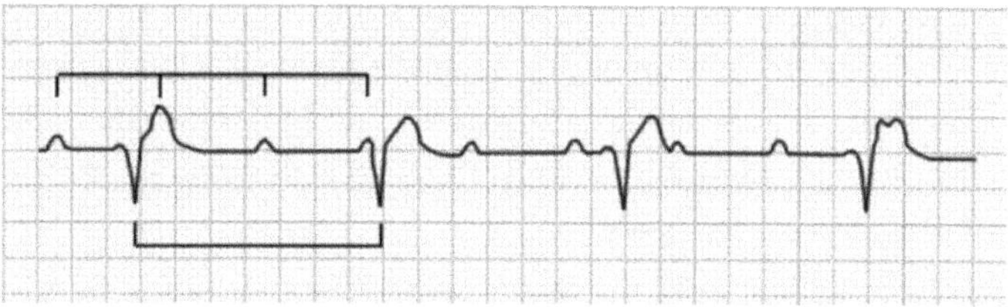

■ **Figure 13.7** Complete Heart Block. There are more P waves than QRS complexes, and there is no association between P and QRS complexes as demonstrated by varying PR intervals. Recognize the P waves buried within the QRS complexes deform the native QRS complex. Importantly, there is ample opportunity for AV conduction to occur.

Describing the atrial rate during AV block is important for two reasons: First, very high atrial rates that fail to conduct 1:1 to the ventricle represent normal AV nodal physiology. For instance, an atrial rate of 300 beats per minute (as seen during atrial flutter) that conducts 4:1 with a ventricular rate of 75 bpm (3 nonconducted consecutive flutter waves) is physiologic and indeed desirable. By comparison, 2:1 AV block during sinus rhythm at an atrial rate of 60 bpm (resulting in a ventricular rate of 30 bpm) is clearly pathologic. Therefore, simply describing the conduction ratio would be incomplete and may give the impression that the individual with 4:1 AV block in atrial flutter has greater pathology. Second, the sinus rate may provide insight into the hemodynamic

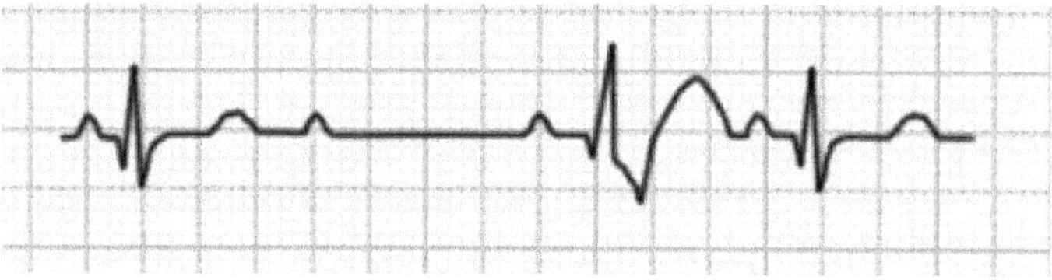

■ **Figure 13.8** High Grade AV Block. The second and third P-wave do not conduct. The wide QRS complex seen after the third P-wave is a ventricular escape complex. The failure of two consecutive P waves makes the diagnosis of high grade AV block.

consequences of the bradycardia that results from complete AV block. Sinus acceleration during complete AV block is often a sign of hemodynamic instability. Conversely, a normal sinus rate could reflect hemodynamically stability, sinus node dysfunction, or the use of β-blocker medications.

Table 13.2 Recommendations for Pacing in Acquired Atrioventricular (AV) Block in Adults (ACC/AHA/HRS 2008)

Class I

1. Indicated for advanced second-degree AV block at any anatomic level associated with bradycardia with symptoms (including heart failure) or ventricular arrhythmias presumed to be due to AV block
2. Indicated for third-degree and advanced second-degree AV block at any anatomic level associated with arrhythmias and other medical conditions that require drug therapy that results in symptomatic bradycardia
3. Indicated for third-degree and advanced second-degree AV block at any anatomic level in awake, symptom-free patients in sinus rhythm, with documented periods of asystole greater than or equal to 3.0 seconds or any escape rate less than 40 bpm or with an escape rhythm that is below the AV node
4. Indicated for third-degree and advanced second-degree AV block at any anatomic level in awake, symptom-free patients with atrial fibrillation and bradycardia with 1 or more pauses of at least 5 seconds or longer
5. Indicated for third-degree and advanced second-degree AV block at any anatomic level after catheter ablation of the AV junction
6. Indicated for third-degree and advanced second-degree AV block at any anatomic level associated with postoperative AV block that is not expected to resolve after cardiac surgery
7. Indicated for third-degree and advanced second-degree AV block at any anatomic level associated with neuromuscular diseases with AV block, such as myotonic muscular dystrophy, Kearns-Sayre syndrome, Erb dystrophy (limb-girdle muscular dystrophy), and peroneal muscular atrophy, with or without symptoms
8. Indicated for second-degree AV block with associated symptomatic bradycardia regardless of type or site of block

9. Indicated for asymptomatic persistent third-degree AV block at any anatomic site with average awake ventricular rates of 40 bpm or faster if cardiomegaly or LV dysfunction is present or if the site of block is below the AV node
10. Indicated for second- or third-degree AV block during exercise in the absence of myocardial ischemia

Class IIa

1. Reasonable for persistent third-degree AV block with an escape rate greater than 40 bpm in asymptomatic adult patients without cardiomegaly
2. Reasonable for asymptomatic second-degree AV block at intra- or infra-His levels found at electrophysiological study
3. Reasonable for first- or second-degree AV block with symptoms similar to those of pacemaker syndrome or hemodynamic compromise
4. Reasonable for asymptomatic type II second-degree AV block with a narrow QRS. When type II second-degree AV block occurs with a wide QRS, including isolated right bundle-branch block, pacing becomes a Class I recommendation.

Class IIb

1. Consider for neuromuscular diseases such as myotonic muscular dystrophy, Erb dystrophy (limb-girdle muscular dystrophy), and peroneal muscular atrophy with any degree of AV block (including first-degree AV block), with or without symptoms, because there may be unpredictable progression of AV conduction disease
2. Consider for AV block in the setting of drug use and/or drug toxicity when the block is expected to recur even after the drug is withdrawn (Level of Evidence: B)

Class III

1. Not indicated for asymptomatic first-degree AV block (Level of Evidence: B)
2. Not indicated for asymptomatic type I second-degree AV block at the supra-His (AV node) level or that which is not known to be intra- or infra-Hisian (Level of Evidence: C)
3. Not indicated for AV block that is expected to resolve and is unlikely to recur (e.g., drug toxicity, Lyme disease, or transient increases in vagal tone or during hypoxia in sleep apnea syndrome in the absence of symptoms) (Level of Evidence: B)

Bifascicular and Trifascicular Block

Bifascicular or trifascicular blocks, when associated with advanced AV blocks, have been found to have high mortality rates and a significant incidence of sudden death.

- Bifascicular block can be
  - RBBB with left anterior fascicular block (LAFB)
  - RBBB with left posterior fascicular block (LPFB)
- Trifascicular block is block documented in all three fascicles at different times
  - Alternating right and LBBB
  - RBBB with LAFB on one ECG and RBBB with LPFB on another ECG
- Bifascicular block with PR prolongation is often incorrectly referred to as "trifascicular" block; however, the prolongation of the PR interval may be due to AV nodal delay rather than delay in the third fascicle. Hence, when encountered, this should simply be described as "bifascicular block with prolonged PR (Figure 13.3)."

Clinical Pearls

- Be sure to think of reversible causes of bradyarrhythmias. Drug toxicities such as digitalis excess or β-blocker or calcium channel blocker overdose are common causes of bradyarrhythmias. Hyperkalemia is also an important and often overlooked cause of bradyarrhythmias.
- Obstructive sleep apnea is an important cause of clinically significant sinus bradycardia and sinus pauses during sleep.
- The presence of suspicious clinical symptoms (e.g., syncope) with bifascicular block with PR prolongation suggests infranodal, pathologic block, and need for further invasive electrophysiologic study or placement of an electronic pacemaker.
- Stokes-Adams attacks refer to sudden, transient episodes of syncope that may be preceded by pallor prior to losing

Table 13.3 Recommendations for Permanent Pacing in Chronic Bifascicular Block

Class I

1. Indicated for advanced second-degree AV block or intermittent third-degree AV block (Level of Evidence: B)
2. Indicated for type II second-degree AV block (Level of Evidence: B)
3. Indicated for alternating bundle-branch block (Level of Evidence: C)

Class IIa

1. Reasonable for syncope not demonstrated to be due to AV block when other likely causes have been excluded, specifically ventricular tachycardia (VT) (Level of Evidence: B)
2. Reasonable for an incidental finding at electrophysiological study of a markedly prolonged HV interval (greater than or equal to 100 milliseconds) in asymptomatic patients (Level of Evidence: B)
3. Reasonable for an incidental finding at electrophysiological study of pacing-induced infra-His block that is not physiological (Level of Evidence: B)

Class IIb

1. Consider in the setting of neuromuscular diseases such as myotonic muscular dystrophy, Erb dystrophy (limb-girdle muscular dystrophy), and peroneal muscular atrophy with bifascicular block or any fascicular block, with or without symptoms (Level of Evidence: C)

Class III

1. Not indicated for fascicular block without AV block or symptoms (Level of Evidence: B)
2. Not indicated for fascicular block with first-degree AV block without symptoms (Level of Evidence: B)

consciousness and seizure-like activity during an attack due to the severe decrease in cardiac output related to an abrupt bradyarrhythmia.

14 ▪ Wide QRS Complex Arrhythmias

JAMES M. YAU, MD
REGINALD T. HO, MD

Wide QRS complex tachycardias (WCTs) frequently present a challenge to physicians, particularly when urgent therapy is required. Accurate rhythm diagnosis is important for both acute and long-term management. WCTs are defined as tachycardias ≥ 100 beats per minute) whose QRS duration exceeds 120 ms. WCTs can be categorized into regular and irregular WCTs (Table 14.1). Regular WCTs can be further subdivided by its QRS morphology in lead V1 into right bundle branch block (RBBB) (terminal positive deflection) and left bundle branch block (LBBB) (terminal negative deflection) tachycardias. This chapter discusses the (1) differential diagnosis of WCTs, (2) a practical approach to diagnosis, and (3) acute and long-term therapies.

Table 14.1 Causes of Wide QRS Complex Tachycardia

Regular
Supraventricular tachycardia with bundle branch block (BBB)
Pre-existing
Rate related (functional)
Monomorphic ventricular tachycardia
Pre-excited tachycardia
Pacemaker-mediated tachycardia
Irregular
Polymorphic ventricular tachycardia
Afib or atrial tachyarrhythmia with variable AV conduction and BBB
Afib or atrial tachyarrhythmia and accessory pathway
Artifact

Differential Diagnosis

Normal ventricular activation results from conduction over a healthy His-Purkinje system (HPS), which manifests the fastest conduction velocity in the heart. Because of simultaneous activation of both ventricles by the rapidly conducting HPS, the normal QRS complex is narrow (generally 80 to 100 ms). Wide QRS complexes are generated when ventricular activation is altered and all (e.g., ventricular tachycardia [VT]) or part (e.g., bundle branch block [BBB]) of the ventricle is activated by slower muscle to muscle conduction.

The differential diagnosis of regular WCTs includes (1) supraventricular tachycardia (SVT) with BBB, (2) VT, (3) pre-excited tachycardia, (4) pacemaker-mediated tachycardia, and (5) hyperkalemia. Any SVT with BBB cause a WCT with either RBBB or LBBB morphology. BBB can either be fixed (preexisting) or functional (rate related) if the SVT encroaches on the bundle branch refractory period. An inability of the bundle branch to sustain 1:1 conduction causes aberration. Bundle branch refractory periods show a direct cycle length dependent relationship (i.e., longer refractory periods at slower heart rates) so that the abrupt onset of a rapid SVT during slow sinus rates (long-short sequence) predispose to aberration. Once established, BBB can persist because of concealed transseptal retrograde penetration from conducting to nonconducting bundle (transseptal linking).

Monomorphic VT is another cause of a regular WCT. Sustained VT is defined as tachycardia lasting ≥ 30 seconds or causing hemodynamic instability. Because most VTs originate from right or left ventricular muscle, QRS complexes are broad and generally manifest LBBB- or RBBB-type morphology, respectively. Certain specific VTs, however, originate from or near the HPS (e.g., bundle branch reentrant tachycardia, idiopathic LV tachycardia) and generate QRS complexes that are typical of aberration.

Pre-excited tachycardias are WCTs associated with antegrade conduction over an accessory pathway (AP). The AP can be an active participant during tachycardia (antidromic atrioventricular reentrant tachycardia) or be passively activated (bystander pre-excited tachycardia). The onset of ventricular activation from its insertion site with the AP results in broad QRS complexes that appear ventricular in origin because of muscle to muscle conduction.

Pacemaker-mediated tachycardias include sensor driven tachycardia (rate-responsive pacing), atrial tracking at the pacemaker upper rate, and pacemaker-mediated endless loop tachycardia (Figure 14.1). The common denominator to all these mechanisms is that the ventricle is paced rapidly causing a WCT. Generally, the presence of pacing stimuli establishes a paced rhythm; however, the stimulus artifact might be small or undetectable during single-lead telemetry, particularly with a bipolar pacing lead configuration. Pacing from the right and left ventricle produces LBBB- and RBBB-type morphology QRS complexes, respectively.

Severe hyperkalemia is a rare cause of a WCT that, if misdiagnosed and if left untreated, could be fatal. The loss of the P wave (sinoventricular rhythm) and the widening of the QRS complex when associated with sinus tachycardia produce a WCT that could be mistaken for slow VT. QRS widening and broad, peaked T waves create an "M pattern" in lead V4 (Figure 14.2).

The differential diagnosis of irregular WCTs includes (1) polymorphic VT, (2) atrial fibrillation (or any atrial tachyarrhythmia with variable conduction) and preexcitation, (3) atrial fibrillation (or any atrial tachyarrhythmia with variable conduction) and BBB, and (4) artifact. QRS complexes during polymorphic VT are wide and change both morphology and axis because the reentrant circuit is not stationary but migrates along the epicardial surface of the ventricle. It can occur in the setting of a long (torsade de pointes) or normal QT interval. QRS complexes during pre-excited atrial fibrillation show variable degrees of preexcitation as conduction fuses over both the HPS and AP. Pre-excited atrial fibrillation in the setting of multiple APs can mimic polymorphic VT. Atrial fibrillation with aberrant conduction also causes an irregular WCT. Atrial flutter with 1:1 AV conduction and changing patterns of RBBB and LBBB can also simulate polymorphic VT. Finally, motion artifact

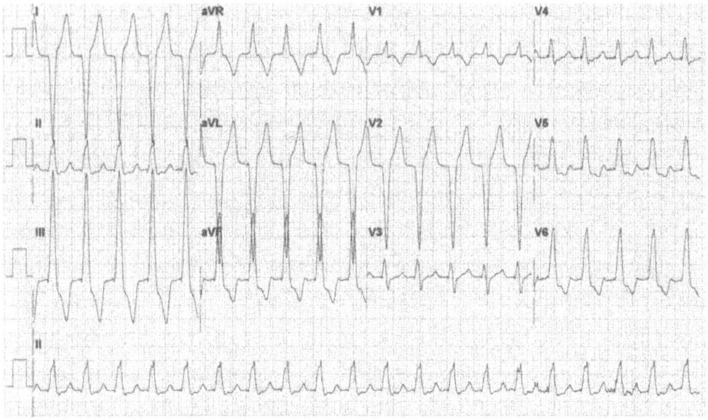

■ **Figure 14.1** 12-lead ECG showing a pacemaker-mediated tachycardia in a patient with a dual-chamber pacemaker.

Source: Goldberger ZD, Rho RW, Page RL. Approach to the diagnosis and initial management of the stable adult patient with a wide complex tachycardia. *Am J Cardiol* 2008;101:1456–1466.

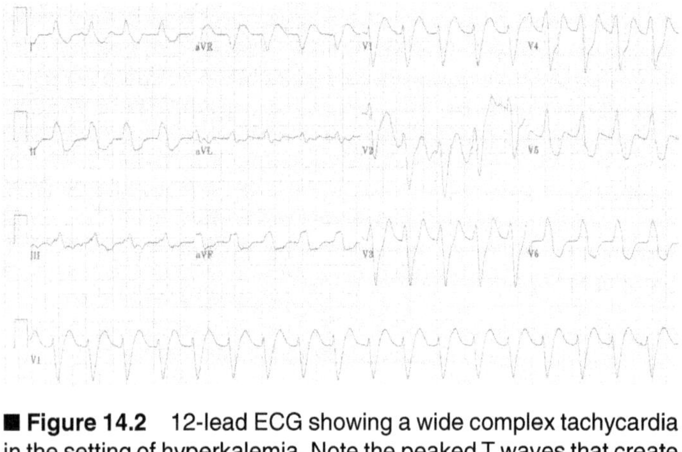

■ **Figure 14.2** 12-lead ECG showing a wide complex tachycardia in the setting of hyperkalemia. Note the peaked T waves that create an "M pattern" in lead V_4.

Source: Adapted from Eckardt L, Breithardt G, Kirchhof P. Approach to wide complex tachycardias in patients without structural heart disease. *Heart* 2006;92:704–711. Gupta AK, Thakur RK. Wide QRS complex tachycardias. *Med Clin North Am* 2001;85(2):245–266.

(e.g., brushing teeth) captured on telemetry can be mistaken for polymorphic VT. Demonstrating that sinus rhythm QRS complexes march through the recording establishes the "WCT" as artifact.

Practical Approach to Diagnosis

Although the 12-lead electrocardiogram (ECG) of the WCT is invaluable for diagnosis, a thorough understanding of the patient's medical history is equally indispensable. Diagnosis is best established by a critical analysis of the 12-lead ECG (or available rhythm strip) coupled with a detailed history and physical examination.

Clinical Diagnosis

Bayesian analysis dictates that the accuracy of a test result is dependent on the pretest probability that the patient actually has that result. The likelihood that a WCT in a young patient without structural heart disease is either an SVT with aberration or a pre-excited tachycardia is high. Conversely, a WCT in an older patient with a history of congestive heart failure and prior myocardial infarction is VT until proven otherwise. Knowledge of the patient's cardiac history (e.g., prior infarction, LV function, and cardiac surgeries) is therefore essential.

Examination findings indicating significant heart disease (e.g., chronic congestive heart failure, ICD implantation) point toward a diagnosis of VT, although such patients are also susceptible to atrial tachyarrhythmias and BBB. The specific examination finding of AV dissociation (cannon A waves in the jugular venous pulsation, variable intensity of the first heart sound) during WCT favors VT. The response of tachycardia to carotid sinus massage (if carotid bruits are absent) can be helpful because pressure to the carotid sinus bulb increases vagal tone and slows both sinus node automaticity and AV nodal conduction. Carotid sinus massage can (1) slow aberrantly conducted sinus tachycardia, (2) induce AV block during aberrantly conducted atrial flutter or tachycardia, (3) terminate aberrantly conducted SVTs (AVNRT, orthodromic AVRT), and (4) induce AV dissociation during VT.

Symptoms, hemodynamic status, and tachycardia rate are often not useful in establishing the diagnosis because of the significant overlap between SVT and VT with these parameters.

12-Lead ECG Diagnosis

Obtaining a baseline 12-lead ECG is critical. A WCT with BBB morphology identical to that during sinus rhythm is likely to be SVT (with the rare exception of bundle branch reentrant tachycardia). A WCT with a BBB width that is narrower than during sinus rhythm is likely to be VT. In the absence of a baseline ECG, there are multiple individual ECG criteria at the physician's disposal to facilitate diagnosis. These criteria primarily differentiate SVT with BBB from VT. These criteria can be divided into four categories: (1) QRS duration, (2) QRS axis, (3) QRS morphology, and the (4) atrioventricular relationship.

Individual ECG Criteria

QRS Duration

Measurements of QRS duration include the width of the intrinsicoid deflection (onset of r wave to nadir of s wave) and QRS complex, both of which are a function of the conduction velocity. Because the entire ventricle is activated by slow muscle to muscle conduction during VT but only partially (after His-Purkinje activation) during BBB, the width of the intrinsicoid deflection (first half of the QRS complex) and QRS complex are wider during VT than SVT with BBB. QRS widths exceeding 140 and 160 ms during RBBB and LBBB tachycardias, respectively, favor the diagnosis of VT.

QRS Axis

Although left anterior fascicular block (LAFB) and left posterior fascicular block (LPFB) cause left superior and right inferior axes, respectively, no hemiblock pattern causes extreme right axis deviation (right superior); therefore, a WCT with a "northwest" axis favors VT (Figure 14.3). An axis shift more than 40° from sinus rhythm also suggests VT.

QRS Morphology

BBB causes specific morphologic alterations of the QRS complex. Morphologic criteria are based on the premise that any deviation from the "typical BBB pattern" argues for VT. For RBBB WCT, a "typical RBBB aberration pattern" (triphasic QRS configuration [rSR' with r < R']) in V1 and r/s ratio > 1 in V6 favors SVT. A monophasic or biphasic R, qR, or Rsr' (R > r') in V1 and r/s ratio < 1 in V6 suggests VT. During "typical LBBB aberration pattern," the intrinsicoid deflection is narrow and a q wave is absent in V6 (because of the loss of normal left to right septal forces) (Figure 14.4); therefore, a LBBB WCT with an initial r wave > 30 ms, an onset of r wave to nadir of S wave > 60 ms, and notching of the downslope of the S wave (indicating scar) in V1 and a q wave in V6 favor ventricular tachycardia (VT). Concordance is an unusual pattern where precordial QRS complexes are either predominantly negative (negative concordance) or positive (positive concordance) and strongly supports VT. Negative concordance indicates origin

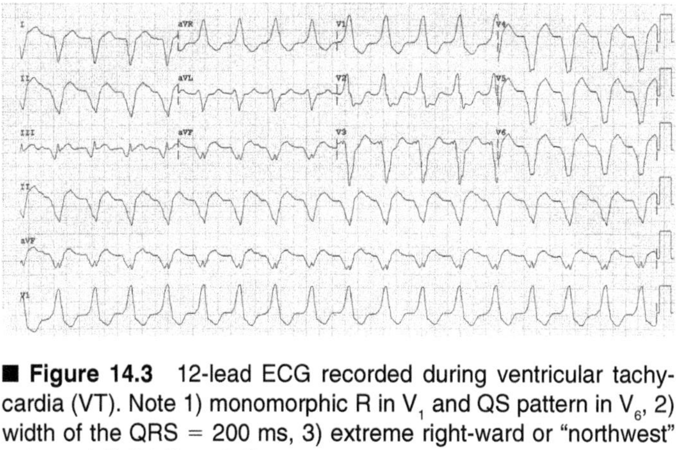

■ **Figure 14.3** 12-lead ECG recorded during ventricular tachycardia (VT). Note 1) monomorphic R in V_1 and QS pattern in V_6, 2) width of the QRS = 200 ms, 3) extreme right-ward or "northwest" axis, and 4) AV dissociation.

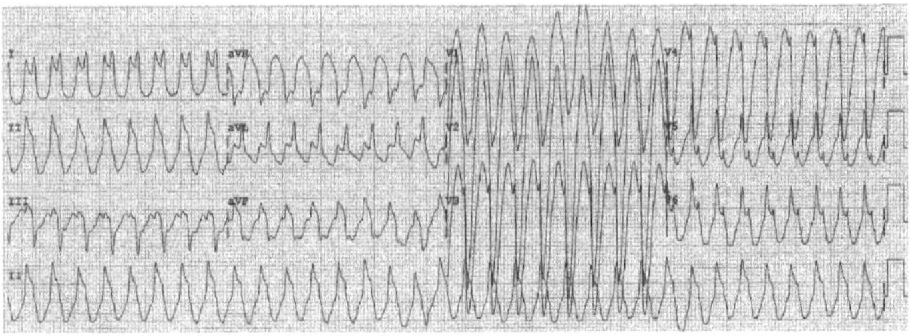

■ **Figure 14.4** 12-lead ECG of a patient in atrial flutter with 1:1 conduction and LBBB aberration.

of tachycardia from the LV apex and is specific for VT. Positive concordance indicates origin of tachycardia from the LV base and is observed with both a basal VT (Figure 14.5) or pre-excited tachycardia (as accessory pathways insert into the ventricle near the mitral annulus) (Figure 14.6).

Atrioventricular Dissociation

The presence of AV dissociation indicates that the atrium is not "driving" the ventricle and is quite specific for VT (Figures 14.3 and

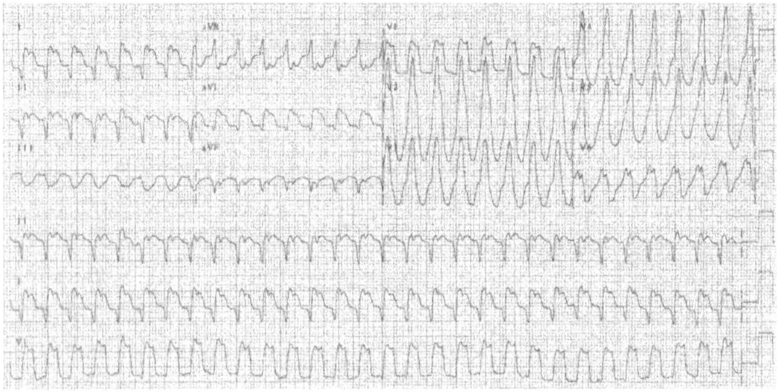

■ **Figure 14.5** 12-lead ECG recorded during ventricular tachycardia. There is positive concordance as all the QRS complexes in the precordial leads are predominantly positive.

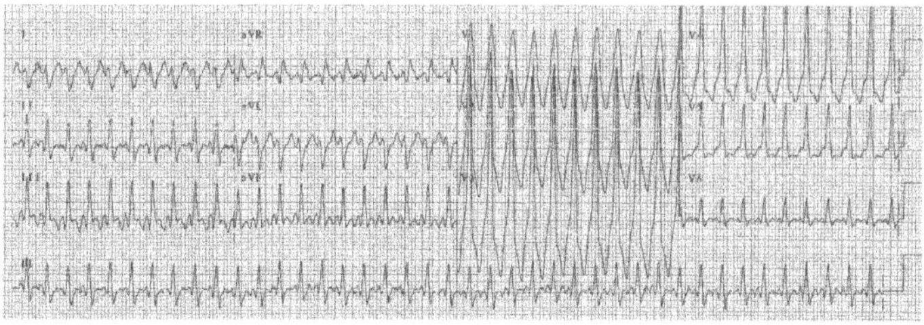

■ **Figure 14.6** 12-lead ECG recorded during a preexcited tachycardia. Note there is positive concordance of the QRS complexes in the precordial leads that resembles ventricular tachycardia.

14.7). ECG manifestations of AV dissociation are (1) P waves marching through QRS complexes, (2) fusion beats, and (3) capture beats. Although AV dissociation can occur with certain SVTs (AVNRT or junctional tachycardia with upper common final pathway block, antidromic tachycardia using a nodofascicular pathway), these are quite rare. Both fusion and capture complexes (Figure 14.7) occur when a sinus impulse conducts to the ventricle during

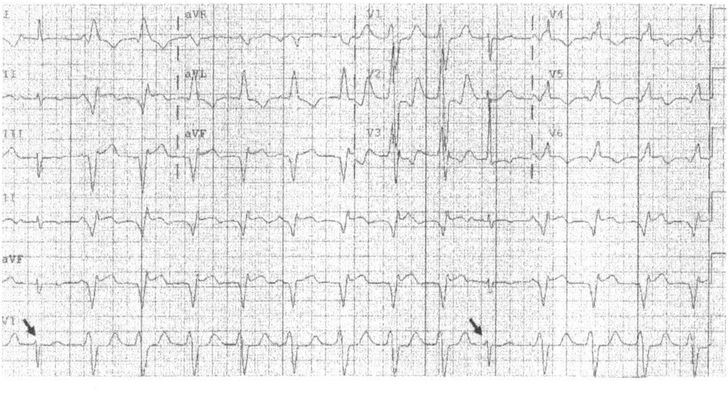

■ **Figure 14.7** 12-lead ECG recorded during "slow" ventricular tachycardia. Note 1) the initial R = 80 ms, 2) qR in lead V6, and 3) captured beats that represent normal ventricular activation via the His-Purkinje system (the narrow QRS complexes indicated by the arrows).

ongoing (generally slow) VT. Activation of the ventricle by both the sinus conducted and tachycardia complex results in a fused QRS complex intermediate in morphology between the two beats. Activation of the ventricle only by the sinus conducted complex generates a QRS morphology identical to that during sinus rhythm (capture complex).

12-Lead ECG Algorithms

A diagnosis of a WCT is best established not by analysis of any single criterion but rather collectively as a group. Various algorithms have been proposed using individual criteria in a stepwise fashion to arrive at the correct diagnosis, one of which is the Brugada algorithm (Figure 14.8). Individual qualifying criteria in the Brugada algorithm were designed to be relatively insensitive but very specific for VT with the sensitivity of the algorithm increased by the use of multiple criteria. The first qualifying criterion for VT (absence of an r/s complex in any precordial leads) is elegantly worded, as it identifies VT with positive and negative concordance, as well as precordial "qR" patterns. The second qualifying criteria for VT (r/s interval $>$ 100 ms) takes advantage of slow muscle to muscle conduction during VT that contrasts the rapid initial His-Purkinje activation during BBB. The third criterion (presence of AV dissociation) is very specific for VT, as SVT with AV dissociation is rare. The last criterion is the V1/V6 morphologic criterion when diagnosis still remains uncertain. Brugada et al. also proposed an algorithm to differentiate pre-excited tachycardia from VT. ECG diagnosis alone can be difficult because in both cases the ventricles are activated by slow muscle to muscle conduction. Because accessory pathways insert at the base of the ventricle and AP-mediated tachycardias demonstrate an obligatory 1:1 AV relationship, the following criteria favor VT: (1) predominantly negative QRS complexes in the precordial leads V4 to V6 (indicating origin from the apex of the heart), (2) the presence of QR complex in one or more of the precordial leads V2 to V6 (indicating the presence of myocardial scar), and (3) AV dissociation.

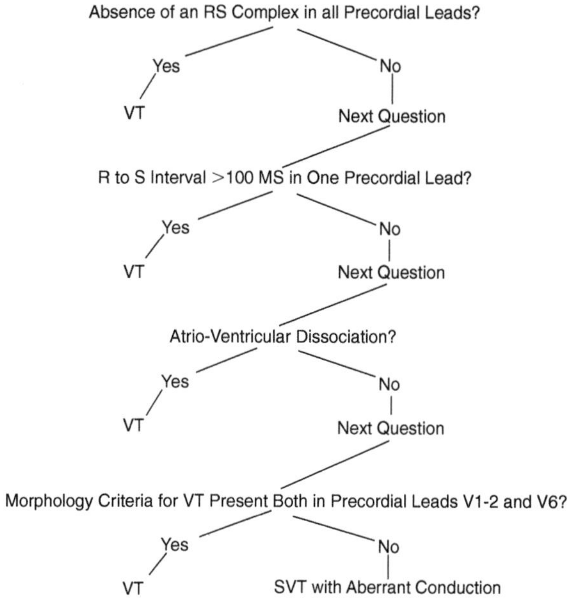

■ **Figure 14.8** The Brugada criteria for differentiation SVT with aberration from VT.

Source: Brugada P, *Circulation.* 1991;83:5.

Treatments

Acute Therapy

The initial and most important step is assessing the hemodynamic status of the patient, as outlined in the ACLS protocol. Emergent defibrillation is required for unresponsive, pulseless patients in a WCT. Management of a stable patient in VT includes (1) synchronized cardioversion after appropriate sedation or (2) intravenous (IV) amiodarone or procainamide (both of which treat SVT and VT if diagnosis is unclear). Intravenous amiodarone and procainamide dosing is as follows:

- Amiodarone bolus (150 mg IV infused over 10 minutes) followed by an infusion of 1 mg/min for 6 hours and then 0.5

mg/min. A rapid infusion of 150 mg every 10 minutes may be repeated as needed (maximum of 2.2 g in 24 hours).
- Procainamide load (17 mg/kg intravenously infused over 30 minutes) followed by an infusion of 1 to 4 mg/min. Procainamide should be used with caution in patients with cardiac and renal dysfunction.

Therapy specific for idiopathic LV VT is IV verapamil. Torsade de pointes should be treated with intravenous magnesium and possible isoproterenol infusion or transvenous pacing (to increase the ventricular rate and shorten the QT interval).

Management of the stable patient with WCT caused by SVT includes (1) vagal maneuvers (carotid sinus massage, valsalva, adenosine) to terminate tachycardia, (2) intravenous β-blocker or calcium channel blocker, (3) intravenous procainamide, or (4) synchronized cardioversion. Adenosine is given as a 6 mg IVP and followed by a 12-mg intravenous dose if unsuccessful. A second 12-mg dose could also be given if needed.

Long-Term Therapy

Long-term treatment of a WCT depends on its diagnosis. Insertion of an ICD is recommended for patients with hemodynamically unstable VT or VT in the setting of structural heart disease. Idiopathic VTs (VT without structural heart disease) and SVTs can be managed with either drug therapy or catheter ablation.

15 ■ Narrow QRS Complex Arrhythmias

Matthew Stopper, MD
Daniel Frisch, MD

- Cardiac arrhythmias refer to impulse formation that originates outside of the sinus node. They may be classified as either wide complex or narrow complex based on the width of the QRS complex on 12-lead electrocardiogram (ECG). The narrow complex tachycardias (NCTs) include arrhythmias with a QRS complex < 120 ms with an origin within or above the atrioventricular (AV) node and ventricular activation via the normal His-Purkinje system. Sources of origin include the sinus node (SN), atrial tissue (including areas of connection with thoracic veins), AV node, His bundle, or combinations of these structures.
- The term supraventricular tachycardia (SVT) refers to a group of paroxysmal NCTs that have sudden onset and termination, have a regular cycle length, and may be recurrent and episodic. SVT includes AV nodal reciprocating tachycardia (AVNRT), AV reciprocating tachycardia (AVRT), and atrial tachycardia (AT), including focal, multifocal (e.g., multifocal atrial tachycardia [MAT]), reentrant (e.g., SN reentry tachycardia [SNRT]), and triggered mechanisms. Sinus tachycardia (ST) and inappropriate sinus tachycardia (IST) are generally more incessant without sudden onset or termination. Atrial fibrillation (AF) and atrial flutter (AFL) may be either paroxysmal or incessant, although they are described as having sudden onset and termination if these arrhythmias are symptomatic in a given individual. Although they are SVTs, AF and AFL are not generally included under the SVT umbrella because of their characteristic and recognizable 12-lead ECG patterns of irregularly

irregular ventricular activity and "saw tooth" flutter waves, respectively (Table 15.1).

Epidemiology

- AF and AFL are the most common of all arrhythmias, affecting 2.2 million people in America and accounting for one

Table 15.1 Differential Diagnosis and Mechanisms for Narrow Complex Tachycardias

NCT	Mechanism(s)
Sinus tachycardia (ST)	Normal physiology
Inappropriate sinus tachycardia (IST)	Enhanced abnormal automaticity
Sinoatrial reentry tachycardia (SNRT)	Reentry
Atrial fibrillation (AF)	Enhanced abnormal automaticity/reentry
Atrial flutter (A. Flutter)	Reentry with the circuit generally confined to atrial tissue
Atrial tachycardia	Enhanced abnormal automaticity, reentry, or triggered activity
Multifocal atrial tachycardia (MAT)	Enhanced abnormal automaticity
AV nodal reciprocating tachycardia (AVNRT)	Reentry via dual pathways within the AV node without atrial or ventricular tissue contributing to the circuit
Atrioventricular reciprocating tachycardia (AVRT)	Reentry via an accessory pathway with atrial tissue, the AV node, His bundle, ventricular tissue, and accessory pathway all being obligate parts of the circuit
Junctional ectopic tachycardia (JET)	Enhanced abnormal automaticity

third of hospitalizations for heart rhythm disturbances and a per patient cost of approximately $3,600 and at least 7.9 billion total dollars annually.

- AF and AFL tend to present in older patients with structural heart disease.
- Rates tend to be slower on average than other NCTs (usually < 155 beats per minute).

- The prevalence of SVT in the general population is 2.25/1,000 persons with an incidence of 35/100,000 person-years.
  - AVNRT is the most common SVT (60%), followed by AVRT (30%) and AT (10%). Rare arrhythmias such as junctional ectopic tachycardia (JET) or variant accessory-pathway mediated tachycardias (e.g., nodofascicular tachycardias) account for a much smaller percentage.
  - SVT tends to present at younger ages in patients without known structural heart disease (mean age of 37 years).
  - AVNRT is more common in women (70%), with a mean age of onset at 32 years.
  - Accessory pathway-mediated SVT (AVRT) is more common in young men (mean age of 23 years).
  - Older age and structural heart disease make AT more likely.

Mechanisms

- Reentry, triggered activity, and enhanced automaticity are the electrophysiological mechanisms responsible for all arrhythmias, including the NCTs, with some NCTs having more than one mechanism contributing to their initiation and/ or maintenance.
  - Reentry describes a phenomenon produced when an electrical impulse repetitively propagates through a circuit of myocardial tissue. The specific set of circumstances required to produce a reentrant tachycardia is as follows:

        - There must be two distinct limbs of the circuit separated by a functional or anatomic obstacle but connected proximally and distally.
        - At least one limb of the circuit must be able to conduct in a retrograde direction.
        - The limbs must have different electrophysiological properties. There must be a condition producing transient unidirectional block in one limb of the pathway with sufficiently slow conduction in the other limb (slow limb) to allow recovery such that retrograde conduction in the previously blocked limb may occur. This retrograde conduction must in turn be slow enough to allow recovery of the slow limb of the circuit, allowing the impulse to "reenter" the slow limb and propagate in a continuous circuit (Figure 15.1).
    - Triggered activity occurs when disturbances during repolarization known as afterdepolarizations are of sufficient magnitude to exceed threshold and "trigger" an early action potential.
    - Enhanced automaticity occurs when cells exhibit enhanced phase 4 diastolic depolarization and an increased firing rate. When the rate exceeds that of the SN, the cells will overdrive the SN and may produce tachycardia. This phenomenon may be observed in cells with pacemaker function such as the AV node or in myocardial cells that do not normally have pacemaker function in the setting of injury of ischemia.

General Diagnostic Approach

- Initially, a determination should be made as to the hemodynamic stability of the patient and whether signs or symptoms are present that would require emergent treatment of the tachycardia such as hypotension, shock, dyspnea, chest discomfort, or altered level of consciousness. If the patient is

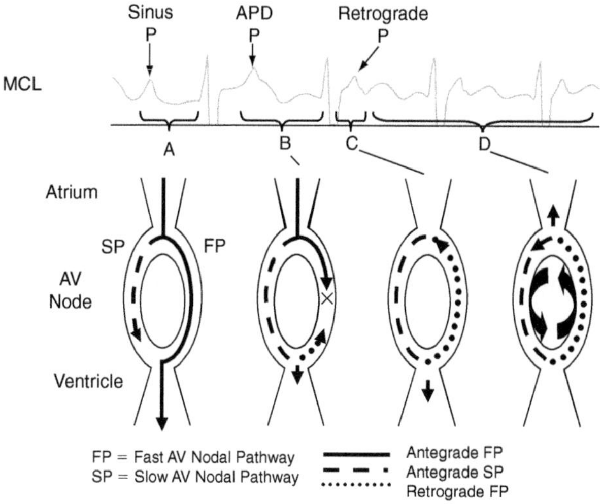

■ **Figure 15.1** Schematic and tracing of dual pathway physiology and initiation of AVNRT. **(A)** Normal Sinus Rhythm with ventricular activation via the fast pathway. **(B)** An Atrial premature depolarization comes early enough to block in the fast pathway, but conducts to the ventricle via the slow pathway and a markedly prolonged PR interval. **(C)** The fast pathway has now recovered, and the impulse is able to return to the atria retrograde via the fast pathway. **(D)** Perpetuation of AVNRT.

unstable, then advanced cardiac life support (ACLS) protocols are appropriate. If the patient is stable, then a systematic approach is useful to discern the involved sites and mechanisms of arrhythmia.

- History and physical exam
  - Common symptoms include "irregular heart beat," palpitations or "skipped beats," lightheadedness, dyspnea, fatigue, chest discomfort, presyncope, and rarely syncope.
  - Important historical factors include the rapidity of onset and/or termination, the number of episodes, and if the tachycardia is incessant, symptoms of congestive heart failure.

  - A physical exam should initially be focused on the hemodynamic stability of the patient and signs of structural heart disease and congestive heart failure. If the patient is stable, some clues on history and physical may suggest specific diagnoses.
  - Tachycardias that result in a lack of AV synchrony or near simultaneous contraction of the atria and ventricles and thus atrial contraction against closed AV valves will produce atrial stretch and possible symptoms of polyuria due to release of atrial natriuretic peptide. Such patients may also complain of pulsations in the neck and exhibit pronounced single jugular venous pulsations or the "frog sign" on physical exam. These findings may be suggestive of AVNRT or AVRT.
- A 12-lead ECG or failing that a rhythm strip should be obtained whenever the patient's hemodynamic status permits. The 12-lead ECG will often narrow or yield a definitive diagnosis (Table 15.2). A comparison to the patient's baseline 12-lead ECG, if available, is helpful and may point to a particular etiology by displaying changes in P-wave and QRS axis and morphology such as the presence of a manifest extranodal accessory pathway (i.e., pre-excitation).
- Regularity of the tachycardia should be determined.
  - If the tachycardia is irregularly irregular (i.e., no pattern of regular ventricular activation), the rhythm is likely AF or MAT.
    - AF will lack any discernible or organized atrial activity.
    - MAT will display at least three distinct P-wave morphologies and is commonly seen in patients with severe pulmonary pathology.
    - AFL with variable AV conduction may have an irregular appearance; however, there is commonly a pattern to the tachycardia as the R-R intervals will be multiples of the underlying flutter wave frequency. AFL with fixed AV conduction will be regular and will be diagnosed based

Table 15.2 Steps and Clues for Diagnosis of SVT Based on 12-Lead ECG

Evaluation in All Patients
Identify the P wave if possible
Determine the P wave axis
Determine the P wave morphology
Determine the P wave relationship to the QRS
Determine the RP and PR intervals
Examine closely for QRS alternans
When Definitive Diagnosis Is Not Evident
Obtain an old ECG
Run a long 12-lead rhythm strip ECG
Maximize ECG gain to accentuate P waves (20 mm/mV)
Maximize ECG paper speed to accentuate P waves (50 mm/s)
Use vagal maneuvers and adenosine
Search for any zones of transition
Search for any perturbation in cycle length or QRS
Search for any perturbation in RP or PR interval
Note the influence of BBB, AV block, or VPDs on the SVT

on identification of the flutter (F) waves typical of this rhythm.

- P-wave morphology—If the tachycardia is regular, the next step is to identify atrial activity with special attention to P-wave morphology, timing, and relationship to the QRS complexes. If P waves are not evident on the tracing, vagal maneuvers (e.g., carotid sinus massage) or administration of short-acting AV nodal blocking agents such as adenosine may help identify atrial activity and/or terminate the tachycardia. Given the rates of some tachycardias, the P waves may be fused with the QRS complex or T wave; therefore, one must be vigilant in searching for high-frequency deflections superimposed on these portions of the tracings. A comparison to baseline sinus rhythm ECGs can be useful.

- Normal sinus P waves are directed leftward and inferiorly (i.e., + in I, II, and AVF) and biphasic in V1, lasting no longer than 0.12 sec in lead II.
- P waves during tachycardia identical to a patient's normal sinus P waves suggest ST, IST, or SNRT, as the initiating impulse must be at or near the patient's SN.
- P waves that are inverted in leads II and AVF suggest retrograde activation of the atria from either the AV node or an extranodal accessory pathway and are characteristic of AVNRT and AVRT.
  - In typical AVNRT, the atrial activation is via a retrograde fast AV nodal pathway, and thus, the P wave may be fused with the QRS complex and may resemble an r' in V1 or a small terminal s wave in II, III, and AVF. Because atrial activation occurs in the midline, P waves are often narrower than SN-derived impulses (see Figure 15.2).
- In AT, the P-wave morphology will be determined by the site of origin of the ectopic focus in the atria. If the focus is near the SN, the P-wave morphology will be similar to the sinus P wave. Likewise, if the focus is low in the atria and near the AV node, the P waves may be similar to the retrograde P waves characteristic of AVNRT. Furthermore, by analyzing the P-wave morphology in V1 and AVL, a determination as to the chamber of origin can generally be made. A P wave that is positive in V1 and negative in AVL suggests a left atrial origin to the tachycardia, whereas the converse is generally true for an AT with a right atrial focus.

- Vagal maneuvers—When atrial activity can not be readily identified, maneuvers and medications aimed at causing transient slowing or block in the AV node may aid in making

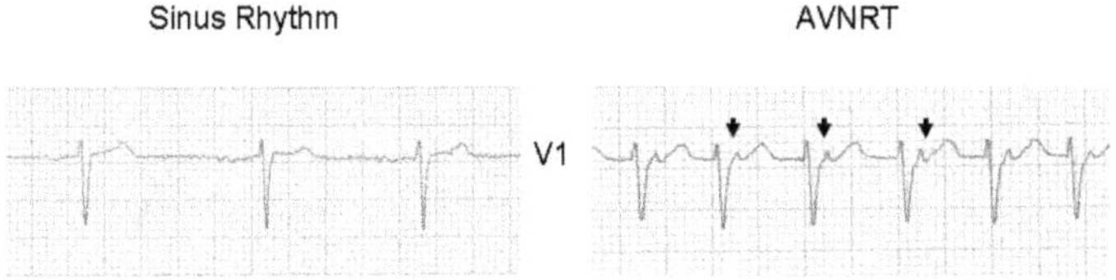

■ **Figure 15.2** Examples of the same patient in Sinus Rhythm and during typical AVNRT. The retrograde activation of the atria via the fast pathway is manifest on the 12 lead ECG as "retrograde" P-waves in the terminal portion of the QRS complex—often referred to as "pseudo S waves" in lead II, and a "pseudo r" (arrows) in V1.

the diagnosis. In cases in which the reentrant circuit relies on AV nodal conduction, interrupting AV nodal conduction will often terminate the tachycardia. These maneuvers should be done during a continuous 12-lead ECG recording, as subsequent analysis may reveal a diagnosis. Physiologically, all vagal maneuvers cause transient slowing of the rate of SN depolarization and cause slower conduction and longer refractory periods in the AV node. Vagal maneuvers and adenosine may have no effect on the tachycardia, may cause transient slowing or block with eventual recovery of prior ventricular rate and conduction, or may terminate the arrhythmia. Even if the tachycardia does not break, the response to vagal maneuvers or adenosine may help narrow the differential diagnosis (see Table 15.3). These interventions should be done with proper monitoring, nearby resuscitative equipment, and the patient in the supine position, as abrupt changes in blood pressure and heart rate may occur.

- Effective vagal maneuvers include carotid sinus massage (CSM), the Valsalva maneuver, and coughing.
  - CSM is accomplished by placing two fingers over the carotid bulb, which is usually located inferiorly to the angle of the jaw at the level of the thyroid cartilage. Firm constant pressure is then applied for 5 to 10 seconds.

Table 15.3 Effect of Vagal Maneuvers and Adenosine on NCTs

Rhythm	Effect of Vagal Maneuvers or Adenosine
Sinus tachycardia	Gradual, temporary slowing of HR
Atrial tachycardia	AV block or rarely termination
AVNRT	Possible termination
AVRT	Possible termination
Atrial fibrillation	Slowing or no effect
Atrial flutter	Persistent flutter waves with AV block

  - CSM is generally well tolerated but is contraindicated in the setting of a carotid bruit, history of stroke or transient ischemic attack, recent myocardial infarction, and history of ventricular tachycardia or fibrillation.
  - If CSM is initially unsuccessful, it may be repeated on the contralateral side.
- The Valsalva maneuver is accomplished by placing the patient in the supine position and having him or her attempt to exhale forcefully at a normal tidal volume (i.e., without a deep breath before the maneuver) against a closed glottis. This straining should be held for 10 seconds, after which the patient should resume normal respirations.
  - An adequate Valsalva maneuver should result in distended neck veins, marked increased tension in the abdominal muscles, and flushing of the face.
- Adenosine may be used if vagal maneuvers fail to treat or diagnose the underlying rhythm.
- Adenosine is a potent A1 receptor agonist with a half life of less than 10 seconds in the circulation. If given peripherally, it is given as an initial, rapid 6-mg bolus followed by a rapid saline flush with the patient in the supine position under continuous monitoring. If the

initial dose fails, two repeat doses of 12 mg may be given several minutes apart.

- Caution should be used if adenosine is being given through a central venous catheter, in patients with asthma, or in heart transplant patients due to autonomic denervation. A reduced initial dose of 1 to 3 mg should be used in these situations.
- Side effects of adenosine include prolonged sinus pauses, prolonged high-grade AV block, facial flushing, hypotension, and in 10% to 15% of patients, atrial fibrillation. Atrial fibrillation from adenosine is usually transient but may carry more risk if there is an accessory pathway capable of rapid conduction from the atria to the ventricles.

• P-wave timing and RP relationship—After the P wave has been identified using the previously mentioned techniques, a determination should be made as to where the P wave falls relative to the QRS complex in the associated cardiac cycle. In a short R-P tachycardia, the P wave falls closer to the prior QRS complex. The P wave falls closer to the after QRS complex in long R-P tachycardia (see Figure 15.3).
  - Short R-P tachycardias are either due to rapid retrograde activation of the atria, as in typical AVNRT and AVRT, or prolonged antegrade activation of the ventricles, as in AT with delayed AV conduction.
  - Long R-P tachycardias are either due to delayed retrograde activation of the atria, as in atypical AVNRT and PJRT (i.e., AVRT via a slowly conducting accessory pathway), or normal/accelerated antegrade activation of the ventricles, as in AT with normal AV conduction.
  - When the P wave is equidistant from the QRS complexes, either atrial flutter, AVNRT with 2:1 AV conduction, or AT with 2:1 AV conduction should be considered.

• RP variation and block

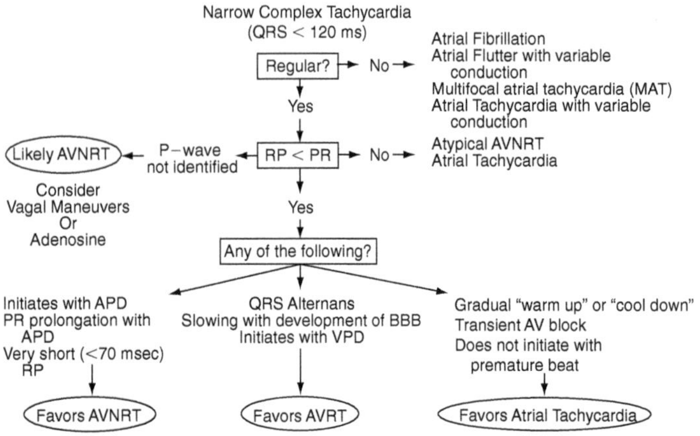

■ **Figure 15.3** Algorithm for diagnosing NCT. AVNRT—Atrio ventricular-node reciprocating tachycardia. AVRT—Atrioventricular reciprocating tachycardia

- The presence of AV dissociation or AV block excludes the possibility of AVRT as the atria and ventricles are obligate parts of the tachycardia circuit and block in either of these structures will terminate the tachycardia.
- In AT, atrial depolarization drives ventricular activation (i.e., the P wave drives the QRS but is not mechanistically tied to it); therefore, spontaneous variations in RP interval with relatively fixed PR intervals favor the diagnosis of AT. If spontaneous variations in P-wave timing precede variations in QRS timing, AT is the most likely diagnosis.

• Initiation, termination, and the development of bundle branch block
  - Initiation with a premature beat favors reentry as the tachycardia mechanism. The implication is that there is block in the usual faster antegrade pathway, conduction down a slower antegrade pathway, and time for recovery for a retrograde pathway to occur (either the initially blocked pathway or another pathway capable of retrograde conduction).

  - AVNRT is typically initiated with an atrial premature depolarization (APD) with subsequent PR prolongation (or "jump") with the initiating P wave having different morphology than subsequent P waves (see Figure 15-1).
  - AVRT is typically initiated with a ventricular premature depolarization (VPD).
  - Slowing of the tachycardia cycle length with the development of bundle branch block is a specific finding for AVRT via an accessory pathway ipsilateral to the blocked bundle. In this case, the cycle length slows because of block in the ipsilateral bundle branch requiring antegrade conduction to occur over the contralateral bundle branch to complete the reentrant circuit.
  - AT often starts in the absence of an APD and without PR prolongation. If the mechanism is increased automatically, there may be a gradual "warm up" or increase in rate after initiation and a gradual slowing or "cool down" before termination.
  - If the tachycardia ends with a P wave (i.e., atrial activation), the diagnosis is likely AVRT or AVNRT. For AT to terminate in this fashion, it would require the unlikely scenario of termination of the tachycardia with simultaneous and unrelated block in the AV node.
- QRS alternans—Although insensitive, the presence of QRS alternans greater than 1 mm in an SVT that has been present for at least 10 seconds at a rate less than 180 BPM is highly specific for AVRT.

Treatment

General Considerations

- Whenever possible, arrhythmia-specific acute and chronic treatment should be initiated. Initial consideration should be given to ruling out sinus tachycardia with another or primary cause of hypotension such as septic shock or hypovolemia

(i.e., gastrointestinal bleeding). Again, a 12-lead ECG is invaluable for establishing a diagnosis.
- If the tachycardia appears to be the primary driver of hemodynamic instability, vagal maneuvers may be briefly tried, followed by IV adenosine. If immediate therapy is required, direct current cardioversion (DCCV) should not be delayed.
- Longer acting intravenous agents such as calcium channel blockers (diltiazem or verapamil) or β-blockers (metoprolol) may be employed for rate control in the hemodynamically stable patient, but care should be used if both agents are used concomitantly, as bradycardia and hypotension may result.

Diagnosis and Management of Specific Arrhythmias

Sinus Tachycardia

- Sinus tachycardia is an increase in the sinus rate to greater than 100 impulses per minute secondary to an appropriate stimulus. Generally, the SN increases its rate of firing in response to exercise or adrenergic arousal. Pathologic stimuli that increase SN firing include fever, hypovolemia, sepsis, and thyrotoxicosis. Prescribed or illicit stimulants such as caffeine, theophylline, cocaine, and amphetamines may also cause sinus tachycardia.
- When sinus tachycardia is suspected, a vigilant search for the underlying cause is essential. After the underlying pharmacologic or pathologic stimulus is identified, the tachycardia should resolve.

Inappropriate Sinus Tachycardia

- Inappropriate sinus tachycardia is an increase in the rate of SN firing that is out of proportion to any underlying intrinsic or extrinsic physiologic stimulus. The P wave is identical to the P wave in sinus rhythm, and occult systemic causes of sinus tachycardia such as thyrotoxicosis or pheochromocytoma must be carefully excluded.

- The onset of tachycardia is nonparoxysmal, and often there is nocturnal resumption of normal SN firing rates.
- Treatment is aimed at symptom control, and β-blockers are generally first-line therapy.

Atrial Fibrillation

- Atrial fibrillation is an atrial arrhythmia caused by disorganized and chaotic electrical activity within the atrial tissue. As the electrical activity is generally of low amplitude, atrial activity may be difficult to detect on surface ECG, but the arrhythmia is immediately recognizable by the irregularly irregular ventricular response. Depending on the health of the AV node and concomitant drugs that may block or slow AV nodal conduction, the ventricular rate may range considerably (Figure 15.4).
- Clinically, it is useful to classify AF in one of four ways:
  - Paroxysmal (PAF)—AF that has occurred more than once, but terminated spontaneously within 7 days of onset.
  - Persistent—AF that has lasted for more than 7 days but less than a year without spontaneous termination.

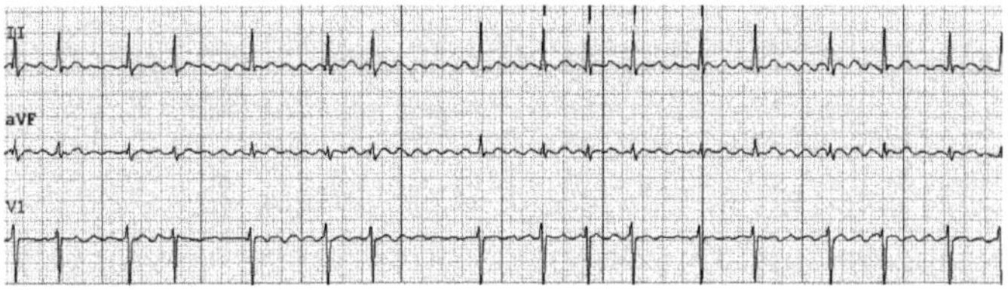

■ **Figure 15.4** Coarse Atrial Fibrillation. Note the chaotic atrial activity evident by the finely undulating baseline. While the baseline resembles flutter waves, there is significant variation in morphology, no fixed relationship with the QRS complexes, and an irregularly irregular QRS pattern.

  - Long-standing persistent—AF that has lasted more than a year without spontaneous termination.
  - Permanent—AF that has lasted for more than 1 year or AF in which either cardioversion has failed or a decision has been made not to restore sinus rhythm.
- Risk factors for the development of AF include advancing age, valvular disease, congestive heart failure, left atrial enlargement, and systemic hypertension.
- Treatment of AF generally centers on acute management with either subsequent attempts at rhythm control (i.e., medications to prevent recurrence of AF), rate control, and prevention of thromboembolism from stasis and clotting of blood in the mechanically discoordinated atria. There is no clear survival advantage to either a rate control or rhythm control strategy and the chosen strategy will depend on the clinical characteristics, symptoms, and preferences of each individual patient.
- Approach to newly discovered AF (see Figure 15.5).
  - All patients with newly diagnosed AF should have a thorough history and physical, with particular attention to symptoms, whether the duration AF is less than 48 hours, greater than 48 hours, or unknown. A 12-lead ECG and blood tests for thyroid, liver, and kidney dysfunction should be obtained, whereas a transthoracic echocardiogram to identify valvular or structural heart disease may elucidate predisposing structural heart disease for AF and supply important information for subsequent management and pharmacotherapy/anticoagulation.
  - After AF has been discovered and potential systemic causes have been determined and treated, a decision should be made whether to pursue a strategy that aims to control the ventricular rate but allow the AF to continue versus a strategy that seeks to convert the rhythm back to sinus rhythm. The need for anticoagulation is dictated by the patient's long-term risk of thromboembolism versus their risk of

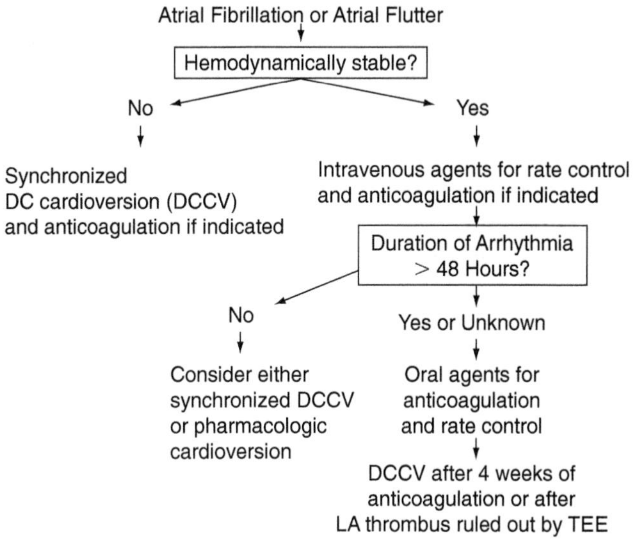

■ **Figure 15.5** Algorithm for restoration of sinus rhythm in patients with atrial fibrillation and atrial flutter.

significant bleeding and is independent of the strategy used and of the type of AF (e.g., paroxysmal or persistent).

- Cardioversion
- AF of less than 48 hours duration is generally not thought to have existed long enough for acute thrombus to form in the atria (particularly the left atrial appendage); therefore, if occurrence of AF is certain to be within this time window, cardioversion can be performed without anticoagulation or TEE before or after the cardioversion.
- Urgent DCCV—If the patient is hemodynamically unstable, immediate synchronized DCCV should be considered. Higher initial voltages increase the chances of successful DCCV, as do anterior/posterior positioning of the cardioversion pads.
    - If the onset of AF has been less than 48 hours, immediate DCCV may be performed without delay for

anticoagulation. Subsequent anticoagulation may be based on the patient's long-term risk of thromboembolism (TE).

- If the onset of AF is longer than 48 hours or is unknown but the patient requires immediate DCCV for hemodynamic instability, concomitant bolus and infusion of unfractionated heparin should be administered with a partial thromboplastin time of 1.5 to 2.0 times the upper limit of normal. Thereafter, warfarin should be administered for goal INR of 2.0 to 3.0 for at least 3 to 4 weeks and longer if indicated.

- Nonurgent cardioversion—If the patient has significant symptoms or has difficulty with rate control, it is reasonable to attempt either pharmacologic or direct-current CV. Regardless of the mode of cardioversion, consideration must be given to the duration of AF and need for anticoagulation.
  - If the duration of AF is greater than 48 hours or unknown, the patient should be anticoagulated with warfarin for at least 3 to 4 weeks prior to any attempt at cardioversion with continuation for at least 4 weeks after successful cardioversion.
  - Alternatively, a transesophageal echocardiogram may be performed to exclude the clot in the left atrial appendage. The patient still should be therapeutically anticoagulated at the time of cardioversion with a subsequent 4 weeks of warfarin therapy at goal INR of 2.0 to 3.0.
  - Pharmacologic cardioversion may be accomplished with agents such as ibutilide, dofetilide, flecainide, propafenone, or amiodarone.
    - Ibutilide, dofetilide, flecainide, and propafenone must be initiated in the hospital and are generally reserved for patients without structural or ischemic heart disease. Ibutilide may be used in patients with mildly depressed LV systolic function, and dofetilide may be used in patients with severe LV dysfunction. Only ibutilide is available in an intravenous form in the United States.

Concomitant use of β-blockers or calcium channel blockers is generally used to avoid rapid ventricular rates if the AF is converted to AFL by these agents.

- Amiodarone may be initiated for the pharmacologic conversion of AF in patients with known structural or ischemic heart disease. Although amiodarone is less proarrhythmic than the previously mentioned agents, its long-term use may be limited by various toxicities, including liver, thyroid, or pulmonary side effects.

- Rate control
  - In the hemodynamically stable patient with AF, the initial management is often aimed at controlling the ventricular rate.
  - Often intravenous calcium channel blockers (verapamil, diltiazem) or β-blockers (metoprolol, esmolol) are the initial agents of choice for rate control. Digoxin may be considered if a patient's blood pressure cannot tolerate other agents. Attention should be paid to comorbidities that may limit the use of these medications. β-Blockers may adversely affect patients with reactive airway disease; calcium-channel blockers may exacerbate peripheral edema, and digoxin may lead to toxic effects in patients with renal dysfunction.
  - For chronic rate control, oral calcium channel blockers and β-blockers are the agents of choice. Various short- and long-acting formulations are available. Digoxin may be considered orally for long-term management of resting heart rate but is a poor rate control agent when used alone.
  - If pharmacotherapy is insufficient at controlling rate and symptoms or if the side effects of pharmacotherapy are intolerable, AV nodal ablation with subsequent permanent pacemaker placement may be considered.
- Maintenance of sinus rhythm
  - In appropriate patients who are symptomatic while in AF, antiarrhythmics agents may be used chronically after

cardioversion to help maintain sinus rhythm. The use of these agents must be carefully considered as they often have either significant potential toxicity or proarrhythmic effects.

- Amiodarone and to a lesser extent the β-blockers bisoprolol and atenolol have been shown to prevent the recurrence of AF and are generally safe in patients with heart failure, left ventricular hypertrophy, and coronary disease. Amiodarone, however, has many associated extracardiac toxicities.
- Dofetilide, disopyramide, sotalol, flecainide, and propafenone have also been shown to reduce the recurrence of AF. Although these agents have fewer extracardiac toxicities, they often cannot be used with concomitant coronary disease, and care must be taken to avoid their potential proarrhythmic effects.

- When antiarrhythmic agents are unsuccessful and patients are symptomatic, catheter ablation may be considered. This procedure, which attempts to modify the left atrium to make it unable to support atrial fibrillation, centers around the electrical isolation of the pulmonary veins. Although techniques, patient selection, and evidence are being accumulated, patients best suited for the procedure are those without LA dilation who have paroxysmal AF.
- Anticoagulation and prevention of thromboembolism
- As noted previously, the degree and mode of anticoagulation should be based on the risk of thromboembolism balanced against a given patient's risk of bleeding and not the type of AF nor the type of rhythm-control strategy employed.
  - Current recommendations are that any patient without a contraindication and more than one moderate risk factor for TE should be anticoagulated with warfarin with an INR of 2.0–3.0 (see Figure 15.6).

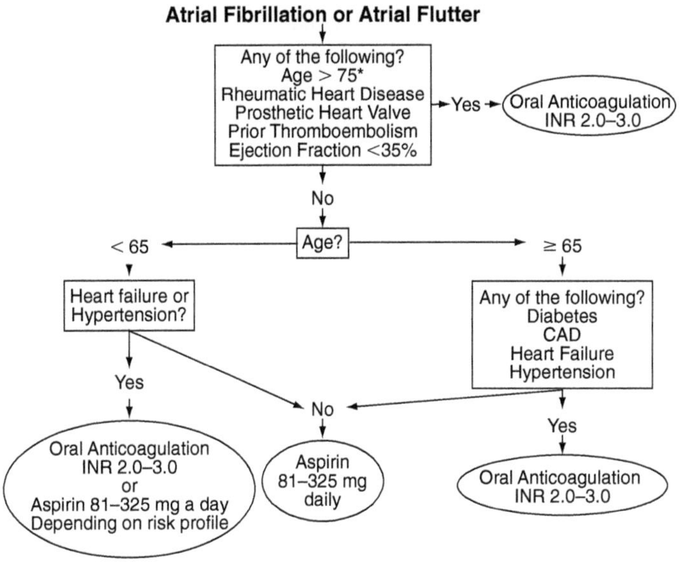

■ **Figure 15.6** Algorithm for anticoagulation in atrial fibrillation and atrial flutter. *Aspirin 81–325 mg a day is reasonable option for men age > 75 with no other risk factors or heart disease.

- In patients who are low risk for TE or in whom there is a contraindication for warfarin therapy, aspirin at doses from 81 to 325 mg are reasonable.
- In patients who have exactly 1 moderate risk factor for TE, either warfarin or aspirin at the previously mentioned doses may be initiated. Other risk factors as well as patient and physician preference may help guide decisions in this category.

Atrial Flutter

- Typical atrial flutter, or more specifically cavo-tricuspid-isthmus–dependent atrial flutter, is an organized atrial arrhythmia in which a circuit navigates the tricuspid annulus and causes rapid regular atrial depolarizations, often at atrial rates between 250 and 350 beats per minute.

- Counterclockwise flutter—In the prototypic form, the arrhythmia is sustained by a counterclockwise re-entry circuit around the tricuspid annulus requiring passage through a narrow strip of atrial tissue between the tricuspid annulus and inferior vena cava (i.e., the cavo-tricuspid-isthmus). This pattern of recurrent atrial activation leads to the typical flutter or F wave, which has a negative deflection in the inferior frontal leads and positive deflection in V1. Typically, the flutter waves are also negative in V6 (see Figure 15.7).
- Clockwise flutter—In the less common cavo-tricuspid-isthmus–dependent atrial flutter, clockwise flutter, the anatomic circuit is unchanged, but the direction of rotation around the tricuspid annulus is reversed, leading to predominantly positive F waves in the inferior frontal leads and a negative deflection in V1.
- Atypical flutter—Atrial flutter that does not circulate around the tricuspid annulus is considered atypical. The circuit may be in a different part of the tricuspid annulus or in the left atrium.

• Treatment—The treatment and recommendations for AFL are similar to AF. An attempt should be made to achieve ventricular rate control using calcium channel blockers or β-blockers. As the inputs into the AV node are more regular

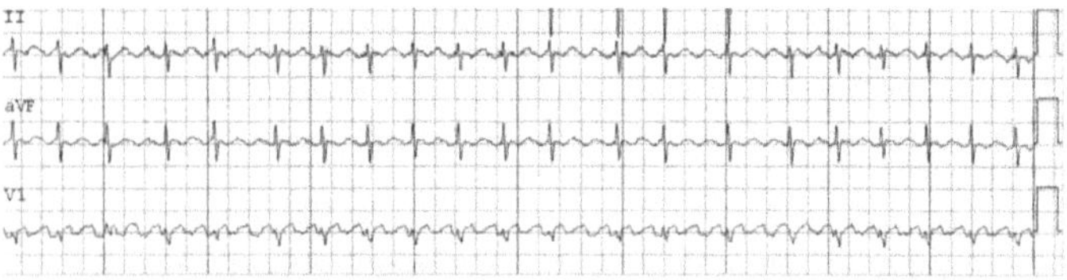

■ **Figure 15.7** Typical counterclockwise isthmus dependent atrial flutter with variable conduction. Note the negative f-wave in lead II, and the positive F-wave in V1.

with AFL because of the well-defined anatomic circuit, the ventricular rate can be more difficult to control than in AF.

- DCCV—For hemodynamically unstable patients, immediate DCCV should be performed. Lower energies (50 to 100 J) are often successful at terminating AFL.
- Maintenance of sinus rhythm—The same pharmacologic agents recommended for the maintenance of sinus rhythm in AF may be used in AFL. Caution must be used, however, as the Vaughn-Williams class IC agents (flecainide, propafenone), as they may slow the rate of flutter and allowing one to one ventricular activation with rates in excess of 200 beats per minute. If IC agents are used, they must be combined with AV nodal blockade with either a calcium channel blocker or β-blocker.
- Anticoagulation—The recommendations with regard to anticoagulation are the same as listed previously for anticoagulation in AF.
- Catheter ablation—As the underlying mechanism for most AFL is a well-defined anatomic pathway in the right atrium, catheter ablation is safe and highly successful at terminating flutter and preventing recurrence. This is accomplished by placing ablation lesions between the tricuspid annulus and the inferior vena cava or cavotricuspid isthmus. Catheter ablation may be considered as first-line therapy even for a first episode of well tolerated AFL. Unfortunately, up to 50% of patients who undergo successful catheter ablation of AFL will develop AF within 2 years.

MAT

- MAT is an irregular tachycardia that is often seen in patients with severe underlying pulmonary disease or electrolyte abnormalities. The characteristic ECG reveals an irregular NCT with at least three different P-wave morphologies.

- Treatment of MAT is generally aimed at optimizing the underlying pulmonary insult or electrolyte disturbance.
    - Rate control—Calcium channel blockers such as diltiazem and verapamil are the mainstays of treatment for MAT, as β-blockers often cannot be used because of underlying pulmonary disease.
    - Rhythm control—Antiarrhythmic medications are generally not effective in this arrhythmia, and there is no role for either DCCV or catheter ablation, as the rapid atrial activity may arise from multiple sites within either the left or right atrium.

Atrial Tachycardia

- Atrial tachycardia is a regular NCT that arises from an ectopic focus in either the left or right atrium (see Figure 15.8). The underlying electrophysiologic mechanism may be due to re-entry, triggered activity, or increased abnormal automaticity. Though re-entry may be the mechanism, the circuit is usually small and does not involve the AV node or ventricles. Despite this, a subset of atrial tachycardias will be sensitive to adenosine or vagal maneuvers.
- Treatment—Although AT may be either paroxysmal or incessant, treatment is aimed at either controlling the rate through AV blockade or suppression of the underlying ectopic focus.
    - Rate control—Either β-blockers or calcium channel blockers may be used in attempts to achieve ventricular rate reduction through AV nodal blockade, although this is often difficult to properly achieve. In some cases, β-blockers or calcium channel blockers may be successful in terminating and suppressing the tachycardia.
    - DCCV—DCCV is generally not effective in durable maintenance of sinus rhythm but may be attempted if a patient is hemodynamically unstable.

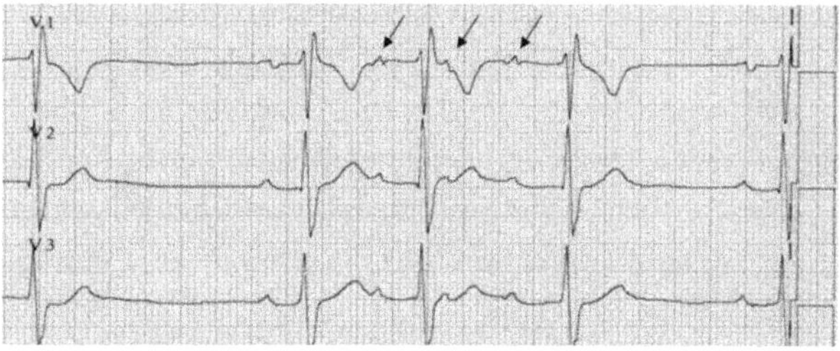

■ **Figure 15.8** Sinus bradycardia with a brief burst of atrial tachycardia. Note the altered O-wave morphology (arrows), variable R-P interval, and 2:1 AV block.

- Suppression—Classes IA (e.g., procainamide, disopyramide), IC (e.g., flecainide, propafenone), or III (e.g., amiodarone, sotalol) antiarrhythmic drugs may be used in an attempt to suppress the focus of tachycardia. As AT is often a manifestation of structural heart disease, amiodarone is often the preferred agent given the other agents' propensity to be proarrhythmic.
- Catheter ablation—In most cases of drug refractory AT, the ectopic focus of tachycardia can be identified and ablated with high success rates, regardless of the underlying electrophysiologic mechanism.

AV Nodal Reciprocating Tachycardia

- AV nodal reciprocating tachycardia (AVNRT) is the most common form of PSVT. The electrophysiologic mechanism is a re-entry circuit that involves distinct functional limbs within the AV node often in the absence of discrete anatomic pathways. These pathways have different electrophysiologic properties (i.e., a "fast pathway" and "slow pathway") allowing for perpetuation of the circuit.
- The atria and ventricles are bystanders in AVNRT, and their sequence of initiation will depend on whether the antegrade limb of the circuit is the fast or slow pathway.

- Typical AVNRT—In the most common form of AVNRT, the slow pathway serves as the antegrade limb, and the fast AV nodal pathway serves as the retrograde limb. The atria and ventricles are activated nearly simultaneously; therefore, the surface ECG will manifest retrograde P waves that are either buried within the QRS complex or a short RP tachycardia (< 80 ms).
- Atypical AVNRT—In this rarer form of AVNRT, fast pathway serves as the antegrade limb of the circuit and the slow pathway the retrograde limb; therefore, the atria are activated after the ventricles and the surface ECG will manifest retrograde P waves with a long RP interval.

- Treatment for either typical or atypical AVNRT is aimed at both acutely and chronically altering the electrophysiologic characteristics of the tachycardia circuit and thereby terminating the tachycardia and preventing recurrence.
  - Acute treatment—After AVNRT has been identified, acute management may proceed rapidly from vagal maneuvers (e.g., Valsalva maneuver or CSM—assuming no contraindications) to intravenous adenosine. Short-acting intravenous β-blockers and calcium channel blockers may in some cases terminate the tachycardia. If these interventions are unsuccessful and the patient is or becomes hemodynamically unstable, DCCV may be considered per ACLS protocol.
  - Chronic treatment—Chronic treatment is aimed at altering the electrophysiologic properties of the AV node either with pharmacotherapy or anatomic alterations. In patients with infrequent and relatively asymptomatic episodes, the patient may be taught to perform vagal maneuvers, and there may be no need for either long-term pharmacotherapy or invasive interventions.
    - Catheter ablation of the "slow pathway" is first-line therapy for patients with documented AVNRT; however,

this procedure carries a small risk of complete AV block requiring a permanent pacemaker. The long-term "cure" rate exceeds 90% to 95%.

- Alternatively, pharmacologic therapy may be effective.
  - Long-acting oral calcium channel blockers, β-blockers, or digoxin may be effective in preventing recurrence.
  - Because most patients with AVNRT lack structural or coronary heart disease, class IC agents such as flecainide and propafenone may be considered and are effective. As previously discussed, if these agents are to be used, one must consider adding a calcium channel blocker or β-blocker to prevent 1:1 conduction over the AV node should atrial flutter occur. For the same reasons, and the typically young age at which AVNRT presents, amiodarone can generally be avoided.

AV Reciprocating Tachycardia

- AV reciprocating tachycardia (AVRT) is a form of PSVT mediated by an accessory AV pathway, which allows electrical communication between the atria and ventricles. The mechanism of the tachycardia is a reentry circuit, which involves the atria, AV node, His-Purkinje system, ventricles, and the accessory pathway. Typically, the accessory pathway functions as the retrograde limb of the circuit, but rarely it may be the antegrade limb.
  - Accessory pathways may have a multitude of electrophysiologic properties and anatomic locations. Commonly, however, accessory pathway function is "all or none," unlike the AV node, which displays decremental properties. Some pathways may be able to conduct in an antegrade or retrograde manner (i.e., from the atrium to the ventricle or from the ventricle to the atrium, depending on the circumstance). Likewise, the baseline ECG may exhibit

evidence of ventricular "pre-excitation" or a delta-wave if the pathway allows conduction from the atrium to the ventricle. This finding, along with syncope or symptomatic arrhythmia, defines the Wolff-Parkinson-White syndrome (WPW). If the pathway only allows conduction from the ventricles to the atria, there will be no manifestation on baseline ECG, as the pathway will be "concealed" unless AVRT ensues.

- Direction of re-entry circuit—As some accessory pathways will allow conduction in either direction, the QRS morphology and properties of AVRT will depend on the direction of the re-entry circuit and mechanism of ventricular depolarization.
  - Orthodromic AVRT—As some accessory pathways will allow conduction in either direction, the re-entry circuit may propagate antegradely in the common way through the AV node and use the His-Purkinje system for ventricular activation and thereby result in an NCT (see Figure 15.9).
  - Antidromic AVRT—Conversely, if the reentry circuit is reversed and the atria are activated from retrograde conduction through the AV node and the ventricles via the accessory pathway and slow myocyte to myocyte spread, the QRS complex will be wide. Ventricular tachycardia must be excluded.
  - P-wave morphology and timing—In orthodromic AVRT, the P-wave morphology and timing will be determined by the anatomic location characteristics of the accessory pathway. Generally, AVRT results in a short RP tachycardia (though not as short as typical AVNRT), and the P wave is generally negative in the inferior leads. The exact morphology will change, however, if the accessory pathway is located anteriorly versus posteriorly and around the tricuspid valve versus mitral valve. In

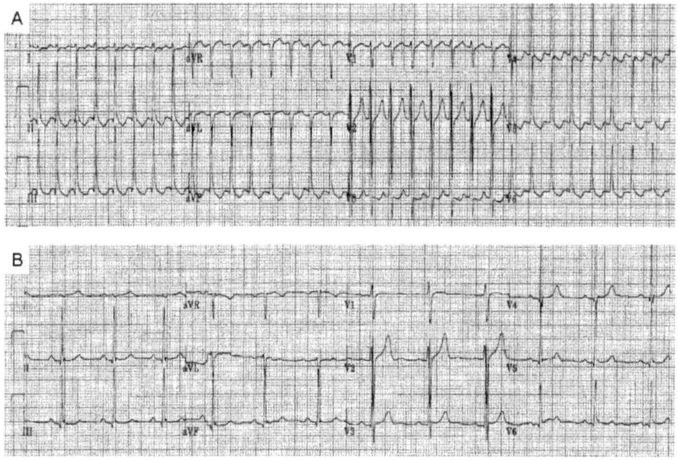

■ **Figure 15.9** 12 lead ECGs of a patient with a concealed accessory pathway confirmed at EP study. A. Orthodromic AVRT. B. Same patient with sinus rhythm, Note the absence of pre-excitation.

some cases, a slowly conducting accessory pathway near the AV node can lead to AVRT with a long RP interval, which is known as permanent junctional reciprocating tachycardia PJRT.

- Treatment—As in AVNRT, treatment is aimed at terminating the tachycardia and preventing recurrence. As the tachycardia relies on both the accessory pathway and AV node for perpetuation, alteration of the electrophysiologic properties of either may accomplish this goal. As opposed to AVNRT, however, care must be taken when using agents that block conduction through the AV node, as this can cause rapid activation of the ventricles via the accessory pathway and cause malignant and life threatening ventricular arrhythmias.

- Acute treatment—Vagal maneuvers and CSM may be employed both to aid in the diagnosis and to treat AVRT acutely. Calcium channel blockers or β-blockers may be useful, but care must be taken, as noted previously here, given their ability to block conduction in the AV node. Adenosine, in general, should be avoided if AVRT is suspected given the possibility of inducing AF. Should this occur and the accessory pathway is capable of rapid conduction from the atria to the ventricles, very rapid and irregular ventricular activation may occur and precipitate ventricular fibrillation. Procainamide should be considered when pre-excited AF is observed.
- Chronic treatment—Chronic treatment is generally aimed at slowing conduction in the accessory pathway. This may be accomplished by either oral pharmacotherapy or catheter ablation.
  - Catheter ablation of the accessory pathway is preferable if the arrhythmia is frequent, symptomatic, or poorly tolerated.
  - Drugs such as flecainide, propafenone, sotalol, and amiodarone may be used for long-term prophylaxis of AVRT.
  - If AVRT is infrequent and well tolerated and there is no evidence of ventricular pre-excitation (i.e., no delta wave on 12-lead ECG), single-dose calcium channel blockers or β-blockers may be prescribed when the arrhythmia occurs—also known as the "pill in the pocket" approach.

Focal Junctional Tachycardia/Junctional Ectopic Tachycardia (JET)

- Focal junctional tachycardia occurs when rapid depolarizations form a focus in the AV node or His-Purkinje system. This arrhythmia is rare in adults, and the mechanism is thought to be due to either increased abnormal automaticity or triggered activity. There is often AV dissociation, as the atria may continue to be activated by the SN during the tachycardia, and typically, the tracing may exhibit sinus P waves, which are "in sync" with the QRS complexes or "isorhythmic AV dissociation." This arrhythmia may be responsive to β-blockade, and if incessant catheter, modification of the AV node may be considered.

16 ▪ Medical Management of Peripheral Artery Disease

Li Shien Low, MD
Danielle Duffy, MD

Definitions

- The term "peripheral arterial disease" (PAD) encompasses a diverse group of disorders that lead to progressive stenosis, occlusion, or aneurysmal dilation of the aorta and its noncoronary branch arteries, including the carotid, upper-extremity, visceral, and lower-extremity arterial branches. The most common systemic pathophysiological processes that leads to PAD is atherosclerosis, although degenerative diseases (e.g., Marfan's syndrome), dysplastic disorders (e.g., fibromuscular dysplasia), vascular inflammation (arteritis), in situ thrombosis, and thromboembolism should also be considered in the initial differential diagnosis.
- The most recent Atherosclerotic Peripheral Vascular Disease Interdisciplinary Working Group commissioned by the American Heart Association now recommends the term "peripheral artery disease" to describe disease that affects the lower- or upper-extremity arteries.
- For the purposes of this chapter, we use the term PAD to represent atherosclerotic disease, and we focus on the diagnosis and management of lower-extremity PAD.
- In patients with PAD, the classic symptom is intermittent claudication, which is defined as muscle discomfort in the lower limb that is reproducible with exercise and relieved by rest within 10 minutes. The muscle discomfort may be described as fatigue, aching, or cramping. These symptoms are most commonly in the calves but may also affect the thighs or buttocks.

Epidemiology and Risk Factors

- According to the results from the National Health and Nutrition Examination Survey (1999–2000) using an ankle-brachial index (ABI) < 0.90 as the definition of PAD, the prevalence of PAD among individuals aged 40 years and older was 4.3%, and the prevalence of PAD among individuals aged 70 years and older was 14.5%.
- There is a slightly higher prevalence of PAD in males compared with females in the younger age range; however, there is little gender difference in prevalence with advancing age. In terms of ethnic groups, the prevalence of PAD is highest among non-Hispanic blacks.
- Obtaining an accurate measurement of the incidence and prevalence of PAD is challenging, as only a fraction of patients with PAD has classic lower-extremity symptoms; therefore, the index of suspicion for PAD must be high in order to make the diagnosis.
- The main risk factors for PAD strongly correlate with established atherosclerotic disease and risk factors, including smoking history, diabetes, hypertension, dyslipidemia, hyperhomocysteinemia, elevated C-reactive protein, and chronic kidney disease (glomerular filtration rate [GFR] < 60 ml/min).
- Given the overlap of risk factors, patients with PAD are at high risk for having coexisting coronary artery disease (CAD) and cerebrovascular disease. In fact, cardiovascular ischemic events are more common than limb ischemic events.
- Patients with lower-extremity PAD are at a 20% to 60% increased risk for having a myocardial infarction with a twofold to sixfold increased mortality caused by cardiovascular events.
- Based on epidemiologic studies and clinical trials, patients with PAD have an annual mortality rate ranging from 4% to

6% from a combination of myocardial infarction, stroke, and vascular events. Mortality is highest among patients with the most severe disease, especially those who have undergone a revascularization procedure or amputation.

- The prognosis of the limb depends on the extent of disease, with the best predictors of progression to critical limb ischemia (CLI) being an ABI < 0.5 and the presence of diabetes mellitus. CLI is characterized by the development of rest pain, new wounds, or gangrene. Approximately 50% of patients with CLI will require revascularization (see the section on CLI later here).
- Despite a significantly increased cardiovascular risk, the PARTNERS study showed that PAD is underdiagnosed and that patients are treated less intensively than those with known cardiovascular disease, which can result in nonfavorable outcomes, increased costs of long-term care, and impaired quality of life.

Vascular History and Physical Examination

- Asymptomatic individuals aged 50 years or older with any atherosclerotic risk factor or any adult age 70 years or older should undergo a complete vascular review of symptoms and comprehensive pulse examination.
- Additionally, any individual with lower-extremity symptoms warrants a vascular history, review of symptoms, and physical examination.
- Vascular history and review of symptoms
  - Family history of abdominal aortic aneurysm or other vascular disease in a first-degree relative
  - Exertional walking impairment or claudication symptoms, including fatigue, aching, numbness or pain in the lower extremities. Occlusive disease in the iliac arteries may produce hip, buttock, and thigh pain, as well as calf pain. Occlusive disease in the femoral and popliteal arteries is

usually associated with calf pain. Occlusive disease in the tibial arteries may produce calf pain or, more rarely, foot pain and numbness.

- Poorly healing wounds or ulcers on the legs or feet
- Rest pain in the lower leg or foot, especially if exacerbated by elevation
- Other causes of exertional leg pain ("pseudoclaudication") should be distinguished from true claudication. These etiologies include venous occlusive disease, chronic compartment syndrome, lumbar disc disease, spinal stenosis, osteoarthritis, Baker's cyst, or inflammatory muscle disease.

- Vascular physical examination
  - Bilateral arm blood pressures, noting any significant (> 10 to 15 mm Hg) asymmetry. The arm with the higher pressure should be used for all subsequent readings. The presence of a subclavian or axillary arterial stenosis should be considered on the side with the lower pressure and requires further evaluation.
  - Inspection of the feet and legs for signs of PAD, which include pale color, cool temperature, breakdown of skin integrity, distal hair loss, trophic skin changes, hypertrophic nails, and/or the presence of ulcerations
  - Palpation of pulses for intensity: carotids, abdominal aorta (note the maximal diameter), brachial, radial, ulnar, femoral, popliteal, dorsalis pedis, and posterior tibial. Allen's test can be performed to assess blood supply to the hand.
  - Pulses should be graded according to the following scale: 0, absent; 1, diminished; 2, normal; and 3, bounding. An especially prominent or widened pulse at the femoral and/or popliteal location should raise the suspicion for an aneurysm.
  - Auscultation for bruits of the carotid arteries, femoral arteries, and flanks (for renal artery stenosis).

  - The finding of diminished distal pulses may overestimate the presence of PAD.
- If the suspicion for PAD is high based on risk factors identified, signs of arterial insufficiency on exam, or symptoms of intermittent claudication, proceed with further testing, starting with the ABI (Figure 16.1).

Diagnostic Testing Modalities

- ABI
  - ABI is the standard test for the diagnosis of lower-extremity PAD.
  - An ABI should be performed in patients with risk factors for PAD and any patient with symptoms of intermittent claudication (Figure 16.1).
  - Using lower-extremity contrast angiography as the gold standard, the sensitivity of an ABI of < 0.9 for detecting a stenosis of 50% or greater ranges from 79% to 95% and the specificity ranges from 96% to 100%. The positive and negative predictive values are 90% and 99%, respectively, with an accuracy of 98%.
  - The ABI quantitatively assesses the severity of disease and can be followed over time for progression of disease or in response to therapy.
  - The ABI is performed by measuring the systolic blood pressure from both brachial arteries and from both the dorsalis pedis and posterior tibial arteries after the patient has been at rest in the supine position for 10 minutes. Lower-extremity systolic pressures are recorded with the cuff on the lower calf (just above the ankle) using a handheld Doppler instrument over the dorsalis pedis or posterior tibial artery. If the arm blood pressures are not equal, the higher blood pressure is used for the ABI calculations. Pulse wave reflection in healthy individuals causes the ankle pressure to be 10 to 15 mm Hg higher than the

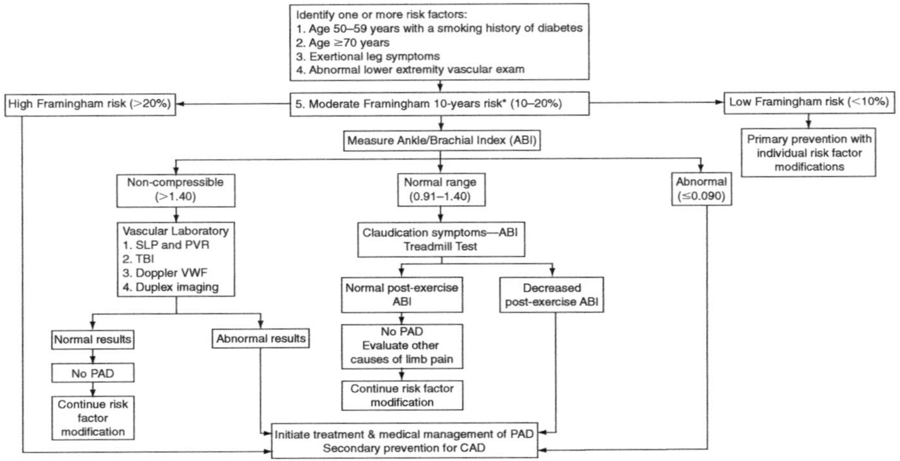

■ **Figure 16.1** Approach to the diagnosis of peripheral artery disease. A Framingham 10-year cardiovascular risk score should be calculated for all patients with 2 or more cardiovascular risk factors (smoking, hypertension, low HDL, family history of premature coronary disease, age ≥ 45 for men or ≥ 55 for women). Abbreviations: SLP, segmental limb pressure; PVR, pulse volume recording; TBI, toe-brachial index; VWF, velocity waveform. *An online Framingham risk calculator can be found at: http://hp2010.nhlbihin.net/atpiii/calculator.asp?usertype=prof

Source: Adapted and reprinted from Norgren L, et al. for the TASC II Working Group. Intersociety Consensus for the Management of Peripheral Arterial Disease (TASC II). *Eur J Vasc Endovasc Surg.* 2007;33:S1–S70, with permission from Elsevier.

brachial arterial systolic pressure, and thus, the normal ankle-arm brachial index systolic blood pressure ratio is greater than 1. Calculated ABI values should be recorded to 2 decimal places. The ABI should be measured in both legs.

  - An abnormal ABI value is less than 0.90. ABI values between 0.41 and 0.90 are considered to be mildly to moderately diminished. ABI values that are less than or equal to 0.40 are severely decreased. The presence of a severely decreased ABI identifies individuals who are at particularly high risk for the subsequent development of rest pain, ischemic ulceration, or gangrene.
  - For patients with symptoms that strongly suggest lower-extremity PAD but a normal or high ABI, further vascular testing should be performed (Figure 16.1). A "normal" value could be due to collateral circulation, and a value > 1.40 could be due to noncompressible vessels, which are more common in the older patients, patients with diabetes, and patients with renal disease.
  - An abnormal ABI provides important prognostic and risk stratification information. An ABI < 0.9 is associated with a twofold to sixfold increased risk of cardiovascular mortality; as such, these patients should be treated aggressively to prevent cardiovascular disease. It has also been proposed that for each decrease in ABI of 0.10 there is a 10% increase in the relative risk for a major vascular event.

- Treadmill exercise testing and postexercise ABI
  - Treadmill ABI is a useful test to diagnose PAD when the resting ABI is normal, but symptoms of intermittent claudication are present.
  - Patients with claudication symptoms from an isolated larger vessel (e.g., iliac) stenosis may have a normal resting ABI, but with exercise, the stenosis will become hemodynamically significant and can be detected by a decrease in the ABI immediately after exercise.

  - A postexercise ABI will also help to distinguish claudication from pseudoclaudication.
  - To perform a postexercise ABI, the resting ABI is measured before exercise. The patient then walks on a treadmill until claudication symptoms occur. The standard protocol has the patient walk at 2 mph at a 10% to 12% grade until symptoms occur or a maximum of 5 minutes. The ankle pressure is again measured immediately after exercise. The resting brachial pressure is used in the calculation.
  - A decrease in ABI of 15% to 20% after exercise is diagnostic of PAD.
  - A treadmill walking test (without ABI measurement) gives an objective measure of a patient's functional impairment and any improvement obtained in response to claudication interventions. During the test, clinicians or technicians should record the time of onset of leg symptoms, total walking time, and the presence of any cardiovascular or other limiting symptoms.
  - An exercise treadmill test should also be performed prior to undergoing an exercise or rehabilitation program for PAD in order to provide objective data and to demonstrate safety.
  - If a patient cannot perform a treadmill or walking test because of other comorbidities, active pedal plantar flexion by performing heel raises from a standing position can be performed as the alternative form of exercise.
- Segmental pressure measurements or segmental limb pressures (SLPs)
  - SLPs measure the arterial pressures at various levels of the lower extremity with blood pressure cuffs placed sequentially along the limb.
  - This technique allows localization of an individual hemodynamically significant large-vessel occlusive arterial stenosis and gives a noninvasive assessment of its magnitude and severity.

  - SLPs are obtained by placing a sphygmomanometer cuff at various points along the leg and measuring the systolic pressure of the major artery under the cuff with a Doppler probe over one of the pedal arteries. In most vascular laboratories, these blood pressure cuffs are placed at the upper thigh, the lower thigh, the upper calf, and the lower calf above the ankle.
  - The location of an occlusive lesion is apparent from the pressure gradient between the different cuffs. In general, a gradient of greater than 20 mm Hg between adjacent segments represents a physiologically important focal stenosis.
  - As with the ABI, segmental pressure measurements may be artifactually elevated or uninterpretable in patients with noncompressible vessels.
- Segmental plethysmography or pulse volume recordings (PVRs)
  - PVRs are often used in combination with segmental limb pressures to increase the diagnostic accuracy for PAD, especially in patients with diabetes who have calcified arteries and falsely elevated (noncompressible) segmental limb pressures.
  - PVRs can also be used to monitor arterial flow after revascularization procedures.
  - Arterial inflow in the lower extremities is pulsatile, which leads to detectable changes in lower-extremity limb volume between systole and diastole. These changes can be detected and graphically recorded by plethysmography.
  - The magnitude of the pulse volume provides an index of large-vessel patency and correlates with blood flow. Any sequential diminution in pulsatility (upstroke and amplitude) signifies the presence of a flow-limiting stenosis in the more proximal arterial segment. Pulsatility is usually a qualitative measurement, with normal values determined by the individual vascular laboratory.

  - To perform PVR, limb cuffs are placed segmentally along the leg at selected locations and connected to a plethysmograph, which produces a pulse volume recording.
  - PVR waveforms are obtained by inflating the cuffs to approximately 60 to 65 mm Hg, which is sufficient to detect volume changes without resulting in arterial occlusion.
  - SLPs or PVR measurements alone are 85% accurate when compared with angiography in detecting and localizing significant occlusive lesions. When used together, the accuracy approaches 95%.
  - The pulse volume recording gives prognostic information regarding the risk of limb amputation. The presence of a low pulse volume correlates with other signs of limb jeopardy and an adverse limb prognosis.
- Toe-brachial index (TBI)
  - The TBI is useful in patients with noncompressible tibial arteries (ankle pressure $\geq$ 250 mm Hg or ABI $>$ 1.40), which is often seen in the older population or those with diabetes or renal disease.
  - The toe pressures give an accurate measurement of distal limb systolic pressure in vessels that do not usually become compressible.
  - TBI is performed by applying a small occlusion cuff with a flow sensor (plethysmographic detection device) on the proximal portion of the first or second toe.
  - Toe pressure is normally 30 mm Hg less than ankle pressure, and thus, an abnormal TBI diagnostic for lower-extremity PAD is $<$ 0.70.
  - False-positive results with the TBI are low.
  - A major limitation is the presence of ulceration, lesions or loss of tissue, which are especially common in diabetic patients.
- Continuous-wave Doppler ultrasound

- Continuous wave Doppler ultrasound is used to obtain velocity waveforms.
- Doppler ultrasound allows for the initial diagnosis of disease location and severity as well as the monitoring of disease progression and the effects of revascularization.
- This technique is useful for localizing stenoses even in patients with poorly compressible arteries or a normal ABI.
- When assessed over the tibial artery, a reduced or absent forward flow velocity is highly accurate for detecting PAD or isolated tibial artery occlusive disease as can occur in patients with diabetes.
- The Doppler waveforms progress from a normal triphasic pattern to a biphasic and ultimately monophasic waveform in patients with significant PAD.
- A decrease in the "pulsatility index" of the velocities from the more proximal to more distal segments implies presence of occlusive disease in between. The degree of decline of this index is proportional to the severity of disease.
- The usefulness is maximized when combined with visualization of the arterial wall through duplex imaging (see the Duplex ultrasound section later here).

• Duplex ultrasound
  - Duplex ultrasound can be used to diagnose the anatomic location and degree of stenosis through images of the vessel (either black and white or color).
  - This imaging technique can evaluate arterial pathology other than atherosclerotic stenosis, such as aneurysms, arterial dissection, popliteal artery entrapment, lymphoceles, and soft tissue masses.
  - Duplex ultrasound can also be used to obtain a quantitative assessment of peak systolic velocities within or beyond the stenosis compared with upstream segments.
  - In addition, it can be used to visualize the presence or absence of turbulence and the preservation of pulsatility.

- The sensitivity and specificity are both 90% to 95% for the diagnosis of a stenosis greater than 50% from the iliac to the popliteal arteries.
- This technique is dependent on the ability to visualize the vessel; therefore, accuracy is diminished if visualization is less than adequate due to technical reasons.
- Duplex ultrasound can also be used for routine surveillance after bypass surgery with a venous conduit and to identify an arterial lesion that is suitable for revascularization.

- Magnetic resonance angiography (MRA)
  - MRA is useful for determining the anatomic location and degree of stenosis.
  - MRA is also useful for selecting patients who are candidates for endovascular intervention, for treatment planning prior to intervention or invasive angiography, and for assessing suitability of lesions for endovascular approaches.
  - Contrast-enhanced MRA with gadolinium has a sensitivity and specificity of > 93% for the diagnosis of PAD when compared with invasive angiography.
  - MRA provides rapid, high-resolution, three-dimensional images, which allows visualization of eccentric lesions.
  - This imaging technique does not require the use of iodinated contrast and does not expose the patient to radiation.
  - Calcium in the vessel does not produce artifact, but metallic alloy (nonnitinol) stents can produce artifact.
  - MRA could possibly overestimate the degree of stenosis because of turbulence.
  - MRA cannot be used in patients with pacemakers/defibrillators, other contraindications to MRI, or severe claustrophobia.
- Computed tomographic angiography (CTA)

- CTA may be used to diagnose the anatomic location and presence of a significant stenosis.
- Multidetector CTA (MDCTA) allows for rapid imaging of the entire lower extremity and abdomen in one breath hold, giving a faster scan time than MRA.
- The sensitivity and specificity of MDCTA for PAD are 89% to 99% and 83% to 100%, respectively. Only limited direct comparisons to MRA are currently available.
- The major limitations include the need for use of iodinated contrast, significant use of radiation, and artifact from calcium and/or stents.
- Some advantages of CTA over invasive angiography include the ability to rotate images in space for evaluation of eccentric stenoses, and imaging of the tissue surrounding stenoses to evaluate for compressive causes.
- The potential disadvantages compared with invasive angiography include lower special resolution and the potential for venous opacification to obscure arterial filling.
- To date, CTA has not been adequately studied for following patients after revascularization.

- Angiography
  - Invasive angiography is considered the "gold-standard" imaging modality for defining both the normal anatomy and vascular pathology of the arteries of the lower extremities from the level of the renal arteries to the pedal arteries.
  - Angiography is currently the only universally accepted method for guiding percutaneous peripheral interventional procedures.
  - Digital subtraction angiography techniques allow for enhanced imaging capabilities by eliminating artifact from bony structures and soft tissue.
  - Angiography is used when revascularization is being considered to stratify patients before intervention.

- This technique gives inflow and outflow patterns and allows characterization of the lesion(s).
- The procedure is invasive and therefore carries more than minimal risk. Risks of invasive angiography include the risks of vascular access (bleeding, infection, vessel injury) and the risks of catheter manipulation (atheroemboliza-tion, dissection, perforation).
- Angiography does require iodinated contrast so caution, hydration, and consideration of n-acetylcysteine for renal protection are needed for those patients at higher risk of contrast-induced nephrotoxicity (renal insufficiency, diabetes, dehydration, and low cardiac output). Certain patients may also be allergic to the contrast agent and require additional caution and preparation with preproce-dure steroids.
- Patients should be followed closely after this procedure.

Treatment of Lower-Extremity PAD

- Risk factor modification
  - The main modifiable risk factors for PAD include current cigarette smoking, diabetes, hypertension, and dyslipidemia.
  - The main goal of risk factor modification is to reduce the long-term risk of cardiovascular and cerebrovascular events.
  - Smoking cessation can help to reduce progression of vascular disease; therefore, smoking cessation counsel-ing should be performed at all visits. The use of behavior modification therapies, nicotine replacement therapy, and/or pharmacologic therapy (e.g., bupropion or varenicline) should be considered on an individual basis.
  - The aim is for optimal diabetes control with a goal hemo-globin A1C of $< 7\%$.

- In diabetics, meticulous foot care is also necessary in order to recognize and initiate early treatment of any foot and lower-extremity ulcers or wounds.
- Optimal blood pressure should be targeted with a goal of < 140/90 in nondiabetics and < 130/80 in diabetics and individuals with chronic renal disease. Choice of antihypertensive agents should follow current guidelines and is left up to the discretion of the treating physician; of note, β-blockers are not contraindicated. Additionally, in the HOPE trial of ramipril versus placebo in high-risk vascular patients, there was a 22% relative-risk reduction in myocardial infarction, stroke, and death from cardiovascular causes in the ramipril arm; therefore, angiotensin-converting enzyme inhibitors should be considered as part of the antihypertensive regimen if appropriate.
- The low-density lipoprotein (LDL) cholesterol goal should be < 100 mg/dl in all patients with a target of < 70 mg/dl for the highest risk patients (e.g., multiple vascular beds involved). First-line therapy for LDL-C reduction is HMG coenzyme-A reductase inhibitors (statins), which have shown consistent and statistically significant reductions in total cardiovascular, cerebrovascular, and coronary events in high-risk patients. Additional therapies such as ezetemibe, niacin, fibrates, or bile acid sequestrants should be added as clinically indicated to achieve the LDL-C goal.

• Exercise and lower-extremity PAD rehabilitation
  - According to the most recent guidelines, initial therapy for all patients with PAD and intermittent claudication should be a supervised exercise rehabilitation program.
  - In fact, exercise-induced clinical benefits are superior to those achieved by drug therapies.
  - The overall goals of therapy are to increase pain-free walking distance, duration, speed, muscle workload, and functional status.

- A meta-analysis from the Cochrane Collaboration comparing exercise with usual care or placebo showed an average of 50% to 200% improvement in walking ability, with a mean increase in walking time of greater than 5 minutes.
- With a formal exercise training program, claudication symptoms should improve gradually in as early as 4 to 8 weeks and progressively over 12 weeks.
- Treadmill and track walking are the most effective exercises for claudication.
- A standard training program guides patients in exercise for at least 30 to 45 minutes per session, 3 sessions per week for a minimum of 12 weeks.
- At each training session, the patient should walk to the highest level of tolerable claudication pain.
- The general guidelines for an exercise rehabilitation session are as follows:
  - Set a speed and grade on the treadmill that will elicit claudication symptoms within a 3- to 5-minute period.
  - Ask patients to walk at this workload until they experience claudication pain of near-maximal severity. They should then rest to allow the symptoms to dissipate before restarting.
  - The exercise–rest–exercise pattern should be repeated throughout the session, with the rehabilitation personnel titrating up the grade and speed of the treadmill as the weeks progress and the patient augments his or her walking capacity to ensure there is always a stimulus of claudication pain.
  - As patients' exercise capabilities improve and cardiac demand increases, it is important for the supervising personnel to monitor for cardiac signs and symptoms such as angina, arrhythmia, and/or electrocardiogram changes.

- In addition to improving claudication symptoms, regular exercise also helps to prevent and treat established atherosclerotic disease and risk factors such as glucose intolerance, diabetes, hypertension, hyperlipidemia, hypertriglyceridemia, and low levels of HDL cholesterol. Increased physical activity can also decrease the risk of multiple other medical conditions unrelated to cardiovascular disease such as osteoporosis, colon cancer, breast cancer, psychiatric disorders as well as increases event-free survival.

- Pharmacologic therapies for PAD
  - Medical therapy for claudication
    - Cilostazol (100-mg tablet twice daily)
      - Cilostazol was approved by the Food and Drug Administration in 1999 for the treatment of intermittent claudication.
      - It is a phosphodiesterase type III inhibitor that increases intracellular concentrations of cAMP, thus inhibiting platelet aggregation, the formation of arterial thrombi, and vascular smooth muscle proliferation.
      - A meta-analysis of placebo-controlled trials found a 50% increase in maximal walking distance after an average treatment period of 6 months compared with 21% with placebo. In addition, patients also reported improvements in quality of life and functional status based on validated questionnaires.
      - Cilostazol is not advised for patients with heart failure.
      - It is also contraindicated in patients with moderate to severe renal or hepatic impairment.
      - The most common side effects include headache, dizziness, gastrointestinal complaints (diarrhea), peripheral edema, and palpitations.

            - Cilostazol is recommended by the 2006 American College of Cardiology (ACC)/American Heart Association (AHA) guidelines based on strong evidence as effective and useful therapy for the relief of claudication symptoms.
            - A 3-month therapeutic trial is reasonable to evaluate for improvement in symptoms; clinical improvement can be seen within 2 to 4 weeks of cilostazol initiation.
        - Pentoxifylline (400-mg tablet three times daily)
            - In 1984, pentoxifylline was approved by the Food and Drug Administration and was the first drug approved for the treatment of peripheral arterial disease.
            - It is a methylxanthine derivative. Proposed mechanisms of action include decrease in blood and plasma viscosity, increase in blood cell deformability, lowering of plasma fibrinogen concentrations, inhibition of neutrophil adhesion and activation, and antiplatelet effects.
            - Although a meta-analysis of pentoxifylline does show a statistically significant net benefit, the drug demonstrated only a small effect in improving walking capacities when compared with cilostazol.
            - The most common side effects include: sore throat, rhinitis, and gastrointestinal complaints (dyspepsia, nausea, and diarrhea).
            - ACC/AHA guidelines do not universally recommend this therapy for the relief of intermittent claudication due to conflicting evidence and/or opinions on its efficacy.
    - Antiplatelet therapy
        - All patients with atherosclerotic lower-extremity PAD should be treated with antiplatelet therapy to reduce the risk of cardiovascular and cerebrovascular morbidity and mortality. It is an effective long-term secondary preventive modality for vascular events in high-risk patients.

    - Aspirin (75 to 325 mg daily)
        - Aspirin is strongly recommended to reduce the risk of myocardial infarction, stroke, and vascular mortality.
        - In a large meta-analysis by the Antithrombotic Trialists' Collaboration, there was a significant reduction in the combined endpoint of nonfatal myocardial infarction, nonfatal stroke, and vascular death with aspirin compared with placebo. Indeed, in the subset of patients with PAD, similar benefits were found: a 23% reduction in vascular events in those with intermittent claudication, 22% in patients with peripheral arterial grafts, and 29% in those who had peripheral angioplasty.
    - Clopidogrel (75 mg daily)
        - Clopidogrel is recommended as an effective alternative to aspirin.
        - In the CAPRIE trial (Clopidogrel versus Aspirin in Patients at Risk of Ischemic Events), a subgroup analysis of patients with PAD showed that clopidogrel had an absolute risk reduction of 1.15% and a relative risk reduction of 23.8% for fatal and nonfatal vascular events compared with aspirin 325 mg.
        - Combination therapy with clopidogrel and aspirin is not generally recommended, as the combination has not been shown to be superior to aspirin alone.
- Revascularization
    - A detailed description of revascularization procedures is beyond the scope of this chapter.
    - In general, determining the need for revascularization should be based on the potential procedural risks versus benefits.
    - Patients with intermittent claudication should have significant functional impairment with a reasonable likelihood of symptomatic improvement and absence of other disease that would limit exercise even if claudication is improved before being referred for evaluation for revascularization.

- Revascularization can also be considered for patients with intermittent claudication if there is continued limitation to quality of life after appropriate exercise and pharmacologic therapy.
- In patients with critical limb ischemia or acute limb ischemia, there is increased urgency for revascularization for limb salvage (see the following sections).

Critical Limb Ischemia

- Definition
  - CLI is defined as limb pain that occurs at rest or impending limb loss that is caused by severe compromise of blood flow to the affected extremity.
  - The term "critical limb ischemia" should be used for all patients with chronic ischemic rest pain, ulcers, or gangrene due to objectively proven arterial occlusive disease. Patients with CLI have resting perfusion that is inadequate to sustain viability in the distal tissue bed.
  - The term CLI implies chronicity and should be distinguished from acute limb ischemia (discussed later here).
  - Ischemic rest pain most commonly occurs below an ankle pressure of 50 mm Hg or a toe pressure less than 30 mm Hg.
  - The patients at highest risk for the development of CLI are nondiabetics with an ABI < 0.4 or any diabetic with PAD.
- Presentation
  - Patients with CLI usually present with limb pain at rest, with or without trophic skin changes or tissue loss. Pain is often worse when the patient is supine and may lessen when the limb is in the dependent position.
  - Individuals with diabetes may present with severe CLI and tissue loss but without pain because of concomitant neuropathy.
  - CLI is usually due to diffuse or multisegmental vascular disease.

    - CLI may be the first symptom of PAD.
- Implications
    - If the limb is left untreated, CLI would likely lead to a major limb amputation within 6 months.
    - In addition to dire limb consequences, CLI is associated with significantly increased intermediate-term morbidity and mortality.
    - Patients with chronic CLI have a mortality of approximately 25% in the first year after presentation.
    - The burden of cardiovascular disease is particularly high in this subset of patients with CLI, and thus, aggressive prevention strategies are warranted to reduce cardiovascular risk.
- Diagnostic evaluation
    - The initial diagnostic evaluation of patients with CLI should attempt to confirm the diagnosis, localize the lesion(s), and assess the severity. In addition, an assessment of the patient's endovascular or operative risk is critical.
    - Patients who are endovascular or surgical candidates should have imaging of the lower-limb arteries.
    - A detailed coronary assessment should be considered in selected patients in whom coronary ischemic symptoms would otherwise warrant evaluation if CLI were not present.
- Treatment and follow-up
    - For all patients with CLI, referral to a vascular specialist is indicated to expedite treatment, prevent further deterioration, and reverse the ischemic process if possible through revascularization procedures.
    - The primary goals of treatment are to relieve pain, heal ischemic ulcers, prevent limb loss, improve patient function, and prolong survival.
    - If there is evidence of skin ulcerations or limb infection with underlying CLI, antibiotics should be prescribed.

In addition, referral to a wound care specialist should be made promptly.
- Given the overlap of CLI and concomitant CAD, it is necessary to perform continued assessment of cardiovascular risk and aggressive cardiovascular risk factor modification.
- Patients with a prior history of CLI should be followed biannually by a vascular specialist.

Acute Limb Ischemia

- Definition
  - Acute limb ischemia (ALI) arises when a rapid or sudden decrease in limb perfusion threatens tissue viability.
  - ALI can be due to thrombosis after an atherosclerotic plaque rupture, thrombosis of a lower-extremity bypass graft, or embolism from the heart or a proximal arterial aneurysm. When an embolic occlusion affects a vascular bed not previously conditioned by collaterals, the resulting ischemic syndrome is typically severe.
- Presentation
  - Patients with ALI present with sudden onset or sudden worsening of lower-extremity pain.
  - The hallmark clinical symptoms and physical examination signs of ALI are the "5 Ps": pain, pulselessness, pallor, paresthesia, and paralysis.
- Implications
  - The most critical consideration is if the limb is viable, viable but immediately threatened, or nonviable. This distinction will direct all further management.
  - Mortality rates for ALI range from 15% to 20%.
- Diagnostic evaluation
  - Patients should be asked about prior vascular procedures and of conditions associated with a high risk of systemic embolization such as atrial fibrillation, severe dilated cardiomyopathy, left ventricular aneurysm, atheromatous

plaque in the aorta or proximal limb arteries, or mural thrombus of an aortic aneurysm.

- ABI should be performed immediately; the finding of absent flow signals in the foot arteries is highly consistent with the diagnosis of ALI.
- If ALI is thought to be reversible, the patient should undergo arteriography to determine the best endovascular or surgical option. CTA or MRA may also be used to diagnose and delineate the extent of disease.

- Treatment and follow-up
  - The initial goal of therapy is to prevent thrombus propagation and worsening ischemia.
  - All patients with suspected ALI should have immediate referral to or consultation with a vascular specialist.
  - In addition, immediate systemic anticoagulation, usually with intravenous unfractionated heparin, is recommended.
  - Catheter-directed thrombolytic therapy is the initial treatment of choice if there are no contraindications and the clinical conditions allow.
  - Other endovascular and surgical revascularization procedures should be considered if the limb is profoundly ischemic and/or thrombolytic therapy is not an option.
  - Long-term anticoagulation with warfarin is indicated for at least 3 to 6 months or longer for patients with documented thromboembolism.

17 ▪ Peripheral Artery Disease

Geno J. Merli, MD, FACP, FHM
George Tzanis, MD

Introduction

Peripheral artery disease (PAD) is a chronic arterial occlusive disease of the lower extremities caused by atherosclerosis. The National Heart Lung and Blood Institute estimates that approximately 5% of U.S. adults older than 50 years and about 12% to 20% of adults older than 65 years have lower-extremity atherosclerosis labeled as PAD. Autopsy studies of accidental deaths show that American adolescents have pathological signs of subclinical atherosclerosis. With increasing age and traditional atherosclerotic risk factors, these lesions tend to progress in all large- and medium-sized vessels. Patients with PAD in the lower extremities have a 3- to 6-fold increased rate of cardiovascular mortality compared with patients of the same age without PAD. More importantly, the risk of future cardiovascular events in patients with PAD is at least comparable and is likely to be greater than the risk faced by those with established coronary artery disease.

Recently, Cacoub et al. published data from the Reduction of Atherothrombosis for Continued Health Registry that demonstrated that patients with PAD do not achieve risk factor control as frequently as individuals with established coronary artery or cerebral vascular disease. Modification of risk factors is associated with a reduction in major cardiovascular events in a 1-year follow-up. This chapter uses an evidence-based data classification in order to better define the prevalence of PAD, risk factors, and approaches to assessment and management of PAD (Table 17.1).

Table 17.1 Classification of Recommendations

- Class I—Conditions for which there is evidence for and/or general agreement that a given procedure or treatment is beneficial, useful, and effective
- Class II—Conditions for which there is conflicting evidence and/or a divergence of opinion about the usefulness/efficacy of a procedure or treatment
  - Class IIa—Weight of evidence/opinion is in favor of usefulness/efficacy
  - Class IIb—Usefulness/efficacy is less well established by evidence/opinion
- Class III—Conditions for which there is evidence and/or general agreement that a procedure/treatment is not useful/effective and in some cases may be harmful

Level of Evidence:

- Level of Evidence A: Data derived from multiple randomized clinical trials or meta-analysis
- Level of Evidence B: Data derived from a single randomized trial or nonrandomized studies
- Level of Evidence C: Only consensus opinion of experts, case studies, or standard of care

Source: Adapted from Hirsch AT, Haskal ZJ, Hertzer NR, et al. ACC/AHA 2005 Practice Guidelines for the Management of Paitents with Peripheral Arterial Disease (Lower Extremity, Renal, Mesenteric, and Abdominal Aorta). *Circulation* 2006;1131:1474–1547.

Prevalence, Risk Factors, and Burden of PAD

Based on epidemiologic projections, 27 million people in Europe and North America have PAD, of which 10.5 million are symptomatic and 16.5 million are asymptomatic. Three recent studies, the Prevention of Progression of Arterial Disease and Diabetes (POPADAD), the Minnesota Regional PAD Screening Program, and the PAD Awareness, Risk and Treatment: New Resources for Survival Program (PARTNERS), have demonstrated high PAD detection rates of 20.1%, 26.5%, and 29%, respectively, when specific populations at risk for PAD were screened. The PARTNERS program was a national survey designed to evaluate the prevalence of PAD and other cardiovascular diseases, assess the rate of physician and patient awareness of PAD diagnosis, and evaluate risk factor profiles and treatment with antiplatelet agents. This study found the prevalence of PAD to be 29% in the population of patients older than 70 years and/or older than 50 years with co-morbidities such as smoking or diabetes. All of these studies highlight the fact that within the high-risk population PAD remains underdiagnosed.

The best described independent risk factors for PAD are identical to those for coronary atherosclerosis. Advanced age, smoking, and diabetes are strongly associated with PAD. In one study, 50% of patients with diabetes were found to have PAD. Other PAD risk factors include hypertension, hyperlipidemia, hyperhomocysteinemia, and C-reactive protein.

Tobacco use is highly associated with risk for PAD. Smokers developing PAD have symptoms 10 years earlier than nonsmokers. In a prospective analysis of 2,174 patients older than 40 years, the prevalence of PAD was found to be 4.3%. Correcting for age and other confounding factors, current smoking was strongly associated with increased PAD risk. The risk of PAD increases in a powerful dose-dependent manner with the number of cigarettes smoked per day and number of years smoked. In the Framingham Offspring Study, nearly 3,300 patients with a mean age of 59 years were examined between 1995 and 1998. The prevalence of PAD was 3.9%. Controlling for confounding variables, smoking was associated with an odds ratio of 2.0 (confidence interval, 1.1 to 3.4) for PAD.

Hypertension is associated with systemic atherosclerosis and cardiovascular morbidity, which makes it a risk factor for PAD. Despite the lack of strong evidence that blood pressure control reduces a patient's risk for PAD, experience with other forms of atherosclerosis suggests that keeping the blood pressure within a normal range should be the therapeutic approach.

Lipid abnormalities that are associated with lower-extremity PAD include elevated total and low-density lipoproteins, decreased high-density lipoproteins, and hypertriglyceridemia. The risk of developing lower-extremity PAD increases by approximately 5% to

10% for each 10 mg per dL rise in total cholesterol. In epidemiological studies, total cholesterol levels are generally higher in patients with intermittent claudication than in those without lower-extremity PAD. Similarly, levels of LDL are higher and HDL levels are lower in patients with lower-extremity PAD than in age-matched controls. Elevated levels of triglycerides have been reported to be associated with lower-extremity PAD in some studies but not others. Dyslipidemias are associated with systemic atherosclerosis, and the use of lipid-reducing agents is recommended by the National Cholesterol Education Program-Adult Treatment Panel III guidelines in patients at risk for PAD.

Diabetes mellitus increases the risk of PAD by 2 to 4 fold. In the Framingham Heart Study, diabetes increased the risk of intermittent claudication by 3.5 fold in men and 8.6 fold in women. The risk of developing PAD is proportional to the severity and duration of diabetes. There is evidence that good glycemic control reduces the risk for macrovascular complications, including PAD; however, aggressive glycemic control may be less helpful after the onset of the macrovascular complications. The risk of developing chronic limb ischemia is also greater in diabetics than in non-diabetics. Diabetics with lower-extremity PAD are 7 to 15 fold more likely to undergo a major amputation than nondiabetics with PAD. Diabetics with other risk factors, such as smoking or dyslipidemia, are at particularly high risk for PAD.

Elevated levels of C-reactive protein, which are markers of systemic inflammation, are associated with PAD. Among previously healthy people participating in the Physicians' Health Study, there was a 2.1-fold increased risk of developing lower-extremity PAD in those men whose C-reactive protein concentrations were in the highest quartile. This study also noted that C-reactive protein levels were higher in individuals who subsequently developed lower-extremity PAD and highest in those who ultimately required vascular surgery. In this study population, levels of soluble intercellular adhesion molecule-1, a leukocyte adhesion molecule that is upregulated by inflammatory cytokines, were independently associated with the future development of PAD.

Clinical Diagnosis

(See Figure 17.1)

History

The patient's history is a valuable first step in the assessment of PAD, but it must be remembered that the history in patients with PAD does have some limitations, with only 10% having classic claudication symptoms, 50% with a variety of symptoms, and 40% asymptomatic. Claudication is characterized by cramping, tightness, tiredness, or aching in the lower extremities that is brought on by exercise and relieved with rest. The walking distance to the onset of claudication symptoms as well as the time for resolution should be recorded. This not only helpful with the differential diagnosis of PAD but is useful in assessing therapeutic interventions. Patients with PAD sometimes report leg fatigue, numbness, heaviness, or weakness. Erectile dysfunction can also be a symptom of PAD. The history can offer clues to the location of arterial occlusion based on the muscle groups just distal to the obstruction. For example, claudication in the buttock or hip may be from the aortoiliac system, whereas symptoms in the foot originate from the tibial or peroneal artery. The history can also be helpful in differentiating PAD from pseudoclaudication caused by spinal stenosis. In this latter group, the symptoms experienced in the extremity are usually tingling, weakness, or clumsiness that may or may not be brought on by exercise. These patients will have leg pain on standing that is relieved by sitting or changing position. They frequently comment that leaning forward makes their legs feel better. In addition there is a history of low back pain, usually a tingling.

Clinical Points

1. Individuals at risk for lower-extremity peripheral arterial disease
   a. Age less than 50 years, with diabetes and one other atherosclerosis risk factor (smoking, dyslipidemia, hypertension, or hyperhomocysteinemia)
   b. Age 50 to 69 years and history of smoking or diabetes

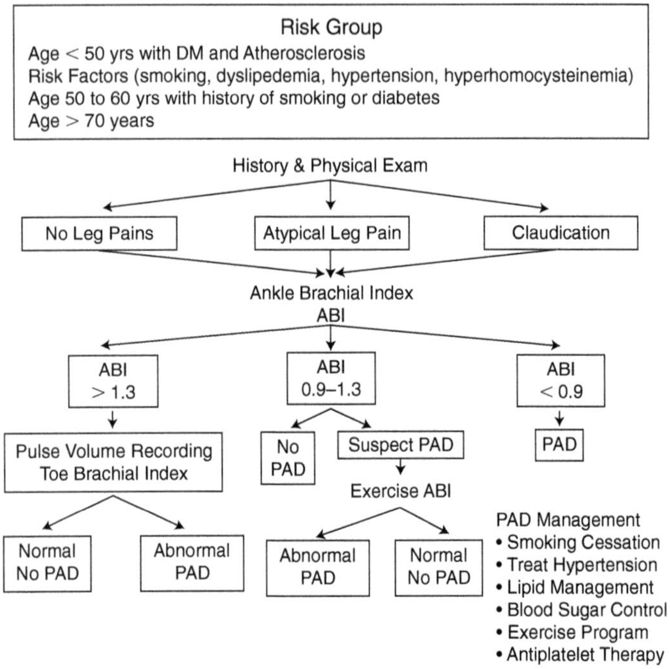

■ **Figure 17.1** Initial Evaluation of PAD

Source: Adapted from Hirsch AT, et al. *Circulation* 2006;1131:1474–1547.

c. Age 70 years and older
d. Leg symptoms with exertion (suggestive of claudication) or ischemic rest pain
e. Abnormal lower-extremity pulse examination
f. Known atherosclerotic coronary, carotid, or renal artery disease

2. Individuals at risk for lower-extremity PAD should undergo a vascular review of symptoms to assess walking impairment, claudication, ischemic rest pain, and/or the presence of non-healing wounds (Class I, Level of Evidence C).

3. Individuals at risk for lower-extremity PAD should undergo a comprehensive pulse examination and inspection of the feet (Class I, Level of Evidence C).
4. Individuals over 50 years of age should be asked if they have a family history of a first-order relative with and abdominal aortic aneurysm (Class I, Level of Evidence C).

Source: American Heart Associate, Inc.

Physical Examination

Because atherosclerosis is a systemic disease, the physical examination should begin with blood pressure measurement in both arms and notation of any interarm asymmetry, palpation and auscultation of the carotids, vertebrals, and abdominal aorta, and evaluation for cardiac murmurs or arrhythmias. The lower extremities should be inspected for the obvious appearance of ulcers, gangrene, edema, atrophy, thickened nails, loss of hair, dry skin, and cool temperature. Palpation of pulses and auscultation of bruits can assist in determining the site or severity of occlusive disease. This can be correlated with the location of claudication symptoms. Pulses are graded as 0 absent, 1 diminished, 2 normal, and 3 bounding. The congenital absence of a dorsalis pedis pulse has been reported to between 4% and 32%, whereas the absence of a posterior tibial pulse is always abnormal. The sensitivity, specificity, and predictive values of traditional clinical pulse examination for PAD were compared in the San Diego Lipid Research Clinics Program Prevalence Study population. The study demonstrated that claudication and an abnormal femoral pulse were very specific for PAD diagnosis (95% to 99%) but were not sensitive (< 20%). The absence of a dorsalis pedis pulse was fairly sensitive (50%) but less specific (73.1%) and had a very low positive predictive value (17.7%). The optimal combination of sensitivity (71.2%) and specificity (91.3%) and moderate positive predictive value (48.7%) was found with an abnormal posterior tibial pulse. According to these findings, the use of the posterior tibial alone would miss a diagnosis of PAD in about 30% of patients, and fewer than half of patients with the abnormal pulse would actually have PAD. Although the physical examination provides important qualitative information and is critical to overall patient treatment, additional noninvasive testing ensures the diagnosis and aids in risk stratification of patients with suspected PAD.

Clinical Points

1. Measurement of blood pressure in both arms and notation of any interarm asymmetry.
2. Palpation of the carotid pulses and notation of the carotid upstroke and amplitude and presence of bruits.
3. Auscultation of the abdomen and flank for bruits.
4. Palpation of the abdomen and notation of the presence of the aortic pulsation and its maximal diameter.
5. Palpation of pulses at the brachial, radial, ulnar, femoral, popliteal, dorsalis pedis, and posterior tibial sites. Performance of Allen's test when knowledge of hand perfusion is needed.
6. Auscultation of both femoral arteries for the presence of bruits
7. Pulse intensity should be assessed and recorded numerically as follows: 0 absent, 1 diminished, 2 normal, and 3 bounding.
8. The shoes and socks should be removed, the feet inspected, the color, temperature, and integrity of the skin and intertriginous areas evaluated, and the presence of ulcerations recorded.
9. Additional findings suggestive of severe PAD, including distal hair loss, trophic skin changes, and hypertrophic nails, should be sought and recorded.

Peripheral Artery Disease Testing

(See Figure 17.1)

Ankle Brachial Index

The ankle brachial index (ABI) is a simple, inexpensive, noninvasive test that correlates well with angiographic disease severity and functional symptoms. In the normal circulation, systolic blood pressure is amplified down the lower limbs such that the ankle systolic blood pressure is slightly greater than or equal to the brachial systolic blood pressure. When the measured ankle systolic blood pressure is divided by the brachial systolic blood pressure, the normal ratio is between 0.9 and 1.3. In PAD the ankle systolic blood pressure falls below the brachial systolic blood pressure, with ABI dropping below 1.0. The interpretation of the ABI is as follows: normal, 0.90 to 1.3; mild, < 0.89 to > 0.60; moderate, < 0.59 to > 0.40; and severe, < 0.39. Studies evaluating the diagnostic accuracy of the ABI have demonstrated that it can differentiate between normal and angiographically diseased limbs with a sensitivity of 97% and a specificity of 100%, and the resting ABI is a significant predictive variable for the severity of angiographic disease.

The major limitation of the ABI to establish the diagnosis of PAD is that calcified tibial peroneal arteries may be rendered noncompressible, especially in patients with diabetes, resulting in an erroneously high ABI. The ABI is dependent on the brachial pressure being a true measure of central systolic pressure. This may not be the case in patients with bilateral subclavian artery stenosis, occasionally seen in patients with diabetes or advanced vascular disease.

An exercise ABI should be completed when patients have symptoms indicative of PAD but a normal ABI. The normal response to exercise is decreased peripheral vascular resistance and increased blood flow to the active extremities, manifested by increased ABI during exercise and subsequent recovery. An ABI that decreases 20% after exercise indicates PAD. Normal results on ABI after exercise suggest another cause for the patient's symptoms.

When the ABI is greater than 1.3 in a population that has a high probability of PAD, such as long-standing diabetes, end-stage renal disease on dialysis, and old age, the peripheral arteries have medical calcification. This results in an inaccurate assess of PAD. In such individuals, diagnostic assessment can be completed by measuring the toe systolic pressure and calculating the toe brachial index. A toe brachial index of less than 0.7 is considered diagnostic for PAD. The toe pressure measurement remains a sensitive diagnostic test in such patients because digital arteries are usually spared the calcinosis that alters compressibility of the more proximal arteries.

Clinical Points

1. The resting ABI should be used to establish the lower-extremity PAD diagnosis in patients with suspected lower-extremity PAD, defined as individuals with exertional leg symptoms, with nonhealing wounds, who are 70 years and older, or who are 50 years and older with a history of smoking or diabetes (Class I, Level of Evidence C).
2. The ABI should be measured in both legs in all new patients with PAD of any severity to confirm the diagnosis of lower extremity PAD and establish a baseline (Class I, Level of Evidence B).
3. The toe brachial index should be used to establish the lower-extremity PAD diagnosis in patients in whom lower-extremity PAD is clinically suspected but in whom the ABI test is not reliable because of noncompressible vessels, especially in patients with long-standing diabetes or advanced age (Class I, Level of Evidence B).
4. Exercise treadmill testing with measurement of pre-exercise and postexercise ABI values are recommended to provide diagnostic data that are useful in differentiating arterial claudication from non-arterial claudication (pseudoclaudication) (Class I, Level of Evidence B).

Pulse Volume Recordings and Doppler Waveform Analysis

Pulse volume recordings can be used in patients when the ABI cannot be calculated or arterial calcification results in a nondiagnostic ABI such as long-standing diabetes, chronic renal failure, or old age. The measurement of segmental pressures and pulse volume recordings can localize occlusions of limb segments by comparing the difference in the systolic blood pressures and the magnitude and contour of pulse volumes to segments located most proximally and distally to the site of occlusion. When used in combination, segmental pressures and pulse volume recordings have demonstrated 95% accuracy as compared with angiography. An alternative to pulse volume recordings is Doppler velocity waveform analysis, in which a continuous-wave Doppler probe is used over multiple arterial segments to detect the blood flow velocity and the velocity patterns. Within each pulse cycle, the probe can detect the quality and magnitude of the triphasic flow pattern (forward, reverse, and late forward flow) to detect any pressure or flow reducing lesions. Disadvantages of Doppler velocity waveform analysis include a high dependence on operator technique and the inability to pinpoint the artery being studied. Doppler velocity waveform analysis and pulse volume recordings are useful in assessing diabetic patients with incompressible arteries, as false elevations in the ABI and segmental pressures are expected.

Clinical Points

1. Pulse volume recordings are reasonable to establish the initial lower-extremity PAD diagnosis and assess localization and severity (Class IIa, Level of Evidence B).
2. Pulse volume recordings can be used to follow the status of lower-extremity revascularization procedures (Class IIa, Level of Evidence B).

Duplex Ultrasound

When it is necessary to localize occlusions more precisely than arterial segments or to characterize more fully the severity and morphologic features of occlusions, ultrasonic duplex scanning is a noninvasive preliminary alternative to angiography. Duplex ultrasound has other important clinical uses in patient patients with PAD. These include evaluation of aneurysm, arterial dissection, popliteal artery entrapment syndrome, lymphoceles, and assessment of soft tissue masses. The sensitivity and specificity for the diagnosis of stenoses greater than 50% diameter from the iliac arteries to the popliteal arteries are each approximately 90% to 95%. Duplex ultrasound can be used for preintervention decision making by predicting whether a patient has anatomy suitable for angioplasty with an accuracy of 84% to 94%. In addition, duplex ultrasound has been used for postrevascularization surveillance of graft patency. Vein grafts fail because of the development of stenoses either within the body of the graft, at the anastomosis, or upstream or downstream from the graft. Duplex ultrasound surveillance studies allow detection of these stenotic areas before they occlude.

Clinical Points

1. Duplex ultrasound of the extremities is useful to diagnose the anatomic location and degree of stenosis of PAD (Class I, Level of Evidence A).
2. Duplex ultrasound is recommended for routine surveillance after femoral-popliteal or femoral-tibial-pedal bypass with a venous conduit. Minimum surveillance intervals are approximately 3, 6, and 12 months and then yearly after graft placement (Class I, Levels of Evidence A).

Digital Subtraction Arteriography

Digital subtraction arteriography (DSA) is the gold standard, but it is invasive and associated with risks, including bleeding, allergic reactions, and contrast nephropathy. Its use has been replaced by the computed tomographic angiography and magnetic resonance angiography.

Clinical Point

1. Digital subtraction angiography is recommended for contrast angiographic studies because this technique allows for enhanced imaging capabilities compared with conventional unsubtracted contrast angiography.

Computed Tomographic Angiography

Computed tomographic angiography (CTA) requires an intravenous injection of iodinated contrast, which opacifies the arteries. The angiographic image is constructed from multiple cross-sectional images and then presented as a maximum intensity projection, similar to the appearance of standard arteriography. The images are three dimensional and can be rotated in space so that eccentric lesions may be observed. This is an advantage over DSA. Unlike magnetic resonance angiography, CTA can be used in patients with pacemakers, defibrillators, metal clips, stents, and prosthesis.

Clinical Points

1. CTA of the extremities may be considered to diagnose the anatomic location and presence of significant stenosis in patients with lower-extremity PAD (Class IIb, Level of Evidence B).
2. CTA of the extremities may be considered as a substitute for MRA for those patients with contraindications to magnetic resonance angiography (MRA) (Class IIb, Level of Evidence B).

Magnetic Resonance Angiography

Magnetic Resonance Angiography (MRA) may be used as the primary diagnostic imaging technique instead of digital subtraction arteriography, especially in patients at high risk for complications of contrast. A meta-analysis of MRA compared with catheter angiography demonstrated that the sensitivity and specificity of MRA for detection of stenosis greater than 50% were both in the range of 90% to 100%, with greatest accuracy when gadolinium-enhanced MRA was used. The most current studies report similar results, with agreement between MRA and catheter angiography of 91% to 97%. Gadolinium-enhanced MRA has also been compared with color duplex ultrasound and demonstrated that MRA had a sensitivity of 98% versus 88% and a specificity of 96% versus 95% in patients greater than 50% stenotic lesions. The addition of gadolinium to MRA is contraindicated in patients with renal impairment. MRA cannot be used in patients with pacemakers, defibrillators, prosthetic joints, mechanical heart valves, stents, surgical clips, and aneurysm clips.

Clinical Points

1. MRA of the extremities is useful to diagnose anatomic location and degree of stenosis of PAD (Class I, Level of Evidence A).
2. MRA of the extremities should be performed with gadolinium enhancement (Class I, Level of Evidence B).

Medical Management of the Vascular Patient

Risk factors for developing PAD include advanced age, cigarette smoking, diabetes mellitus, hyperlipidemia hypertension, and increased homocysteine levels. These must be modified to prevent not only the development but also the progression of PAD when diagnosed (see Figure 17.1).

Smoking

Observational studies have found that the risk of death, myocardial infarction, and amputation is substantially greater in those individuals with PAD who continue to smoke than those who stop smoking. Smokers with PAD have significantly worse claudication, reduced peripheral circulation, and worse exercise tolerance than non-smokers with PAD. Strategies to achieve smoking cessation include physician advice coupled with frequent follow-up visits, nicotine replacement therapy, and buproprion; these have achieved a 5%, 16%, and 30% success rate, respectively. Continued smoking in patients with PAD who require a revascularization procedure have a 3- to 4.7-fold increase in graft failure and an increased risk for amputation. This risk factor must a major focus in the management of the patient with PAD.

Clinical Point

1. Individuals with lower-extremity PAD who smoke cigarettes or use other forms of tobacco should be advised by each of their clinicians to stop smoking and should be offered comprehensive smoking cessation interventions, including behavior modification therapy, nicotine replacement therapy, or buproprion (Class I, Level of Evidence B).

Diabetes Mellitus

Aggressive glucose management is the mainstay of diabetic care in clinical practice, but this approach has not been shown to decrease the risk of adverse cardiovascular events in patients with PAD. A retrospective analysis of the Diabetes Control and Complications Trail, a study of patients with type I diabetes, found that intensive insulin therapy reduced the risk of lower-extremity PAD events, such as claudication, peripheral revascularization, or amputation, by 22%, but that result did not achieve statistical significance. In the United Kingdom Prospective Diabetes Study, patients with type II diabetes mellitus were randomized to aggressive treatment with sulfonylureas or insulin versus conventional treatment. Patients were treated over a period of 10 years. Intensive treatment reduced the risk of myocardial infarction by 16%, a finding of borderline significance, but it did not decrease the risk of death, stroke, or amputation. Meticulous attention to foot care is necessary to reduce the risk of skin ulceration, necrosis, and subsequent amputation. This includes the use of appropriate footwear to avoid pressure injury, daily inspection and cleansing by the patient, and the use of moisturizing cream to prevent dryness and fissuring. Frequent foot inspection by patients and physicians will enable early identification of foot lesions and ulcerations and facilitate referral for treatment.

Aggressive treatment of diabetes decreases the risk of microvascular events such as nephropathy and retinopathy. Therefore, to reduce the risk of microvascular events, pending prospective trials in patients with diabetes and PAD, its recommended that diabetic patient with PAD be treated aggressively to reduce their glycosolated hemoglobin to less than 7% as per the American Diabetes Association.

Clinical Point

1. Treatment of diabetes in individuals with lower-extremity PAD by administration of glucose control therapies to reduce the hemoglobin A1C to less than 7% can be effective to reduce microvascular complications and potentially improve cardiovascular outcomes (Class IIa, Level of Evidence C).

Hyperlipidemia

The treatment of dyslipidemia reduces the risk of adverse cardiovascular events in patients with atherosclerosis. The Heart Protection Study randomized patients with coronary artery disease, cerebrovascular disease, PAD, and or diabetes mellitus and total cholesterol level greater than 135 mg per dL to simvastatin or placebo. The study included 6,748 patients with PAD, in whom there was a 25% risk reduction over 5 years of follow-up. In the National Cholesterol Education Program Adult Treatment Panel III guidelines, individuals with lower-extremity PAD are designated as either high risk or very high risk, depending on associated risk factors. For individuals with PAD, very high risk can be defined as the presence of established PAD plus (a) multiple major risk factors especially diabetes, (b) severe and poorly controlled risk factors (continued cigarette smoking), or (c) multiple risk factors of the metabolic syndrome (high triglycerides > 200 mg/dL) plus non-HDL cholesterol greater than or equal to 130 mg/dL with low HDL cholesterol. With this finding it is recommended that all patients with PAD and an LDL greater than 100 mg/dL be treated with a statin with an LDL target of less than 100 mg/dL. In patients who are very high risk and have PAD, the LDL target should be less than 70 mg/dL.

Clinical Points

1. Treatment with a hydoxymethyl glutharyl (HMG) coenzyme-A reductase inhibitor (statin) medication is indicated for all patients with PAD to achieve a target LDL cholesterol of less than 100 mg/dL (Class I, Level of Evidence B).
2. Treatment with an HMG coenzyme-A reductase inhibitor (statin) medication to achieve a target LDL cholesterol level of less than 70 mg/dL is reasonable for patients with lower-extremity PAD at very high risk of ischemic events (Class IIa, Level of Evidence B).
3. Treatment with fibric acid derivative can be useful for patients with PAD and low HDL cholesterol, normal LDL cholesterol, and elevated triglycerides (Class IIa, Level of Evidence C).

Hypertension

Treatment of high blood pressure is indicated to reduce the risk of cardiovascular events such as stroke, heart failure, and death. ACE inhibitors reduce the risk of death and nonfatal cardiovascular events in patients with coronary artery disease and left ventricular dysfunction. The Heart Outcomes Prevention Evaluation study randomized patients with coronary artery disease , cerebrovascular disease, PAD, and or diabetes to the ACE inhibitor ramipril or placebo. The study included 4,051 patients with PAD. Ramipril reduced the risk of myocardial infarction, stroke, or vascular death in patients with PAD by approximately 25%. It is recommended that ACE inhibitors be considered as treatment for patients with asymptomatic lower-extremity PAD to reduce the risk of adverse cardiovascular events. Beta blockers are also recommended as a management strategy in the PAD population. A meta-analysis of 11 placebo-controlled studies in patients with intermittent claudication found that beta blockers did not adversely affect walking capacity.

Clinical Points

1. Antihypertensive therapy should be administered to hypertensive patients with lower-extremity PAD to achieve a goal of less than 140 mm Hg over 90 mm Hg for nondiabetics and 130 mm Hg over 80 mm Hg for diabetics and chronic renal disease to reduce the risk of myocardial infarction, stroke, congestive heart failure, and cardiovascular death (Class I, Level of Evidence A).
2. Beta adrenergic blocking drugs are effective antihypertensive agents and are not contraindicated in patients with PAD (Class I, Level of Evidence A).
3. The use of ACE inhibitors is reasonable for symptomatic patients with lower-extremity PAD to reduce the risk of adverse cardiovascular events (Class IIa, Level of Evidence B).
4. ACE inhibitors may be considered for patient with asymptomatic lower-extremity PAD to reduce the risk of adverse cardiovascular events (Class IIa, Level of Evidence C).

Hyper-Homocyteinemia

The B complex vitamins, folic acid, cobalamin (B12), and pyridoxine (B6) have been used as therapy to decrease homocysteine levels. A meta-analysis of 12 trials that included 1,114 people found that folic acid, at doses of 0.5 to 5 mg daily, decreased homocysteine concentrations by 25% and that vitamin B12 at doses averaging 0.5 mg daily decreased homocysteine levels by an additional 7%. Vitamin B6 had no significant benefit. At this time the studies have not demonstrated a clinical benefit in PAD patients with elevated homocysteine.

Clinical Point

The effectiveness of the therapeutic use of folic acid and B12 vitamin supplements in individuals with lower-extremity PAD and homocysteine levels greater than 14 micromoles per liter in not well established (Class IIb, Level of Evidence C).

Exercise

Exercise is an important management strategy in patient with PAD and claudication. Regular walking in a supervised claudication exercise program can be expected to result in an increase in the speed, distance, and duration walked, with decreased claudication symptoms at each workload or distance. A meta-analysis of 21 studies by Gardner and Poehlman included both nonrandomized and randomized trials of exercise training and showed that pain-free walking time improved by an average of 180% and maximal walking time increased by 120% in claudication patients who underwent exercise training. This meta-analysis also provided data to summarize clinical predictors of responsiveness to exercise interventions. The greatest improvements in walking ability occurred when each exercise session lasted longer than 30 minutes, when sessions took place at least three times per week, when the exercise modality used was walking to near-maximal pain, and when the program lasted 6 months or longer. A meta-analysis from the Cochran Collaborative that considered only randomized, controlled trials concluded that exercise improved maximal walking ability by an average of 150%.

The time course of the response to a program of exercise has not been fully established. Exercise-induced clinical benefits have been observed as early as 4 weeks and have been observed to continue to improve after 6 months of participation. Gardner et al. reported that improvements in walking ability after 6 months of supervised exercise rehabilitation three times per week were sustained when patients continued to participate in an exercise maintenance program for an additional 12 months.

Clinicians should recognize that minimal data support the efficacy of the informal "go home and walk" advice that still makes up the most typical exercise prescription for claudication. Although some patients might theoretically achieve benefit from such casual exercise prescriptions, the determinants of success and documentation of efficacy are not yet defined. In contrast, a supervised hospital or clinic program, which ensures that patients are receiving a standardized exercise stimulus in a safe environment, is effective. Exercise-induced improvements in walking ability translates to increases in routine daily activity.

Clinical Points

1. A program of supervised exercise training is recommended as an initial treatment modality for patients with intermittent claudication (Class I, Level of Evidence A).
2. Supervised exercise training should be performed for a minimum of 30 to 45 minutes, in sessions performed at least three times per week for a minimum of 12 weeks (Class I, Level of Evidence A).
3. The usefulness of unsupervised exercise programs is not well established as an effective initial treatment modality for patients with intermittent claudicating (Class IIb, Level of Evidence B).

Pharmacologic Treatment of PAD

Pentoxifylline and cilostazol are two pharmacologic agents approved by the FDA for treating peripheral artery disease patients with lifestyle-limiting claudication. The agents have no effect on preventing secondary atherosclerotic vascular events.

Pentoxifylline is a methylxanthine derivative with hemorheologic properties that have been reported to decrease blood and plasma viscosity, increase erythrocyte and leukocyte deformability, inhibit neutrophil adhesion and activation, and lower plasma fibrinogen concentrations. Meta-analysis of randomized, placebo controlled, double-blind clinical trials have found that pentoxifylline causes a marginal but statistically significant improvement in pain-free and maximal walking distance. Pentoxifylline does not increase the ABI at rest or after exercise. The recommended dose is 400 mg orally three times per day. Adverse effects associated with pentoxifylline include sore throat, dyspepsia, nausea, and diarrhea.

Cilostazol is a phosphodiesterase type 3 inhibitor that increases cyclic adenosine monophosphate, which causes vasodilation and platelet inhibition, but the precise mechanism for it affect in claudication is not known. Cilostazol has been reported to inhibit expression of vascular cell adhesion molecule-1, inhibit expression of vascular smooth muscle cell proliferation, and prevent restenosis in patients with coronary artery disease who underwent percutaneous transluminal coronary angioplasty. Five prospective randomized trials of patients with intermittent claudication found that cilostazol improves maximal walking distance by 40% to 60% compared with placebo after 12 to 24 weeks of therapy. In these studies, 100 mg twice daily was more effective than 50 mg twice daily. A meta-analysis of these trials indicated that cilostazol also improved walking ability and health-related quality of life. The most common side effects of cilostazol include headache, diarrhea, abnormal stools, palpitations, and dizziness. Other phosphodiesterase inhibitors such milrinone and vesnarinone are associated with increased mortality in patients with congestive heart failure and reduce systolic left ventricular function. None of the trials conducted to date have found a significant increase in mortality or major cardiovascular events in patients treated with cilostazol. The Food and Drug Administration has mandated a black-box warning that cilostazol should not be used in patients with heart failure.

Vasodilator prostaglandins such as prostaglandin E1 and derivatives of prostacyclin iloprost and beraprost have been studied as potential therapy for treatment of patients with claudication. These agents have not been found to have significant improvement in walking distance. The nutritional supplements L-arginine, propionyl-L-carnitine, and vitamin E as therapies to improve walking distance in patients with claudication have not been well established. Gingko biloba has been shown to be marginally effective in intermittent claudication, but this has not recommended. Chelation therapy with disodium ethylenediaminetetraacetic acid (EDTA) is used in the treatment of heavy metal poisoning. This therapeutic intervention was used in patients with claudication based on the theory that the EDTA treatment leached calcium out of atherosclerotic plaques, resulting in plaques regression and reduction in stenosis. In four trials there was no improvement in walking distance, and there was no evidence of angiographic improvement in atherosclerotic lesions in the chelation treated patients.

The effect of antiplatelet therapy on cardiovascular events has been systematically reviewed by the Antithrombotic Trialists Collaborative. A meta-analysis comprising 287 studies compared the efficacy of antiplatelet therapy versus control in approximately 135,000 high-risk patients with vascular diseases manifested as acute and previous myocardial infarction, acute and previous stroke, or other high-risk conditions such as PAD. Among those patients with PAD treated with antiplatelet therapy, there was a 22% odds reduction for adverse cardiovascular events, including myocardial infarction, stroke, or vascular death. This analysis included 42 trials comprising 9,716 patients with PAD in who there was a 23% proportional reduction in adverse cardiovascular events. Similar benefits were realized by patients with intermittent claudication, those having peripheral angioplasty, and those having peripheral bypass graft procedures. There was a 23% reduction of vascular events in patients with intermittent claudication, 22% in those with peripheral arterial grafts, and 29% in those undergoing peripheral angioplasty. The Antithrombotic Trialists'

Collaboration meta-analysis also compared the efficacy of different doses of aspirin. The proportional reduction in vascular events was 32% with 75 to 150 mg daily, 26% with 160 to 325 mg daily, and 19% with 500 to 1,500 mg daily, the results being relatively comparable among these dose ranges. There was a significantly smaller 13% reduction in cardiovascular events in patients being treated with less than 75 mg of aspirin per day. The odds ratios for a major extracranial bleed among patients taking 75 to 150 mg of aspirin and those taking 160 to 325 mg of aspirin daily were 1.5 and 1.4, respectively. Higher doses of aspirin result in increased risk of gastrointestinal side effects and bleeding rates. One trial compared the efficacy of aspirin 325 mg daily to the clopidogrel 75 mg daily in 19,185 patients with a history of myocardial infarction, stroke, or PAD. Clopidogrel reduced the risk of adverse cardiovascular events by 8.7%. Among the 6,452 patients with PAD, clopidogrel reduced the risk of myocardial infarction, stroke, or vascular death by 23.8% more than aspirin. The aspirin group the risk of intracranial was 0.35% and gastrointestinal bleeding 1.99%, whereas the clopidogrel group had 0.35% gastrointestinal and a 1.99% intracranial hemorrhage. It is recommended that patients with lower-extremity PAD be treated with antiplatelet therapy to reduce the risk of myocardial infarction, stroke, or vascular death. On the basis of the single comparative trial, clopidogrel appears to be more effective than aspirin in preventing ischemic events in symptomatic PAD patients. To date, there is no evidence to support the efficacy of combined aspirin and clopidogrel versus single antiplatelet agent therapy in patient with lower-extremity PAD. In addition, the Antithrombotic Trialists Collaboration had shown that antiplatelet therapy reduced the risk of arterial occlusion over a 19-month period by 30%.

Clinical Points

1. Pentoxyifylline 400 mg, orally, three times daily may be considered as second-line alternative therapy to cilostazol to improve walking distance in patients with PAD intermittent claudication (Class IIb, Level of Evidence A).

2. Cilostazol 100 mg, orally, twice daily is indicated as an effective therapy to improve symptoms and increase walking distance in patients with lower-extremity PAD and intermittent claudication and without heart failure (Class I, Level of Evidence A).
3. Oral vasodilator prostaglandins such as beraprost and iloprost are not effective medications to improve walking distance in patients with intermittent claudication (Class III, Level of Evidence A).
4. The effectiveness of L-arginine, propionyl-L-carnitine, and vitamin E in improving walking distance has not well established (Class IIb, Level of Evidence B).
5. The effectiveness of ginkgo biloba in improving walking distance is marginal and not well established (Class IIb, Level of Evidence B).
6. Chelation (EDTA) is not indicated for treatment of intermittent claudication and may have harmful adverse effects (Class III, Level of Evidence A).

Acute and Chronic Limb Ischemia

(See Figure 17.2)

Acute Limb Ischemia

Acute limb ischemia occurs when a rapid or sudden reduction in limb perfusion threatens tissue viability. The severity of acute limb ischemia depends on the location and extent of arterial obstruction and the capacity of the collaterals to perfuse the ischemic territory. Acute limb ischemia is often associated with thrombosis caused by atherosclerotic plaque rupture, thrombosis of a lower-extremity bypass graft, or lower-extremity embolism of cardiac origin or a proximal arterial aneurysm. Arterial emboli typically lodge at branch points in the arterial circulation where the caliber of the arterial lumen diminishes. The hallmark clinical symptoms and physical examination signs of acute limb ischemia include the 5 "Ps": pain, pallor, pulseless, paresthesias, and paralysis. The clinical history should determine the onset and course of ischemia as well as concomitant medical disorders that could contribute to

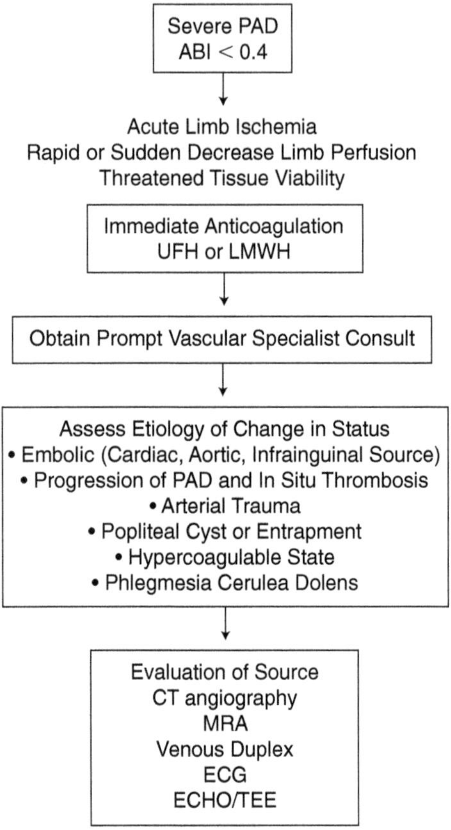

■ **Figure 17.2** Acute Limb Ischemia

Source: Adapted from Hirsch AT, et al. *Circulation* 2006;1131:1474–1547.

the current acute event. The clinical diagnosis of arterial embolism is suggested by the sudden onset or worsening of symptoms, a known embolic source such as atrial fibrillation, dilated cardiomyopathy, left ventricular aneurysm or atherosclerotic aorta disease, the absence of antecedent claudication or other manifestations of obstructive arterial disease or the presence of normal arterial pulses and Doppler systolic blood pressures in the contralateral limb. Persistent pain, sensory loss, and toe muscle weakness are among the most important findings that identify the patient with threatened limb loss. Muscle rigor, tenderness, and pain on passive movement are late signs of advanced ischemia predictive of tissue loss.

The differential diagnosis of acute limb ischemia involves exclusion of conditions that mimic arterial occlusion, identification of nonatherosclerotic causes of arterial occlusion, and differentiation of ischemia caused by an arterial thrombosis from embolism. Conditions that may mimic acute limb ischemia include low cardiac output superimposed on PAD and acute deep vein thrombosis associated with massive leg swelling (phlegmasia cerulea dolens). Acute limb ischemia requires prompt diagnosis and treatment in order to preserve limb viability.

Clinical Points

1. Patients with acute limb ischemia and a salvageable extremity should undergo an emergent evaluation that defines the anatomic level of occlusion and that leads to prompt endovascular or surgical revascularization (Class I, Level of Evidence B).

Chronic Limb Ischemia

Critical limb ischemia is defined as limb pain that occurs at rest or impending limb loss that is caused by sever compromise of blood flow to the affected extremity. The term critical limb ischemia should be used for all patients with chronic ischemic rest pain, ulcers, or gangrene attributable to objectively proven arterial occlusive disease. Unlike patients with claudication, those with chronic limb ischemia have resting perfusion that is inadequate to sustain viability in the distal tissue bed. Atherosclerotic arterial disease that precipitates chronic limb ischemia is most often diffuse or multi-segmental, involving more than one arterial anatomic level (see Figure 17.3).

Patients with chronic limb ischemia present with limb pain at rest, with or without trophic skin changes or tissue loss. The discomfort is often worse when the patient is supine and may lessen

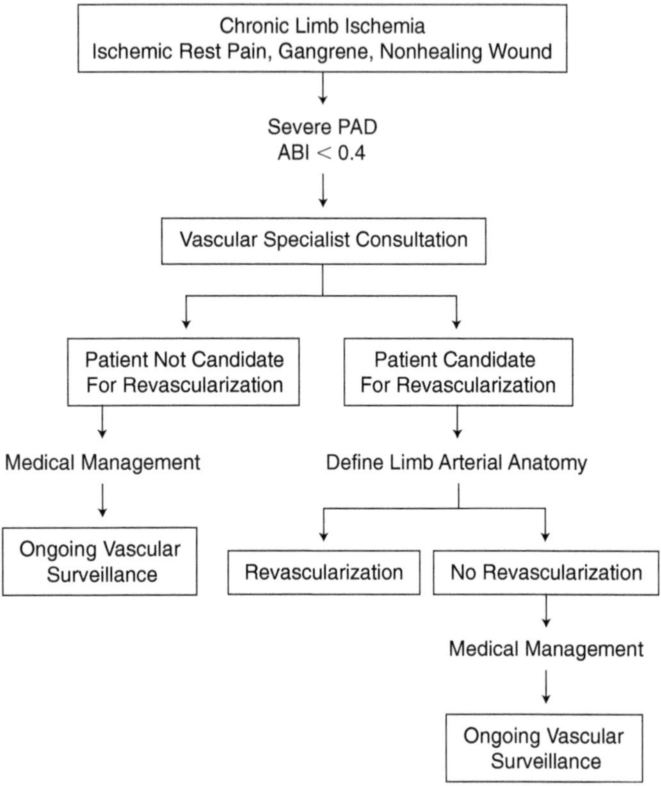

■ **Figure 17.3** Chronic Limb Ischemia

Source: Modified from Hirsch AT, et al. *Circulation* 2006;1131:1474–1547.

when the limb is maintained in the dependent position. It is important in evaluating this patient group to distinguish between ischemia that is acute versus chronic because the diagnostic and therapeutic approaches and prognosis are different. The time course of symptoms and signs in chronic limb ischemia is the important differentiating point in assessing this patient group. This should include evaluation for arterial disease in other vascular beds, global atherosclerosis risk assessment, and evaluation of any specific precipitating factors or events such as trauma, infection, and lower-extremity procedures that may have caused skin ulceration.

Evaluation of patients with chronic limb ischemia requires systemic assessment of pulses and tissue perfusion to identify the level of obstructive lesions and potential involvement of other threatened extremities. Signs of chronic ischemia, including dependent rubor, pallor on elevation of the extremity, and reduce capillary refill, should be confirmed. Distinction should be made between ulcers that are arterial and those that are venous or neuropathic. Arterial ulcers are painful, are located on the toes or foot, and have an irregular boarder with a pinkish base. On the other hand, venous ulcers are mildly painful, are located around the molleolar areas, and have an irregular boarder with a pink base. Neuropathic ulcers are painless, are located on the plantar surface of the foot, and are deep. Treatment of chronic limb ischemia is dependent on increasing blood flow to the affected extremity to relieve pain, heal ischemic ulcerations, and avoid limb loss. Individuals with minimal or no skin breakdown or in whom co-morbid conditions prevent consideration of revascularization can occasionally be treated by medical therapies in the absence of revascularization. Medical care strategies have included the use of antiplatelet agents, anticoagulant medications, intravenous prostanoids, rheologic agents, and maintenance of the limb in a dependent position. None of these clinical interventions has been evaluated adequately or proven to offer predictable improvements in limb outcomes in prospective trials. Critical limb ischemia is associated with a very high intermediate term morbidity and mortality. In the absence of revascularization, most patients with chronic limb ischemia will have amputation within 6 months. Referral to a vascular surgeon is indicated to expedite treatment, prevent further deterioration, and reverse the ischemic process.

Clinical Points

1. Patients with chronic limb ischemia should undergo expedited evaluation and treatment of factors that are known to increase the risk of amputation (Class I, Level of Evidence C).

2. Patients with chronic limb ischemia in whom open surgical repair is anticipated should undergo assessment of underlying cardiovascular risk (Class I, Level of Evidence B).
3. Patients with prior history of chronic limb ischemia or who have undergone successful treatment for chronic limb ischemia should be evaluated at least twice annually by a vascular specialist because of the relatively high incidence of recurrence (Class I, Level of Evidence C).
4. Systemic antibiotics should be initiated promptly in patients with chronic limb ischemia, skin ulcerations, and evidence of limb infection (Class I, Level of Evidence B).
5. Patients at risk for chronic limb ischemia (those with diabetes, neuropathy, chronic renal failure, or infection) who develop acute limb symptoms represent potential vascular emergencies and should be assessed immediately and treated by a specialist competent in treating vascular disease (Class I, Level of Evidence C).

18 ■ Clinical Research

David J. Whellan, MD, MHS, FACC,
Suzanne Adams, RN, MPH
Sue Russell, MFA

- The term "clinical research" refers to medical research in which an investigator or investigators has direct interaction with human subjects.
- Clinical research is thus differentiated from research in animals and from in vivo research, which involves human tissue but is not linked to a living individual. It can also be differentiated from in vitro or basic science research, which in medicine addresses the fundamental biological mechanisms of disease but requires no human interaction.
- The aim of such an investigation is to add to the existing knowledge about a disease and its treatment.
- The two main types of clinical investigations are observational studies and experimental studies.

Observational Studies

- An *observational* study measures variables at a single point in time.
- The investigator chooses a condition or outcome of interest and measures factors that may be related to that outcome.
- An observational study is often the first step toward a cohort study (defined later here).
- Observational studies are generally referred to as either *descriptive* or *analytical.*

Descriptive and Exploratory Studies

- A descriptive study provides descriptive information about a disease, usually on the basis of a single sample (case report) or a small group (case series).

- Exploratory studies are used to develop theories on the basis of observed behaviors. They are intuitive in nature.

Advantages and disadvantages of observational studies are as follows:

- The main advantage of an observational study is that it is relatively inexpensive and quick.
- The disadvantages of observational studies are that they cannot establish causality and do not provide a sufficient basis for generalization.

Examples of observational studies are as follows:

- Concern for privacy in relation to age during physical examination of children: an exploratory study (*Acta Paediatr.* 2009 May 19 [Epub ahead of print])
- Hypertension and cognitive decline in rural elderly Chinese (*J Am Geriatr Soc.* 2009;57:1051–1057)
- Safety and efficacy of ezetimibe in a sample of cardiac transplant patients (*Transplant Proc.* 2008;40:3058–3059)

Analytical Studies

- An analytical study tests a hypothesis with regard to a disease and its causes or treatment.
- Cohort studies, case-control studies, and cross-sectional studies are examples of analytical studies.

Cohort Studies

- In cohort studies, the relative risk is defined as the ratio of the incidence of disease in the exposed group versus the unexposed group.
- Cohort studies can be prospective or retrospective.
- A prospective cohort study follows individuals over time with respect to a specific characteristic, such as a disease, incorporates a control group of individuals who do not have

this characteristic, and compares designated outcomes of the two groups.

- An advantage to prospective cohort studies is that they offer control over subject selection and measurements.
- The disadvantages of prospective cohort studies include the possibility of surveillance bias, which refers to differences in the levels of scrutiny applied to one group compared with another.
- Other disadvantages are potential expense and loss to follow-up.
- A retrospective cohort study uses existing data to identify a baseline measurement in relation to a follow-up measurement also in the past.
- Advantages to retrospective cohort studies are that they establish a sequence of events and offer the possibility of multiple outcomes.
- The disadvantage to retrospective cohort studies is that they offer less control over subject selection and measurements than would be available in prospective studies.

Cross-Sectional Cohort Studies

- A cross-sectional cohort study uses existing data to follow subjects over a specified period of time.
- Cross-sectional cohort studies are used to determine prevalence, describe the natural history of a condition, analyze risk factors for various outcomes, and provide simultaneous assessment of baseline measures and outcomes.
- Cross-sectional cohort studies evaluate the predictive capability of a particular clinical feature, such as a rectal examination, for determining the level of risk for prostate cancer.
- A cross-sectional cohort study uses a sample, provides the ability to generalize, and establishes time–order relationships.
- Advantages of cross-sectional cohort studies include their capacity to establish a sequence of events, the possibility of

studying several different outcomes at a time, and the fact that they yield information on incidence and relative risk of a specified disease.

- Disadvantages of cross-sectional cohort studies are that they require a large sample size, are not feasible for rare outcomes, require a longer period of time than prospective studies, and offer less control over subject selection and measurements.

Case-Control Studies

- Case-control studies are generally retrospective.
- They identify groups of subjects with and without a designated disease and look back in time to find differences in predictor variables that may explain why the cases got the disease and the controls did not. An example of a case-control study might be the incidence of toxic shock syndrome in women who have used a particular variety of tampons or the incidence of pancreatic cancer in habitual coffee drinkers.
- The cases in a case-control study represent the larger population of those with the outcome and should be a clearly delineated, homogeneous population.
- The controls are selected from the same general population from which the cases are selected, but the controls do not have the outcome of interest.
- Several different strategies can be incorporated into the design of case-control studies. For example, these studies can include multiple controls; establish community controls, such as random-digit dialing to accrue subjects; or employ matching and overmatching, as for sickle cell disease.
- The advantages of case-control trials are their usefulness in studying rare conditions, their relative low costs because of short duration, and their ability to provide an association between each predictor and the presence or absence of the designated disease.

- The disadvantages are that they are limited to one outcome variable, do not yield information about how common the disease is or how quickly new cases occur, and are very challenging to design without bias.

Examples of Analytical Studies

Prospective Cohort Studies

- Catheter ablation versus amiodarone plus losartan for prevention of atrial fibrillation recurrence in patients with paroxysmal atrial fibrillation (*Eur J Clin Invest.* 2009 May 27 [Epub ahead of print])
- Retrospective cohort studies
- The contribution of longitudinal comorbidity measurements to survival analysis (*Med Care.* 2009 Jun 16 [Epub ahead of print])
- Cross-sectional cohort studies
- Plasma adiponectin in heart transplant recipients (*Clin Transplant.* 2009;23:83–88)
- Case-control studies
- Lifetime tobacco smoke exposure and breast cancer incidence (*Cancer Causes Control.* 2009 Jun 17 [Epub ahead of print])

Experimental Studies

- An experimental study is one in which the investigator specifies the exposure category for each individual and then follows the individual to detect the effects of the exposure. Experimental trials can be randomized and controlled or controlled but not randomized.

Nonrandomized Controlled Trials

- Nonrandomized controlled trials can detect associations between a treatment and its outcome, but they cannot rule out the possibility that the outcome was due to a third factor linked to both treatment and outcome.

Randomized Controlled Trials

- Randomized controlled trials (RCTs) represent the gold standard of experimental design. In these trials, patients from a well-defined population are randomly assigned to selected treatment groups. RCTs can be therapeutic (comparing treatment methods) or prophylactic (investigating an avenue of disease prevention).
- RCTs compare subjects who differ only with respect to the intervention. They are used to evaluate the efficacy of a treatment under ideal circumstances.
- If entry criteria are rigid enough, there is a high degree of certainty that an extraneous variable cannot influence results; however, this rigidity makes recruitment difficult and limits the generalizability of the study's results.

Randomization and Blinding

- Randomization avoids selection bias, which refers to circumstances when study and control groups are selected in a way that causes them to differ from each other by at least one factor that affects the study's outcomes.
- Randomization equalizes the experimental and comparison groups.
- Each subject has an equal chance to be in any of the groups.
- In a single-blind study, the researcher knows the patient's assigned group but the patient does not.
- In a double-blind study, neither the investigator nor the patient knows the treatment group to which the patient is assigned. The treatment allocations are concealed from the investigator performing the intervention. Computer-generated random allocations are often provided by individuals not involved in data collection.

Endpoints

- An endpoint is a measured outcome that answers a specific clinical question. Types of outcomes include the following:
    - Physiologic
    - Patient centric (quality of life, patient satisfaction)
    - Clinical (mortality, hospitalization, emergency room visits, procedures)
    - Cost

Types of RCTs

- Parallel-design double-blind trials are studies in which patients are assigned to only one treatment group.
- In parallel-design double-blind trials, participants and those administering the intervention remain unaware of the group to which individual subjects are assigned.
- Parallel-design double-blind trials are designed to assess whether one treatment is superior to others.
- Crossover trials are studies in which patients receive more than one treatment under investigation with a specified amount of time in between, called a washout period.
- In crossover trials, participants each serve as their own controls.
- Crossover trials are useful for drug therapy that can be evaluated fairly quickly and for conditions that do not progress rapidly.
- A disadvantage of crossover trials is that subjects may drop out before the second treatment.
- Equivalence and noninferiority trials are comparisons of a new or less expensive treatment against one that is already known to be effective, with the latter referred to as the active control, as opposed to placebo.
- Noninferiority trials incorporate a specific margin within which the new intervention can be deemed to be no worse than the active control.

Analysis of Data in RCTs

- RCTs usually follow the intent-to-treat model, through which patients are analyzed within the group to which they are assigned whether or not they completed the intended intervention.
- Analysis focuses on an estimation of the size of the difference in predefined outcomes among the intervention groups.

Additional Information about Clinical Trials

The FDA Clinical Trial Phases

- Clinical studies are generally considered to test drugs or devices and are organized into four separate phases.
- Phase I studies are conducted in a small number of healthy volunteers and are meant to test the safety of an intervention. These studies may follow trials in animals and focus on the pharmacokinetics of absorption, metabolism, and excretion in humans. This phase also tests for side effects related to dosing levels.
- Phase II studies are meant to test the efficacy of an intervention in patients who actually have the condition. These are usually conducted in individuals who are randomized to receive the intervention being tested versus a control group receiving a placebo or standard care. Often the investigators are blinded to the randomization.
- Phase III studies are also randomized and blinded, but the intervention is tested in much larger numbers of subjects over longer periods of time. Approval for marketing of the drug can be requested when these studies are completed.
- Phase IV studies are often referred to as "postmarketing surveillance," as they are conducted after an intervention

has been approved for use. Here the focus tends to monitor long-term effectiveness, cost-effectiveness, and safety in comparison to other available drugs.

The National Institutes of Health Trial Purposes

- Prevention trials look for better ways to prevent disease in people who have never had the disease or to prevent a disease from returning. These approaches may include medicines, vitamins, vaccines, minerals, or lifestyle changes.
- Screening trials test the best way to detect certain diseases or health conditions.
- Diagnostic trials conducted to find better tests or procedures for diagnosing a particular disease or condition.
- Treatment trials test experimental treatments, new combinations of drugs, or new approaches to surgery or radiation therapy.
- Quality of life trials explore ways to improve comfort and the quality of life for individuals with a chronic illness (also known as supportive care trials).
- Compassionate use trials provide experimental therapeutics prior to final Food and Drug Administration approval to patients whose options with other remedies have been unsuccessful. Usually, case by case approval must be granted by the Food and Drug Administration for such exceptions.
- Quality and practice improvement activities are not always or necessarily recognized as research. Generally, the key is whether the project is intended to develop "generalizable" knowledge versus a focus on internal institutional quality/performance improvement.

References

Chapter 1

Blackburn G. Exercise in prevention of coronary artery disease. In Foody, ed. *Preventive Cardiology.* Humana Press, Totowas, NJ; 2006:145–158.

Bouchard C. Physical activity and prevention of cardiovascular disease: potential mechanisms physical activity and cardiovascular health: a national consensus. Human Kinetics: Chicago, IL;1997;45–57.

Buchsbaum RB, Buchsbaum JC. Tobacco as a cardiovascular risk factor. In Foody, ed. *Preventive Cardiology.* Humana Press; 2006:179–191.

Bullen C. Impact of tobacco smoking and smoking cessation on cardiovascular risk and disease, expert review cardiovascular therapeutics. 2008;6(6):883–895.

Gotto A, Toth P. *Comprehensive Management of High Risk Cardiovascular Patients.* New York: Information Healthcare; 2007:187–238.

Fagard RH. *Diabetes Care,* 2009 Nov; 32 Suppl 2:5429–5431.

Howard BV, Rodriguez BL, Bennett PH, et al. Prevention conference VI: diabetes and cardiovascular disease writing group I. *Circulation* 2002; 105:e132–e137.

Leon Arthur, ed. NIH. Physical activity and cardiovascular health. A national consensus human kinetics. 1997;57–67.

O'Rourke R, Fuszerv, Alexender R, et al. *Hurst's (the Heart) Manual of Cardiology,* 11th ed. New York: McGraw-Hill, 2004:519–532.

Stewart K. The role of exercise training on cardiovascular disease in patients who have type II diabetes. *Cardiol Clin* 2004;22:569–586.

Wong N, Black H, Gavdin J. *Preventive Cardiology: A Practical Approach,* 2nd ed. McGraw-Hill; 2005.

Zarich S. The role of intensive glycemic control in management of patients who have acute MI. *Cardiol Clin* 2005;23:109–117.

Zipes DP, Libby P, Bonow RO, Braunwald E, eds. *Braunwald's Heart Disease: Textbook of Cardiovascular Medicine,* 7th ed. Philadelphia: Saunders; 2005:921–1012.

Chapter 3

Friese RS, Shafi S, Gentilello LM. Pulmonary artery catheter use is associated with reduced mortality in severely injured patients: a National Trauma Data Bank analysis of 53,312 patients. *Crit Care Med* 2006;34:1597–1601.

Graham AS, Ozment C, Tegtmeyer K, Lai S, Braner DAV. Central venous catheterization. *N Engl J Med* 2007;356:e21.

Jacobi J, Fraser GL, Coursin DB, et al. Clinical practice guidelines for the sustained use of sedatives and analgesics in the critically ill adult. *Crit Care Med* 2002;30:119–141.

Kearon C, Kahn S, Agnelli G, Goldhaber S, Raskob GE, Comerota AJ. Antithrombotic therapy for venous thromboembolic disease. *Chest* 2008; 133:454S–545S.

Kollef MH. Current concepts: the prevention of ventilator-associated pneumonia. *N Engl J Med* 1999;340:627–634.

MacIntyre NR, Cook DJ, Ely EW Jr, et al. Evidence-based guidelines for weaning and discontinuing ventilatory support. *Chest* 2001;120: 375S–395S.

McGee DC, Gould MK. Current concepts: preventing complications of central venous catheterization. *N Engl J Med* 2003;348:1123–1133.

Neumar RW, Nolan JP, Adrie C, et al. Post-cardiac arrest syndrome. *Circulation* 2008;118:2452–2483.

Reynolds HR, Hochman JS. Cardiogenic shock: current concepts and improving outcomes. *Circulation* 2008;117:686–697.

Wheeler AP, Bernard GR, Thompson BT, et al. National Heart, Lung, and Blood Institute Acute Respiratory Distress Syndrome (ARDS) Clinical Trials Network. Pulmonary-artery versus central venous catheter to guide treatment of acute lung injury. *N Engl J Med* 2006; 354:2213–2224.

Chapter 4

CIBIS Investigators and Committees. A randomized trial of beta-blockade in heart failure. The Cardiac Insufficiency Bisoprolol Study (CIBIS). *Circulation*; 1994;90(4):1765–1773.

Abraham WT, Adams KF, Fonarow GC, et al. In-hospital mortality in patients with acute decompensated heart failure requiring intravenous vasoactive medications: an analysis from the Acute Decompensated Heart Failure National Registry (ADHERE). *J Am Coll Cardiol* 2005;46(1):57–64.

Adams KF Jr, Fonarow GC, Emerman CL, et al. Characteristics and outcomes of patients hospitalized for heart failure in the United States: rationale, design, and preliminary observations from the first 100,000 cases in the Acute Decompensated Heart Failure National Registry (ADHERE). *Am Heart J* 2005;149:209–216.

Adams KF, Lindenfeld J, Arnold JMO, et al. Executive summary: HFSA 2006 Comprehensive Heart Failure Practice Guidelines. *J Card Fail* 2006;12(1).

Adamson PB, Magalski A, Braunschweig F. Ongoing right ventricular hemodynamics in heart failure: clinical value of measurements derived from an implantable monitoring system. *J Am Coll Cardiol* 2003;41(4):565–571.

Aghababian RV. Acutely decompensated heart failure: opportunities to improve care and outcomes in the emergency department. *Rev Cardiovasc Med* 2002;3:S3–S9.

Ahmed A, Rich MW, Love T, et al. Digoxin and reduction in mortality and hospitalization in heart failure: a comprehensive post hoc analysis of the DIG trial. *Eur Heart J* 2006;27(2):178–186.

Alderman EL, Fisher LD, Litwin P, et al. Results of coronary artery surgery in patients with poor left ventricular function (CASS). *Circulation* 1983;68(4):785–789.

Alla F, Briancon S, Juilliere Y, et al. Differential clinical prognostic classifications in dilated and ischemic advanced heart failure: the EPICAL study. *Am Heart J* 2000;139(5):895–904.

Allman KC, Shaw LJ, Hachamovitch R, Udelson JE. Myocardial viability testing and impact of revascularization on prognosis in patients with coronary artery disease and left ventricular dysfunction: a meta-analysis. *J Am Coll Cardiol* 2002;39(7):1151–1158.

Amabile CM, Spencer AP. Keeping your patient with heart failure safe: a review of potentially dangerous medications. *Arch Intern Med* 2004; 164(7):709–720.

American Heart Association. *Heart Disease and Stroke Statistics—2007 Update.* Dallas, TX: American Heart Association; 2007.

Andersson B, Hamm C, Persson S, et al. Improved exercise hemodynamic status in dilated cardiomyopathy after beta-adrenergic blockade treatment. *J Am Coll Cardiol* 1994;23(6):1397–1404.

Badwhar V, Bolling SF. Mitral valve surgery: when is it appropriate? *Congest Heart Fail* 2002;8(4):210–213.

Baldasseroni S, Opasich C, Gorini M. Left bundle-branch block is associated with increased 1-year sudden and total mortality rate in 5517 outpatients with congestive heart failure: a report from the Italian network on congestive heart failure. *Am Heart J* 2002;143(3):398–405.

Bart BA, Shaw LK, McCants CB Jr. Clinical determinants of mortality in patients with angiographically diagnosed ischemic or nonischemic cardiomyopathy. *J Am Coll Cardiol* 1997;30(4):1002–1008.

Baruch L, Patacsil P, Hameed A, et al. Pharmacodynamic effects of milrinone with and without a bolus loading infusion. *Am Heart J* 2001; 141:266–273.

Beta-Blocker Evaluation of Survival Trial Investigators: a trial of the beta-blocker bucindolol in patients with advanced chronic heart failure. *N Engl J Med* 2001;344:1659.

Blackledge HM, Tomlinson J, Squire IB. Prognosis for patients newly admitted to hospital with heart failure: survival trends in 12,220 index admissions in Leicestershire 1993–2001. *Heart* 2003;89:615–620.

Bounous EP, Mark DB, Pollock BG, et al. Surgical survival benefits for coronary disease patients with left ventricular dysfunction. *Circulation* 1988;78(3 Pt 2):I151–I157.

Bristow MR, O'Connell JB, Gilbert EM, et al. Dose-response of chronic beta-blocker treatment in heart failure from either idiopathic dilated or ischemic cardiomyopathy. Bucindolol Investigators. *Circulation* 1994;89(4):1632–1642.

Carson P, Ziesche S, Johnson G, Cohn JN. Racial differences in response to therapy for heart failure: analysis of the vasodilator-heart failure trials: Vasodilator-Heart Failure Trial Study Group. *J Card Fail* 1999; 5(3):178–187.

Cataliotti A, Malatino LS, Jougasaki M, et al. Circulating natriuretic peptide concentrations in patients with end-stage renal disease: role of brain natriuretic peptide as a biomarker for ventricular remodeling. *Mayo Clin Proc* 2001;76:1111.

Chareonthaitawee P, Gersh BJ, Araoz PA, Gibbons RJ. Revascularization in severe left ventricular dysfunction: the role of viability testing. *J Am Coll Cardiol* 2005;46(4):567–574.

Cleland JG, Dargie HJ, Ball SG, et al. Effects of enalapril in heart failure: a double blind study of effects on exercise performance, renal function, hormones, and metabolic state. *Br Heart J* 1985;54(3):305–312.

Cleland JG, Daubert JC, Erdmann E, et al. The effect of cardiac resynchronization on morbidity and mortality in heart failure. *N Engl J Med* 2005;352:1539.

Cohn JN, Archibald DG, Ziesche S, et al. Effect of vasodilator therapy on mortality in chronic congestive heart failure: results of a Veterans Administration Cooperative Study. *N Engl J Med* 1986;314:1547–1552.

Cohn JN, Fowler MB, Bristow MR, et al. Safety and efficacy of carvedilol in severe heart failure: the U.S. Carvedilol Heart Failure Study Group. *J Card Fail* 1997;3:173–179.

Cohn JN, Johnson G, Ziesche S, et al. A comparison of enalapril with hydralazine-isosorbide dinitrate in the treatment of chronic congestive heart failure. *N Engl J Med* 1991;325(5):303–310.

Cohn JN, Tognoni G. A randomized trial of the angiotensin-receptor blocker valsartan in chronic heart failure. *N Engl J Med* 2001;345: 1667–1675.

Colucci WS, Packer M, Bristow MR, et al., for the U.S. Carvedilol Heart Failure Study Group. Carvedilol inhibits clinical progression in patients with mild symptoms of heart failure. *Circulation* 1996;94:2800–2806.

Cooper LT, Baughman KL, Feldman AM. The role of endomyocardial biopsy in the management of cardiovascular disease: a scientific statement from the American Heart Association, the American College of Cardiology, and the European Society of Cardiology. *Circulation* 2007;116:2216–2233.

Costanzo MR, Saltzberg M, O'Sullivan J, Sobotka P. Early ultrafiltration in patients with decompensated heart failure and diuretic resistance. *J Am Coll Cardiol* 2005;46(11):2047–2051. Epub November 9, 2005.

Cuffe MS, Califf RM, Adams KF, et al. Outcomes of a Prospective Trial of Intravenous Milrinone for Exacerbations of Chronic Heart Failure (OPTIME-CHF) Investigators short-term intravenous milrinone for acute exacerbation of chronic heart failure: a randomized controlled trial. *JAMA* 2002;287:1541–1547.

Desideri A, Cortigiani L, Christen AI, et al. The extent of perfusion-F18-fluorodeoxyglucose positron emission tomography mismatch determines mortality in medically treated patients with chronic ischemic left ventricular dysfunction. *J Am Coll Cardiol* 2005;46(7):1264–1269.

DiPiro JT, Talbert RL, Yee GC, et al. *Pharmacotherapy: A Pathophysiologic Approach.* China: McGraw-Hill Professional; 2008.

Domanski MJ, Mitchell GF, Norman JE. Independent prognostic information provided by sphygmomanometrically determined pulse pressure and mean arterial pressure in patients with left ventricular dysfunction. *J Am Coll Cardiol* 1999;33(4):951–958.

Dormans TP, van Meyel JJ, Gerlang PG, et al. Diuretic efficacy of high dose furosemide in severe heart failure: bolus injection vs. continuous infusion. *J Am Coll Cardiol* 1996;28;376–382.

Doughty RN, Whalley GA, Gamble G, et al. Left ventricular remodeling with carvedilol in patients with congestive heart failure due to ischemic heart disease: Australia-New Zealand Heart Failure Research Collaborative Group. *J Am Coll Cardiol* 1997;29:1060–1066.

Doust JA, Pietrzak E, Dobson A, Glasziou P. How well does B-type natriuretic peptide predict death and cardiac events in patients with heart failure: systematic review. *BMJ* 2005;330(7492):625.

Drazner MH, Hamilton MA, Fonarow G, et al. Relationship between right- and left-sided filling pressures in 1000 patients with advanced heart failure. *J Heart Lung Transplant* 1999;18:1126–1132.

Effect of enalapril on mortality and the development of heart failure in asymptomatic patients with reduced left ventricular ejection fractions; the SOLVD Investigators. *N Engl J Med* 1992;327(10):685–691.

Effect of enalapril on survival in patients with reduced left ventricular ejection fractions and congestive heart failure: the SOLVD Investigators. *N Engl J Med* 1991;325(5):293–302.

Effects of enalapril on mortality in severe congestive heart failure. Results of the Cooperative North Scandinavian Enalapril Survival Study (CONSENSUS): the CONSENSUS Trial Study Group. *N Engl J Med* 1987;316(23):1429–1435.

Epstein AE, DiMarco JP, Ellenbogen KA, et al. ACC/AHA/HRS 2008 Guidelines for Device-Based Therapy of Cardiac Rhythm Abnormalities: a report of the American College of Cardiology/American Heart Association Task Force on Practice Guidelines (Writing Committee to Revise the ACC/AHA/NASPE 2002 Guideline Update for Implantation of Cardiac Pacemakers and Antiarrhythmia Devices) developed in collaboration with the American Association for Thoracic Surgery and Society of Thoracic Surgeons. *J Am Coll Cardiol* 2008;51:e1.

Erhardt L, MacLean A, Ilgenfritz J, et al. Fosinopril attenuates clinical deterioration and improves exercise tolerance in patients with heart failure: Fosinopril Efficacy/Safety Trial (FEST) Study Group. *Eur Heart J* 1995;16(12):1892–1899.

Exner DV, Dries DL, Domanski MJ, et al. Lesser response to angiotensin-converting-enzyme inhibitor therapy in black as compared with white patients with left ventricular dysfunction. *N Engl J Med* 2001;344(18):1351–1357.

Flather MD, Yusuf S, Kober L, et al. Long-term ACE-inhibitor therapy in patients with heart failure or left-ventricular dysfunction: a systematic overview of data from individual patients: ACE-Inhibitor Myocardial Infarction Collaborative Group. *Lancet* 2000;355:1575.

Fonarow GC, Peacock W, Phillips C, et al. Admission B-type natriuretic peptide levels and in-hospital mortality in acute decompensated heart failure. *J Am Coll Cardiol* 2007;49:1943.

Fonarow GC, Abraham WT, Albert NM, et al. Influence of beta-blocker continuation or withdrawal on outcomes in patients hospitalized with heart failure: findings from the OPTIMIZE-HF program. *J Am Coll Cardiol* 2008;52(3):190–199.

Forman D, Butler J, Wang Y. Incidence, predictors at admission, and impact of worsening renal function among patients hospitalized with heart failure. *J Am Coll Cardiol* 2004;43(1):61–67.

Fox K, Ford I, Steg PG, et al. Heart rate as a prognostic risk factor in patients with coronary artery disease and left-ventricular systolic dysfunction (BEAUTIFUL): a subgroup analysis of a randomised controlled trial. *Lancet* 2008;372:817.

Franz W, Agrawal B, Wiewel D, Ketelhut R. Comparison of the antihypertensive effects of carvedilol and metoprolol on resting and exercise blood pressure. *J Mol Med* 2004;0946–2716:S53–S57.

Fukata H, Sane DC, Brucks S, Little WC. Statin therapy may be associated with lower mortality in patients with diastolic heart failure: a preliminary report. *Circulation* 2005;112(3):357–363.

Gackowski A, Isnard R, Golmard JL, et al. Comparison of echocardiography and plasma B-type natriuretic peptide for monitoring the response to treatment in acute heart failure. *Eur Heart J* 2004;25:1788–1796.

Gaffney TE, Braunwald E. Importance of the adrenergic nervous system in the support of circulatory function in patients with congestive heart failure. *Am J Med* 1963;34:320.

Gattis WA, O'Connor CM, Gallup DS, et al. Predischarge initiation of carvedilol in patients hospitalized for decompensated heart failure: results of the Initiation Management Predischarge: Process for Assessment of Carvedilol Therapy in Heart Failure (IMPACT-HF) trial. *J Am Coll Cardiol* 2004;43(9):1534–1541.

Gheorghiade M, Bonow RO. Chronic heart failure in the United States: a manifestation of coronary artery disease. *Circulation* 1998;97:282–289.

Ghio S, Gavazzi A, Campana C, et al. Independent and additive prognostic value of right ventricular systolic function and pulmonary artery pressure in patients with chronic heart failure. *J Am Coll Cardiol* 2001;37:183.

Gilbert EM, Anderson JL, Deitchman D, et al. Long-term beta-blocker vasodilator therapy improves cardiac function in idiopathic dilated cardiomyopathy: a double-blind, randomized study of bucindolol versus placebo. *Am J Med* 1990;88(3):223–229.

Givertz M, Massie B, Fields T, et al. Effects of KW-3902, an adenosine A1-receptor antagonist, on diuresis and renal function in patients with acute decompensated heart failure and renal impairment or diuretic resistance. *J Am Coll Cardiol* 2007;50:1551–1560.

Granger CB, McMurray JJ, Yusuf S, et al. Effects of candesartan in patients with chronic heart failure and reduced left-ventricular systolic function intolerant to angiotensin-converting-enzyme inhibitors: the CHARM-Alternative trial. *Lancet* 2003;362(9386):772–776.

Guazzi M, Brambilla R, Reina G, et al. Aspirin-angiotensin-converting enzyme inhibitor coadministration and mortality in patients with heart failure: a dose-related adverse effect of aspirin. *Arch Intern Med* 2003;163(13):1574–1579.

Hall D, Zeitler H, Rudolph W. Counteraction of the vasodilator effects of enalapril by aspirin in severe heart failure. *J Am Coll Cardiol* 1992;20(7):1549–1555.

Harris KM, Spirito P, Maron MS, et al. Prevalence, clinical profile and significance of left ventricular remodeling in the end-stage phase of hypertrophic cardiomyopathy. *Circulation* 2006;114:216.

Heywood J, Fonarow G, Costanzo M, et al. High prevalence of renal dysfunction and its impact on outcome in 118,465 patients hospitalized with acute decompensated heart failure: a report from the ADHERE database. *J Card Fail* 2007;13(6):422–430.

Ho KK, Pinsky JL, Kannel WB, et al. The epidemiology of heart failure: the Framingham Study. *J Am Coll Cardiol* 1993;22:6A.

Hunt SA, Abraham WT, Chin MH, et al. ACC/AHA 2005 guideline update for the diagnosis and management of chronic heart failure in the adult: a report of the American College of Cardiology/American Heart Association Task Force on Practice Guidelines (Writing Committee to Update the 2001 Guidelines for the Evaluation and Management of Heart Failure): developed in collaboration with the American College of Chest Physicians and the International Society for Heart and Lung Transplantation: endorsed by the Heart Rhythm Society. *Circulation* 2005;112:e154.

Januzzi JL, van Kimmenade R, Lainchbury J, et al. NT-proBNP testing for diagnosis and short-term prognosis in acute destabilized heart failure: an international pooled analysis of 1256 patients: the International Collaborative of NT-proBNP Study. *Eur Heart J* 2006;27:330.

Jong P, Vowinckel E, Liu PP, et al. Prognosis and determinants of survival in patients newly hospitalized for heart failure: a population-based study. *Arch Intern Med* 2002;162:1689–1694.

Klein L, O'Conner C, Leimberger J, et al. Lower serum sodium is associated with worsening heart failure: results from the Outcomes of a Prospective Trial of Intravenous Milrinone for Exacerbations of Chronic Heart Failure (OPTIME-CHF) study. *Circulation* 2005;111:2454–2460.

Konstam MA, Czerska B, Bohm M. Continuous aortic flow augmentation: a pilot study of hemodynamic and renal responses to a novel percutaneous intervention in decompensated heart failure. *Circulation* 2005;112(20):3107–3114. Epub November 2005.

Kotlyar E, Keogh AM, Macdonald PS, et al. Tolerability of carvedilol in patients with heart failure and concomitant chronic obstructive pulmonary disease or asthma. *J Heart Lung Transplant* 2002;21(12): 1290–1295.

Krumholz HM, Parent EM, Tu N, et al. Readmission after hospitalization for congestive heart failure among Medicare beneficiaries. *Arch Intern Med* 1997;157:99–104.

Lee WH, Packer M. Prognostic importance of serum sodium concentration and its modification by converting-enzyme inhibition in patients with severe chronic heart failure. *Circulation* 1986;73(2):257–267.

Leier CV, Webel J, Bush CA. The cardiovascular effects of continuous infusions of dobutamine in patients with severe cardiac failure. *Circulation* 1977;56:468–472.

Liang CS, Sherman LG, Doherty JU. Sustained improvement of cardiac function in patients with congestive heart failure after short-term infusion of dobutamine. *Circulation* 1984;69(1):113–119.

Libby P, Bonow R, Mann D, et al., eds. *Braunwald's Heart Disease: A Textbook of Cardiovascular Medicine*, 8th ed. Philadelphia: Saunders Elsevier; 2008. Available at: http://www.cardiosource.com/books/index.asp

Lindenfeld J, Robertson AD, Lowes BD, et al. Aspirin impairs reverse myocardial remodeling in patients with heart failure treated with beta-blockers. *J Am Coll Cardiol* 2001;38(7):1950–1956.

Logeart D, Thabut G, Jourdain P, et al. A rapid bedside test for B-type peptide predicts treatment outcomes in patients admitted for decompensated heart failure: a pilot study. *J Am Coll Cardiol* 2001;37:386–391.

Maisel AS. B-type natriuretic peptide levels: diagnostic and prognostic in congestive heart failure: what's next? *Circulation* 2002;105:2328–2331.

Maisel AS, McCord J, Nowak RM, et al. Bedside B-type natriuretic peptide in the emergency diagnosis of heart failure with reduced or preserved ejection fraction: results from the Breathing Not Properly Multinational Study. *J Am Coll Cardiol* 2003;41:2010–2017.

Mancini DM, Eisen H, Kussmaul W. Value of peak exercise oxygen consumption for optimal timing of cardiac transplantation in ambulatory patients with heart failure. *Circulation* 1991;83(3):778–786.

Maron BJ, McKenna WJ, Danielson GK, et al. American College of Cardiology/European Society of Cardiology Clinical Expert Consensus Document on Hypertrophic Cardiomyopathy. *J Am Coll Cardiol* 2003;42:1687.

Maron BJ, Towbin JA, Thiene G, et al. Contemporary definitions and classification of the cardiomyopathies: an American Heart Association Scientific Statement. *Circulation* 2006;113:1807.

Maron BJ. Hypertrophic cardiomyopathy: a systematic review. *JAMA* 2002;287:1308.

McMurray JJ, Ostergren J, Swedberg K, et al. Effects of candesartan in patients with chronic heart failure and reduced left-ventricular systolic function taking angiotensin-converting-enzyme inhibitors: the CHARM-Added trial. *Lancet* 2003;362:767.

Mehra MR, Uber PA, Park MH, et al. Obesity and suppressed B-type natriuretic peptide levels in heart failure. *J Am Coll Cardiol* 2004;43(9): 1590–1595.

Metra M, Nodari S, D'Aloia A, et al. Beta-blocker therapy influences the hemodynamic response to inotropic agents in patients with heart failure: a randomized comparison of dobutamine and enoximone before and after chronic treatment with metoprolol or carvedilol. *J Am Coll Cardiol* 2002;40(7):1248–1258.

Mottram PM, Haluska B, Leano R, et al. Effect of aldosterone antagonism on myocardial dysfunction in hypertensive patients with diastolic heart failure. *Circulation* 2004;110(5):558–565. Epub July 26, 2004.

Murphy J, Lloyd M, eds. *Mayo Clinic Cardiology: Concise Textbook.* Canada: Mayo Clinic Scientific Press; 2007.

Nohria A, Mielniczuk LM, Stevenson LW. Evaluation and monitoring of patients with acute heart failure syndromes. *Am J Cardiol* 2005;96(6A):32G–40G.

Packer M, Bristow MR, Cohn JN, et al. The effect of carvedilol on morbidity and mortality in patients with chronic heart failure. *N Engl J Med* 1996;334:1349–1355.

Packer M, Carver JR, Rodeheffer RJ, et al. Effect of oral milrinone on mortality in severe chronic heart failure: the PROMISE Study Research Group. *N Engl J Med* 1991;325(21):1468–1475.

Packer M, Colucci WS, Sackner-Bernstein JD, et al. Double-blind, placebo-controlled study of the effects of carvedilol in patients with moderate to severe heart failure: the PRECISE Trial (Prospective Randomized Evaluation of Carvedilol on Symptoms and Exercise). *Circulation* 1996;94:2793–2799.

Packer M, Gheorghiade M, Young JB, et al. Withdrawal of digoxin from patients with chronic heart failure treated with angiotensin-converting-enzyme inhibitors: RADIANCE Study. *N Engl J Med* 1993;329(1):1–7.

Paulus WJ, Tschope C, Sanderson JE, et al. How to diagnose diastolic heart failure: a consensus statement on the diagnosis of heart failure with normal left ventricular ejection fraction by the Heart Failure and Echocardiography Associations of the European Society of Cardiology. *Eur Heart J* 2007;28(20):2539–2550.

Peacock WF IV, De Marco T, Fonarow GC, et al. Cardiac troponin and outcome in acute heart failure. *N Engl J Med* 2008;358:2117–2121.

Pfeffer MA, Braunwald E, Moye LA, et al. Effect of captopril on mortality and morbidity in patients with left ventricular dysfunction after myocardial infarction: results of the survival and ventricular enlargement trial: the SAVE Investigators. *N Engl J Med* 1992;327(10):669–677.

Pinamonti B, DiLenarda A, Sinagra GF, et al., and the Heart Muscle Disease Study Group. Restrictive left ventricular filling MFVP in dilated cardiomyopathy assessed by Doppler echocardiography: clinical, echocardiographic and hemodynamic correlations and prognostic implications. *J Am Coll Cardiol* 1993;22:808.

Pitt B, Remme WJ, Zannad F, et al. Eplerenone, a selective aldosterone blocker, in patients with left ventricular dysfunction after myocardial infarction. *N Engl J Med* 2003;348(14):1309–1321.

Pitt B, Zannad F, Remme WJ, et al. The effect of spironolactone on morbidity and mortality in patients with severe heart failure: randomized Aldactone Evaluation Study Investigators. *N Engl J Med* 1999;341:709–717.

Pocock SJ, Wang D, Pfeffer MA. Predictors of mortality and morbidity in patients with chronic heart failure. *Eur Heart J* 2006;27(1):65–75. Epub October 11, 2005.

Publication Committee for the VMAC Investigators. Intravenous nesiritide vs nitroglycerin for treatment of decompensated congestive heart failure: a randomized controlled trial. *JAMA* 2002;287:1531–1540.

Rathore SS, Curtis JP, Wang Y, et al. Association of serum digoxin concentration and outcomes in patients with heart failure. *JAMA* 2003; 289(7):871–878.

Rathore SS, Wang Y, Krumholz HM. Sex-based differences in the effect of digoxin for the treatment of heart failure. *N Engl J Med* 2002; 347:1403.

Rudiger A, Gasser S, Fischler M, et al. Comparable increase of B-type natriuretic peptide and amino-terminal pro-B-type natriuretic peptide levels in patients with severe sepsis, septic shock, and acute heart failure. *Crit Care Med* 2006;34(8):2140–2144.

Sackner-Bernstein J, Kowalski M, Fox M, et al. Short-term risk of death after treatment with nesiritide for decompensated heart failure: a pooled analysis of randomized controlled trials. *JAMA* 2005;293:1900–1905.

Sackner-Bernstein J, Skopicki H, Aaronson K. Risk of worsening renal function with nesiritide in patients with acutely decompensated heart failure. *Circulation* 2005;111:1487–1491.

Salpeter S, Ormiston T, Salpeter E. Cardioselective beta-blockers for reversible airway disease. *Cochrane Database Syst Rev* 2002;(4):CD002992.

Shakar SF, Abraham WT, Gilbert EM, et al. Combined oral positive inotropic and beta-blocker therapy for treatment of refractory class IV heart failure. *J Am Coll Cardiol* 1998;31(6):1336–1340.

Sharpe DN, Murphy J, Coxon R, Hannan SF. Enalapril in patients with chronic heart failure: a placebo-controlled, randomized, double-blind study. *Circulation* 1984;70(2):271–278.

Smith GL, Lichtman JH, Bracken MB. Renal impairment and outcomes in heart failure: systematic review and meta-analysis. *J Am Coll Cardiol* 2006;47(10):1987–1996. Epub April 24, 2006.

Solomon SD, Anavekar N, Skali H. Influence of ejection fraction on cardiovascular outcomes in a broad spectrum of heart failure patients. *Circulation* 2005;112(24):3738–3744. Epub December 5, 2005.

Stevenson LW, Perloff JK. The limited reliability of physical signs for estimating hemodynamics in chronic heart failure. *JAMA* 1989;261:884–888.

Storto ML, Kee ST, Golden JA, Webb WR. Hydrostatic pulmonary edema: high-resolution CT findings. *Am J Roentgenol* 1995;165(4):817–820.

Surawicz B, Knilans TK. *Chou's Electrocardiography in Clinical Practice*, 6th ed. Philadelphia: Saunders Elsevier; 2008.

Takkenberg JJ, Czer LS, Fishbein MC, et al. Eosinophilic myocarditis in patients awaiting heart transplantation. *Crit Care Med* 2004;32:888.

Tarakji K, Brunken R, McCarthy P, et al. Myocardial viability testing and the effect of early intervention in patients with advanced left ventricular systolic dysfunction. *Circulation* 2006;113(2):230–237.

Taylor AL, Ziesche S, Yancy C, et al., for the African-American Heart Failure Trial Investigators: combination of isosorbide dinitrate and hydralazine in blacks with heart failure. *N Engl J Med* 2004;351: 2049–2057.

The Cardiac Insufficiency Bisoprolol Study II (CIBIS-II): a randomised trial. *Lancet* 1999;353(9146):9–13.

Underwood SR, Bax JJ, vom Dahl J, et al. Imaging techniques for the assessment of myocardial hibernation: report of a Study Group of the European Society of Cardiology. *Eur Heart J* 2004;25(10):815–836.

Unverferth DV, Magorien RD, Lewis RP, et al. Long-term benefit of dobutamine in patients with congestive cardiomyopathy. *Am Heart J* 1980; 100:622–630.

Uretsky BF, Young JB, Shahidi FE, et al. Randomized study assessing the effect of digoxin withdrawal in patients with mild to moderate chronic congestive heart failure: results of the PROVED trial: PROVED Investigative Group. *J Am Coll Cardiol* 1993;22(4):955–962.

Veenhuyzen GD, Singh SN, McAreavey D, et al. Prior coronary artery bypass surgery and risk of death among patients with ischemic left ventricular dysfunction. *Circulation* 2001;104(13):1489–1493.

Vermes E, Tardif JC, Bourassa MG, et al. Enalapril decreases the incidence of atrial fibrillation in patients with left ventricular dysfunction: insight from the Studies of Left Ventricular Dysfunction (SOLVD) trials. *Circulation* 2003;107(23):2926–2931. Epub May 27, 2003.

Waagstein F, Bristow MR, Swedberg K, et al. Beneficial effects of metoprolol in idiopathic dilated cardiomyopathy: Metoprolol in Dilated Cardiomyopathy (MDC) Trial Study Group. *Lancet* 1993;342:1441–1446.

Weil JV, Chidsey CA. Plasma volume expansion resulting from interference with adrenergic function in normal man. *Circulation* 1968;37:54.

Willenheimer R, van Veldhuisen DJ, Silke B, et al. Effect on survival and hospitalization of initiating treatment for chronic heart failure with bisoprolol followed by enalapril, as compared with the opposite sequence: results of the randomized Cardiac Insufficiency Bisoprolol Study (CIBIS) III. *Circulation* 2005;112(16):2426–2435.

Witteles R, Kao D, Christopherson D, et al. Impact of nesiritide on renal function in patients with acute decompensated heart failure and pre-existing renal dysfunction: a randomized, double-blind, placebo-controlled clinical trial. *J Am Coll Cardiol* 2007;50:1835–1840.

Yancy CW, Fowler MB, Colucci WS, et al. Race and the response to adrenergic blockade with carvedilol in patients with chronic heart failure. *N Engl J Med* 2001;344:1358.

Chapter 5

Aaronson KD, Eppinger MJ, Dyke DB, Wright S, Pagani FD. Left ventricular assist device therapy improves utilization of donor hearts. *J Am Coll Cardiol* 2002;39(8):1247–1254.

Bank AJ, Mir SH, Nguyen DQ, et al. Effects of left ventricular assist devices on outcomes in patients undergoing heart transplantation. *Ann Thorac Surg* 2000;69(5):1369–1374; discussion, 1375.

Copeland JG, Smith RG, Arabia FA. Cardiac replacement with a total artificial heart as a bridge to transplantation. *N Engl J Med* 2004;351(9): 859–867.

Frazier OH, Myers TJ, Westaby S, Gregoric ID. Clinical experience with an implantable, intracardiac, continuous flow circulatory support device: physiologic implications and their relationship to patient selection. *Ann Thorac Surg* 2004;77(1):133–142.

Lower RR, Shumway NE. Studies on orthotopic hemotransplantation of the canine heart. *Surg Forum* 1960;11:18–19.

Mancini DM, Eisen H, Kussmaul W, et al. Value of peak exercise oxygen consumption for optimal timing of cardiac transplantation in ambulatory patients with heart failure. *Circulation* 1991;83(3):778–786.

Mehra MR, Kobashigawa J, Starling R, et al. Listing criteria for heart transplantation: International Society for Heart and Lung Transplantation guidelines for the care of cardiac transplant candidates—2006. *J Heart Lung Transplant* 2006;25(9):1024–1042.

Meyer SR, Modry DL, Bainey K, et al. Declining need for permanent pacemaker insertion with the bicaval technique of orthotopic heart transplantation. *Can J Cardiol* 2005;21(2):159–163.

Miller LW, Pagani FD, Russell SD, et al. Use of a continuous-flow device in patients awaiting heart transplantation. *N Engl J Med* 2007;357(9): 885–896.

Morgan JA, John R, Rao V, et al. Bridging to transplant with the HeartMate left ventricular assist device: the Columbia Presbyterian 12-year experience. *J Thorac Cardiovasc Surg* 2004;127(5):1309–1316.

Parry G, Holt ND, Dark JH, McComb JM. Declining need for pacemaker implantation after cardiac transplantation. *Pacing Clin Electrophysiol* 1998;21(11 Pt 2):2350–2352.

Pham M, Chen J, Berry GJ, Fuster V, et al., eds. *Surgical Treatment of Heart Failure, Cardiac Transplantation, and Mechanical Ventricular Support. Hurst's the Heart* (12th ed.). McGraw Hill; 2007.

Rose EA, Gelijns AC, Moskowitz AJ. Long-term mechanical left ventricular assistance for end-stage heart failure. *N Engl J Med* 2001;345(20): 1435–1443.

Siegenthaler MP, Westaby S, Frazier OH, et al. Advanced heart failure: feasibility study of long-term continuous axial flow pump support. *Eur Heart J* 2005;26(10):1031–1038.

Steinman TI, Becker BN, Frost AE, et al. Guidelines for the referral and management of patients eligible for solid organ transplantation. *Transplantation* 2001;71(9):1189–1204.

Stewart S, Winters GL, Fishbein MC, et al. Revision of the 1990 working formulation for the standardization of nomenclature in the diagnosis of heart rejection. *J Heart Lung Transplant* 2005;24(11):1710–1720.

Taylor DO, Edwards LB, Boucek MM, et al. Registry of the International Society for Heart and Lung Transplantation: twenty-fourth official adult heart transplant report—2007. *J Heart Lung Transplant* 2007;26(8):769–781.

Traversi E, Pozzoli M, Grande A, et al. The bicaval anastomosis technique for orthotopic heart transplantation yields better atrial function than the standard technique: an echocardiographic automatic boundary detection study. *J Heart Lung Transplant* 1998;17(11):1065–1074.

Vogel RA, Shawl F, Tommaso C, et al. Initial report of the National Registry of Elective Cardiopulmonary Bypass Supported Coronary Angioplasty. *J Am Coll Cardiol* 1990;15(1):23–29.

Chapter 6

Dorn GW, Force T. Protein kinase cascades in the regulation of cardiac hypertrophy. *J Clin Invest* 2005;115:527–537.

Foo RS, Mani K, Kitsis RN. Death begets failure in the heart. *J Clin Invest* 2005;115:565–571.

Heineke J, Molkentin JD. Regulation of cardiac hypertrophy by intracellular signaling pathways. *Nat Rev Mol Cell Biol* 2006;7:589–600.

Mudd JO, Kass DA. Tackling heart failure in the twenty-first century. *Nature* 2008;451:919–928.

Chapter 8

Boden WE, O'Rourke RA, Teo KT, et al. Optimal medical therapy with or without PCI for stable coronary artery disease. *N Engl J Med* 2007;356: 1–14.

Gruentzig AR, Senning A, Siegenthaler WE. Nonoperative dilation of coronary-artery stenosis: percutaneous transluminal coronary angioplasty. *N Engl J Med* 1979;301:61–68.

Kern MJ. The Cardiac Catheterization Handbook, 4th ed. Mosby; 2003.

Pijls HJ, et al. *N Engl J Med* 1996;334(26):1703–1708.

U.S. Department of Health and Human Services. NIH/NHLBI. Available at: www.nhlbi.nih.gov.

Chapter 9

Abbott BG, Afshar M, Berger AK, Wackers FJ. Prognostic significance of ischemic electrocardiographic changes during adenosine infusion in patients with normal myocardial perfusion imaging. *J Nucl Cardiol* 2003;10:9–16.

Adenoscan Package Insert, Astellas Pharma US, Inc., revised July 2005.

Beller GA, Zaret A. Contributions of nuclear cardiology to diagnosis and prognosis of patients with coronary artery disease. *Circulation* 2000;101:1465–1478.

Bonow RO, Carabello BA, Chatterjee K, et al. ACC/AHA 2006 Guidelines for the management of patients with valvular heart disease. *J Am Coll Cardiol* 2006;48:1–148.

Cerqueira MD, Weissman NJ, Dilsizian V, et al. Standardized myocardial segmentation and nomenclature for tomographic imaging of the heart: a statement for healthcare professionals from the Cardiac Imaging Committee of the Council on Clinical Cardiology of the American Heart Association. *Circulation* 2002;105:539–542.

Corbett JR, Akinboboye OO, Bacharach SL, et al. Equilibrium radionuclide angiocardiography. *J Nucl Cardiol*, 2006;13(6):e56–e59.

DePuey EG, Garcia AV. Updated imaging guidelines for nuclear cardiology procedures, part 1. *J Nucl Cardiol* 2001;8:G1–G58.

Elhendy AA, Gregory SA, Holly TA, et al. Combined pharmacologic and low-level exercise stress protocols for radionuclide myocardial perfusion imaging. *J Nucl Cardiol* 2009;16:163.

Friedman JD, Berman DS, Borges-Neto S, et al. First-pass radionuclide angiography. *J Nucl Cardiol* 2006;13:e42–e55.

Germano G, Kavanagh PB, Slomka PJ, et al. Quantitation in gated perfusion SPECT imaging: The Cedars-Sinai approach. *J Nucl Cardiol* 2007;14:433–454.

Gibbons RJ, Balady GJ, Bricker JT, et al. ACC/AHA 2002 guideline update for exercise testing: a report of the American College of Cardiology/American Heart Association Task Force on Practice Guidelines (Committee on Exercise Testing), 2002. American College of Cardiology Web Site. Available at: www.acc.org/qualityandscience/clinical/guidelines/exercise/dirIndex.htm.

Hansen CL, Goldstein RA, Akinboboye OO, et al. Myocardial perfusion and function: single photon emission computed tomography. *J Nucl Cardiol* 2007;14:e39–e60.

Hendel RC, Wackers FJTh, Berman DS, et al. American Society of Nuclear Cardiology consensus statement: reporting of radionuclide myocardial perfusion imaging studies. *J Nucl Cardiol* 2006;13:e152–e156.

Henzlova MJ, Cerqueira MD, Taillefer R, et al. Stress protocols and tracers. *J Nucl Cardiol*, 2006;13(6):e80–e90.

Higgins JP, Higgins JA. Review: electrocardiographic exercise stress testing: an update beyond the ST segment. *Int J Cardiol* 2007;116: 285–299.

Jette M, Sidney K, Blumchen G. Metabolic equivalents (METS) in exercise testing, exercise prescription, and evaluation of functional capacity. *Clin Cardiol* 1990;13:555–565.

Klocke FJ, Baird MG, Berman DS, et al. ACC/AHA/ASNC guidelines for the clinical use of cardiac radionuclide imaging: a report of the American College of Cardiology/ American Heart Association Task Force on Practice Guidelines, 2003, American College of Cardiology Web Site. Available at: http://www.acc.org/qualityandscience/clinical/guidelines/radio/index.pdf

Klodas EM, Miller TD, Christian TF, Hodge DO, Gibbons RJ. Prognostic significance of ischemic electrocardiographic changes during vasodilator stress testing in patients with normal SPECT images. *J Nucl Cardiol* 2003;10:4–8.

Libby P, Bonow RO, Mann DL, Zipes DP. *Braunwald's Heart Disease: A Textbook of Cardiovascular Medicine*, 8th ed. Philadelphia: Saunders; 2007.

Machac J, Bacharach SL, Bateman TM. Positron emission tomography myocardial perfusion and glucose metabolism imaging. *J Nucl Cardiol* 2006;13:e121–e151.

Mieres JH, Shaw L, Arai A, et al. Role of noninvasive testing in the clinical evaluation of women with suspected coronary artery disease: consensus statement from the Cardiac Imaging Committee, Council on Clinical Cardiology, and the Cardiovascular Imaging and Intervention Committee, Council on Cardiovascular Radiology and Intervention, American Heart Association. *Circulation* 2005;111:682–696.

Myers J, Prakash M, Froelicher V. Exercise capacity and mortality among med referred for exercise testing. *N Engl J Med* 2002;346:793–801.

Pellikka PA, Roger VL, Oh JK, et al. Safety of performing dobutamine stress echocardiography in patients with abdominal aortic aneurysm ≥ 4 cm in diameter. *Am J Cardiol* 1996;77:413–416.

Persantine Product Monograph, Boehringer Ingelheim Canada Ltd., revised May 20, 2005.

Regadenson package insert, Astellas Pharma US, Inc., revised April 2008.

Santana-Boado C, Candell-Riera J, Castell-Conesa J, et al. Diagnostic accuracy of technetium-99m-MIBI myocardial SPECT in women and men. *J Nucl Med* 1998;39:751–755.

Shaw LJ, Iskandriam AE. Prognostic value of stress gated SPECT. *J Nucl Cardiol* 2004;11:171–185.

Tilkemeier PL, Wackers FJTh. Myocardial perfusion planar imaging. *J Nucl Cardiol* 2006;13:e91–e96.

Chapter 10

Baumgartner H, Hung J, Bermejo J, et al. Echocardiographic assessment of valve stenosis: EAE/ASE recommendations for clinical practice. *J Am Soc Echocardiogr* 2009;22:1–23.

Bonow RO, Carabello BA, Chatterjee K, et al. 2008 Focused update incorporated into the ACC/AHA guidelines for the management of patients with valvular heart disease. *J Am Coll Cardiol* 2008;52:e1–e142.

Devereux R. Left ventricular geometry, pathophysiology and prognosis. *J Am Coll Cardiol* 1995;25:885–887.

Douglas PS, Khanderia B, Stainback RF, et al. 2007 Appropriateness criteria for transthoracic and transesophageal echocardiography. *J Am Coll Cardiol* 2007;50:187–204.

Elefteriades JA. Natural history of thoracic aortic aneurysms: Indications for surgery, and surgical versus nonsurgical risks. *Ann Thorac Surg* 2002;74:S1877–S1880.

Enriquez-Sarano M, Tajik AJ, Schaff HV, et al. Echocardiographic prediction of left ventricular function after correction of mitral regurgitation: results and clinical implications. *J Am Coll Cardiol* 1994;24: 1536–1543.

Fuster V, Ryden LE, Cannom DS, et al. ACC/AHA/ESC 2006 guidelines for the management of patients with atrial fibrillation—executive summary. *Eur Heart J* 2006;27:1979–2030.

Gorcsan J III, Abraham T, Agler DA, et al. Echocardiography for cardiac resynchronization therapy: Recommendations for performance and reporting—a report from the American Society of Echocardiography Dyssynchrony Working Group. *J Am Soc Echocardiogr* 2008;21: 191–213.

Kang DH, Kim JH, Rim JH, et al. Comparison of early surgery versus conventional treatment in asymptomatic severe mitral regurgitation. *Circulation* 2009;119:797–804.

Klein AL, Grimm RA, Murray RD, et al. Use of transesophageal echocardiography to guide cardioversion in patients with atrial fibrillation. *N Engl J Med* 2001;344:1411–1420.

Lang RM, Bierig M, Devereux RB, et al. Recommendations for chamber quantification: a report from the American Society of Echocardiography's Guidelines and Standards Committee and the Chamber Quantification Writing Group. *J Am Soc Echocardiogr* 2005;18:1440–1463.

Marwick TH. Stress echocardiography. *Heart* 2003;89:113–118.

McConnell MV, Solomon SD, Rayan ME, et al. Regional right ventricular dysfunction detected by echocardiography in acute pulmonary embolus. *Am J Cardiol* 1996;78:469–473.

Moller JE, Hillis GS, Oh JK, et al. Left atrial volume: a powerful predictor of survival after acute myocardial infarction. *Circulation* 2003; 107:2207–2212.

Nagueh SF, Appleton CP, Gillebert TC, et al. Recommendations for the evaluation of left ventricular diastolic function by echocardiography. *J Am Soc Echocardiogr* 2009;22:107–133.

Ommen SR, Nishimura RA, Appleton CP, et al. Clinical utility of Doppler echocardiography and tissue Doppler imaging in the estimation of left ventricular filling pressures: a comparative simultaneous Doppler-catheterization study. *Circulation* 2000;102:1788–1794.

Otto CM, Lind BK, Kitzman DW, et al. Association of aortic-valve sclerosis with cardiovascular mortality and morbidity in the elderly. *N Engl J Med* 1999;341:142–147.

Pearson AC, Labovitz AJ, Tatineni S, et al. Superiority of transesophageal echocardiography in detecting cardiac source of embolism in patients with cerebral ischemia of uncertain etiology. *J Am Coll Cardiol* 1991;17:66–72.

Pellikka PA, Nagueh SF, Elhendy AA, et al. American Society of Echocardiography recommendations for performance, interpretation, and application of stress echocardiography. *J Am Soc Echocardiogr* 2007; 20:1021–1041.

Silvestry FA, Kerber RE, Brook MM, et al. ASE recommendations for clinical practice: echo-guided interventions. *J Am Soc Echocardiogr* 2009;22:213–231.

Spirito P, Belone P, Harris KM, et al. Magnitude of left ventricular hypertrophy and risk of sudden death in hypertrophic cardiomyopathy. *N Engl J Med* 2000;324:1778–1785.

Zoghbi WA, Enriquez-Sarano M, Foster E, et al. Recommendations for evaluation of the severity of native valvular regurgitation with two-dimensional and Doppler echocardiography. *J Am Soc Echocardiol* 2003;16:777–802.

Chapter 11

Achenbach S. Computed tomography coronary angiography. *J Am Coll Cardiol* 2006;48:1919–1928.

Einstein AJ, Henzlova MJ, Rajagopalan S. Estimated risk of cancer associated with radiation exposure from 64 slice computed tomography coronary angiography. *JAMA* 2007;298:317–323.

Angelini P. Coronary artery anomalies-current clinical issues: definitions, classifications, incidence, clinical relevance, and treatment guidelines. *Tex Heart Inst J* 2002;29:271–278.

Araoz PA, Eklund HE, Welch TJ, et al. CT and MR imaging of primary cardiac malignancies. *Radiolographics* 1999;19:1421–1434.

Ardehali H, Howard D, Hariri A, et al. A positive endomyocardial biopsy result for sarcoid is associated with poor prognosis in patients with initially unexplained cardiomyopathy. *Am Heart J* 2005;150:459–463.

Baer FM, Theissen R, Schneider CA, et al. Dobutamine magnetic resonance imaging predicts contractile recovery of chronically dysfunctional myocardium after successful revascularisation. *J Am Coll Cardiol* 1998;31:1040.

Bluemke DA, Krupinski EA, Ovitt T, et al. MR imaging of arrhythmogenic right ventricular cardiomyopathy: morphologic findings and interobserver reliability. *Cardiology* 2003;99:153–162.

Breen JF. Imaging of the pericardium. *J Thorac Imaging* 2001;16(1): 47–54.

Budoff MJ, Achenbach S, Blumenthal RS, et al. Assessment of coronary artery disease by cardiac computed tomography: a scientific statement from the American Heart Association Committee on Cardiovascular Imaging and Intervention, Council on Cardiovascular Radiology and Intervention, and Committee on Cardiac Imaging, Council on Clinical Cardiology. *Circulation* 2006;114(16):1761–1791.

Cademartiri F, Schuijf JD, Pugliese F, et al. Usefulness of 64-slice multislice computed tomography coronary angiography to assess in-stent restenosis. *J Am Coll Cardiol* 2007;49:2204.

Deibler AR, Kuzo RS, Vöhringer M, et al. Imaging of congenital coronary anomalies with multislice computed tomography. *Mayo Clin Proc* 2004;79:1017.

Detrano R, Guerci AD, Carr JJ, et al. Coronary calcium as a predictor of coronary events in four racial or ethnic groups. *N Engl J Med* 2008; 358:1336–1345.

Dewey M, Schnapauff D, Teige F, Hamm B. Non-cardiac findings on coronary computed tomography and magnetic resonance imaging. *Eur Radiol* 2007;17:2038.

Ehara M, Kawai M, Surmely JF, et al. Diagnostic accuracy of coronary in-stent restenosis using 64-slice computed tomography: comparison with invasive coronary angiography. *J Am Coll Cardiol* 2007;49:951.

Gerber TC, Stratmann BP, Kuzo RS, et al. Effect of acquisition technique on radiation dose and image quality in multidetector row computed tomography coronary angiography with submillimeter collimation. *Invest Radiol* 2005;40:556.

Greenland P, Labree L, Azen SP, Dougherty DM, Detrano RC. Coronary artery calcium score combined with Framingham score for risk prediction in asymptomatic individuals. *JAMA* 2004;291:210–215.

Hunold P, Vogt FM, Schmermund A, et al. Radiation exposure during cardiac CT: effective dose at multi-detector row CT and electron beam CT. *Radiology* 203;226:145–152.

Hunold P, Schlosser T, Vogt FM, et al. Myocardial late enhancement in contrast-enhanced cardiac MRI: distinction between infarction scar and non–infarction-related disease. *Am J Roentgenol* 2005;184:1420–1426.

Hunold P, Vogt FM, Schmermund A, et al. Radiation exposure during cardiac CT: effective doses at multi-detector row CT and electron-beam CT. *Radiology* 2003;226:145.

Jacobs JE, Boxt LM, Desjardins B, et al. ACR practice guideline for the performance and interpretation of cardiac computed tomography (CT). *J Am Coll Radiol* 2006;3:677.

Jahnke C, Nagel E, Gebker R, et al. Prognostic value of cardiac magnetic resonance stress tests: adenosine stress perfusion and dobutamine stress wall motion imaging. *Circulation* 2007;115:1769.

Kim RJ, Wu E, Rafael A, et al. The use of contrast-enhanced magnetic resonance imaging to identify reversible myocardial dysfunction. *N Engl J Med* 2000;343:1445–1453.

Kim WY, Danias PG, Stuber M, et al. Coronary magnetic resonance angiography for the detection of coronary stenoses. *N Engl J Med* 2001;345:1863–1869.

Kim RJ, Albert TS, Wible JH, et al. Performance of delayed-enhancement magnetic resonance imaging with gadoversetamide contrast for the detection and assessment of myocardial infarction: an international, multicenter, double-blinded, randomized trial. *Circulation* 2008;117:629.

Klein C, Nekolla SG, Bengel FM, et al. Assessment of myocardial viability with contrast-enhanced magnetic resonance imaging: comparison with positron emission tomography. *Circulation* 2002;105:162.

Klem I, Heitner JF, Shah DJ, et al. Improved detection of coronary artery disease by stress perfusion cardiovascular magnetic resonance with the use of delayed enhancement infarction imaging. *J Am Coll Cardiol* 2006;47:1630–1638.

Kolodgie FD, Gold HK, Burke AP, et al. Intraplaque hemorrhage and progression of coronary atheroma. *N Engl J Med* 2003;349:2316–2325.

Kumar A, Abdel-Aty H, Kriedemann I, et al. Contrast-enhanced cardiovascular magnetic resonance imaging of right ventricular infarction. *J Am Coll Cardiol* 2006;48:1969.

Leber AW, Knez A, von Ziegler F, et al. Quantification of obstructive and nonobstructive coronary lesions by 64-slice computed tomography: a comparative study with quantitative coronary angiography and intravascular ultrasound. *J Am Coll Cardiol* 2005;46:147.

Leschka S, Wildermuth S, Boehm T, et al. Noninvasive coronary angiography with 64 slice-section CT: effect of average heart rate and heart rate variability on image quality. *Radiology* 2006;241:378–385.

Mack MJ, Osborne JA, Shennib H. Arterial graft patency in coronary artery bypass grafting: what do we really know? *Ann Thorac Surg* 1998;66: 1055–1059.

Mahnken AH, Seyfarth T, Flohr T, et al. Flat-panel detector computed tomography for the assessment of coronary artery stents: phantom study in comparison with 16-slice spiral computed tomography. *Invest Radiol* 2005;40(1):8–13.

Mahrholdt H, Goedecke C, Wagner A, et al. Cardiovascular magnetic resonance assessment of human myocarditis: a comparison to histology and molecular pathology. *Circulation* 2004;109:1250–1258.

Manzke R, Kohler T, Nielsen T, et al. Automatic phase determination for retrospectively gated cardiac CT. *Med Phys* 2004;31:3345–3362.

McCrohon JA, Moon JC, Prasad SK, et al. Differentiation of heart failure related to dilated cardiomyopathy and coronary artery disease using gadolinium enhanced cardiovascular magnetic resonance. *Circulation* 2003;108:54–59.

Meyer TS, Martinoff S, Hadamitzky M, et al. Improved noninvasive assessment of coronary artery bypass grafts with 64-slice computed tomographic angiography in an unselected patient population. *J Am Coll Cardiol* 2007;49:946.

Mollet NR, Cademartiri F, van Mieghem CA, et al. High-resolution spiral computed tomography coronary angiography in patients referred for diagnostic conventional coronary angiography. *Circulation* 2005;112:2222–2225.

Moon JC, McKenna WJ, McCrohon JA, et al. Toward clinical risk assessment in hypertrophic cardiomyopathy with gadolinium cardiovascular magnetic resonance. *J Am Coll Cardiol* 2003;41:1561–1567.

Morin RL, Gerber TC, McCollough CH. Radiation dose in computed tomography of the heart. *Circulation* 2003;107:917.

Moshage WE, Achenbach S, Seese B, et al. Coronary artery stenoses: three-dimensional imaging with electrocardiographically triggered, contrast agent-enhanced, electron-beam CT. *Radiology* 1995;196:707.

Nagel E, Lehmkuhl HB, Bocksch W, et al. Noninvasive diagnosis of ischemia-induced wall motion abnormalities with the use of high-dose dobutamine stress MRI: comparison with dobutamine stress echocardiography. *Circulation* 1999;763–770.

Nikolaou K, Flohr T, Reiser MF. Flat panel computed tomography of human ex vivo heart and bone specimens: initial experience. *Eur Radiol* 2005;15:329–333.

Pannu HK, Alvarez W Jr, Fishman EK. Beta-blockers for cardiac CT: a primer for the radiologist. *Am J Roentgenol* 2006;186:S341–S345.

Raff GL, Gallagher MJ, O'Neill WW, Goldstein JA. Diagnostic accuracy of noninvasive coronary angiography using 64-slice spiral computed tomography. *J Am Coll Cardiol* 2005;46:552.

Reynen K. Frequency of primary tumors of the heart. *Am J Cardiol* 1996;77:107.

Robinson FC. Aneurysms of coronary arteries. *Am Heart J* 1985;109:129–135.

Ropers D, Pohle FK, Kuettner A, et al. Diagnostic accuracy of noninvasive coronary angiography in patients after bypass surgery using 64-slice spiral computed tomography with 330-ms gantry rotation. *Circulation* 2006;114:2334.

Rosemond W, Flegal K, Friday G, et al. American Heart Association: Heart disease and stroke statistics 2007 update. *Circulation* 2007;115(5): e69–e171.

Schepis T, Gaemperil O, Koepfli P, et al. Comparison of 64-slice CT with gated SPECT for evaluation of left ventricular function. *J Nucl Med* 2006;47:1288–1294.

Semelka RC, Shoenut JP, Wilson ME, et al. Cardiac masses: signal intensity features on spin-echo, gradient-echo, gadolinium-enhanced spin-echo, and TurboFLASH images. *J Magn Reson Imaging* 1992;2:415–420.

Silverman KJ, Hutchins GM, Bulkley BH, et al. Cardiac sarcoidal clinicopathologic study of 84 unselected patients with systemic sarcoidosis. *Circulation* 1979;58:1204–1211.

Smedama JP, Snoep G, van Kroonenburgh MP, et al. Evaluation of the accuracy of gadolinium-enhanced cardiovascular magnetic resonance in the diagnosis of cardiac sarcoidosis. *J Am Coll Cardiol* 2005; 45:1683–1690.

Srichai MB, Junor C, Rodriguez LL, et al. Clinical, imaging, and pathological characteristics of left ventricular thrombus: a comparison of contrast-enhanced magnetic resonance imaging, transthoracic echocardiography, and transesophageal echocardiography with surgical or pathological validation. *Am Heart J* 2006;152:75.

Sugeng L, Mor-Avi V, Weinert L, et al. Quantitative assessment of left ventricular size and function: side-by-side comparison of real-time three-dimensional echocardiography and computed tomography with magnetic resonance reference. *Circulation* 2006;114:654–661.

Wembar M, Garcia MJ, Heuscher DJ, et al. A dynamic approach to identifying desired physiological phases for cardiac imaging using multislice spiral CT. *Med Phys* 2003;40:556–563.

Chapter 12

American College of Cardiology/American Heart Association. ACC/AHA 2006 Guideline Update on Perioperative Cardiovascular Evaluation for Noncardiac Surgery. Focused Update on Perioperative B-blocker Therapy. Available at: www.acc.org/qualityandscience/clinical/guidelines/perio/periobetablocker.pdf

American College of Cardiology/American Heart Association Task Force on Practice Guidelines. ACC/AHA 2007 guidelines on perioperative cardiovascular evaluation and care for noncardiac surgery: a report of the American College of Cardiology/American Heart Association Task Force on Practice Guidelines (Writing Committee to Revise the 2002 Guidelines on Perioperative Cardiovascular Evaluation for Noncardiac Surgery). *J Am Coll Cardiol* 2007;50:e159–e241.

Howell SJ, Sear JW, Foex P. Hypertension, hypertensive heart disease and perioperative cardiac risk. *Br J Anaesth* 2004;92:570–583.

Laine C, Williams S, eds. In the clinic: preoperative evaluation. *Ann Intern Med* 2009;ITC1:2–16.

Le Manach Y, Godet G, Coriat P, et al. The impact of postoperative discontinuation or continuation of chronic statin therapy on cardiac outcome after major vascular surgery. *Anesth Analg* 2007;104:1326–1333.

Lee TH, Marcantonio ER, Mangione CM, et al. Derivation and prospective validation of a simple index for prediction of cardiac risk of major noncardiac surgery. *Circulation* 1999;100:1043–1049.

POISE Study Group. Effects of extended-release metoprolol succinate in patients undergoing non-cardiac surgery (POISE trial): a randomised controlled trial. *Lancet* 2008;371:1839–1847.

Chapter 13

2005 American Heart Association guidelines for cardiopulmonary resuscitation and emergency cardiovascular care. *Circulation* 2005;112:IV1–IV5.

Antunes E, Brugada J, Steurer G, et al. The differential diagnosis of a regular tachycardia with a wide QRS complex on the 12-lead ECG: ventricular tachycardia, supraventricular tachycardia with aberrant intraventricular conduction, and supraventricular tachycardia with anterograde conduction over an accessory pathway. *PACE* 1994;17(9):1515–1524.

Frink R, James T. Normal blood supply to the human his bundle and proximal bundle branches. *Circulation* 1973;47:8–18.

Zipes DP. Second degree AV block. *Circulation* 1979;60:465–472.

Chapter 14

Akhtar M, Shenasa M, Jazayeri M, et al. Wide complex tachycardia: reappraisal of a common clinical problem. *Ann Intern Med* 1988;109(12):905–912.

Belhassen B, Rotmensch HH, Laniado S. Response of recurrent sustained ventricular tachycardia to verapamil. *Br Heart J* 1981;46:679–682.

Brugada P, Brugada J, Mont L, et al. A new approach to the differential diagnosis of a regular tachycardia with a wide QRS complex. *Circulation* 1991;83(5):1649–1659.

Baerman JM, Morady F, DiCarlo LA, et al. Differentiation of ventricular tachycardia from supraventricular tachycardia with aberration: value of the clinical history. *Ann Emerg Med* 1987;16:40–43.

De Luna AB. Basic electrophysiology. In: *Clinical Electrocardiography: A Textbook.* New York: Futura Publishing Co.; 1993:3–37.

Drew BJ, Scheinman MM. ECG criteria to distinguishing between aberrantly conducted supraventricular tachycardia and ventricular tachycardia: practical aspects for the immediate care setting. *PACE* 1995;18: 2194–2208.

Eckardt L, Breithardt G, Kirchhof P. Approach to wide complex tachycardias in patients without structural heart disease. *Heart* 2006;92:704–711.

Goldberger ZD, Rho RW, Page RL. Approach to the diagnosis and initial management of the stable adult patient with a wide complex tachycardia. *Am J Cardiol* 2008;101:1456–1466.

Gray RA, Jalife J, Panfilov A, et al. Nonstationary vortex-like reentrant activity as a mechanism of polymorphic ventricular tachycardia in the isolated rabbit heart. *Circulation* 1995;91:2454–2469.

Griffith MJ, deBelder MA, Linker NJ, et al. Multivariate analysis to simplify the differential diagnosis of broad complex tachycardia. *Br Heart J* 1991;66:166–174.

Gupta AK, Thakur RK. Wide QRS complex tachycardias. *Med Clin North Am* 2001;85(2):245–266.

Kindwall KE, Brown J, Josephson ME. Electrocardiographic criteria for ventricular tachycardia in wide complex left bundle branch block morphology tachycardias. *Am J Cardiol* 1988;61:1279–1283.

Knight BP, Pelosi F, Michaud GF, et al. Physician interpretation of electrocardiographic artifact that mimics ventricular tachycardia. *Am J Med* 2001;110:335–338.

Lau EW, Pathamanathan RK, Ng GA, et al. The Bayesian approach improves the electrocardiographic diagnosis of broad complex tachycardia. *PACE* 2000;23:1519–1526.

Miller JM, Hsia HH, Rothman SA, et al. Ventricular tachycardia versus supraventricular tachycardia with aberration: electrocardiographic distinctions. In: Zipes DP, Jalife J, eds. *Cardiac Electrophysiology: From Cell to Bedside*, 3rd ed. Philadelphia: WB Saunders; 2000:696–705.

Morady F, Baerman JM, DiCarlo LA, et al. A prevalent misconception regarding wide complex tachycardias. *JAMA* 1985;254:2790–2792.

Podrid P, Ganz L. *Approach to the Diagnosis and Treatment of Wide QRS Complex Tachycardias: Up to Date.* Up To Date, Inc., Waltham, MA;2008.

Rosenbaum MB. Classification of ventricular extrasystoles according to form. *J Electrocardiol* 1969;2:289–297.

Stewart RB, Bardy GH, Greene HL. Wide complex tachycardia: misdiagnosis and outcome after emergency therapy. *Ann Intern Med* 1986;104(6):766–771.
Swanick EJ, LaCamera F, Marriott HJL. Morphological features of right ventricular ectopic beats. *Am J Cardiol* 1972;30:888–891.
Tchou P, Young P, Mahmud R, et al. Useful clinical criteria for the diagnosis of ventricular tachycardia. *Am J Med* 1988;84:53–56.
Wellens HJ. Electrophysiology: ventricular tachycardia: diagnosis of broad QRS complex tachycardia. *Heart* 2001;86:579–585.
Wellens HJ, Bar FW, Lie KI. The value of the electrocardiogram in the differential diagnosis of a tachycardia with a widened QRS complex. *Am J Med* 1978;64:27–33.

Chapter 15

Chinitz JS, Gerstenfeld EP, Marchlinkski FE, Callans DJ. Atrial fibrillation is common after ablation of isolated atrial flutter during long-term follow-up. *Heart Rhythm* 2007;4:1029–1033.
Davies AJ, Kenny RA. Frequency of neurologic complications following carotid sinus massage. *Am J Cardiol* 1998;81(10):1256–1257.
Feinberg WM, Cornell ES, Nightingale SD, et al. Relationship between prothrombin activation fragment F1.2 and international normalized ratio in patients with atrial fibrillation: Stroke Prevention in Atrial Fibrillation Investigators. *Stroke* 1997;28:1101–1106.
Fuster V, Ryden LE, Cannom DS, et al. ACC/AHA/ESC 2006 guidelines for the management of patients with atrial fibrillation. *J Am Coll Cardiol* 2006;48(4):149–246.
Glatter KA. Electrophysiologic effects of adenosine in patients with supraventricular tachycardia. *Circulation* 1999;99(8):1034–1040.
Hsieh MH, Chen SA. Catheter ablation of focal AT. In: Zipes DP, Haissaguerre M, eds. *Catheter Ablation of Arrhythmias.* Armonk, NY: Futura Publishing Co.; 2002:185–204.
Josephson ME, Wellens HJ. Differential diagnosis of supraventricular tachycardia. *Cardiol Clin* 1990;8(3).
Kastor JA. Multifocal atrial tachycardia. *N Engl J Med* 1990;322(24): 1713–1717.
Mirvis DM, Goldberger AL. Evaluation of the patient: electrocardiography. In: Libby P, Bonow RO, Zipes, DP, et al., ed. *Braunwald's Heart Disease*, 8th ed. Philadelphia: Saunders Elsevier; 2008:156–157.
Orejarena LA, Vidaillet H, Jr, DeStefano F, et al. Paroxysmal supraventricular tachycardia in the general population. *J Am Coll Cardiol* 1998;31:150–157.

Strickberger SA. Adenosine-induced atrial arrhythmia: a prospective analysis. *Ann Intern Med* 1997;127(6):417–422.

The AFFIRM Investigators. A comparison of rate control and rhythm control in patients with atrial fibrillation. *N Engl J Med* 2002;347 (23):1825–1833.

Trohman RG. Supraventricular tachycardia: implications for the intensivist. *Crit Care Med* 2000;28(10):N129.

Chapter 16

American Diabetes Association. Standards of medical care in diabetes—2007. *Diabetes Care* 2007;30:S4–S41.

Antithrombotic Trialists' Collaboration. Collaborative meta-analysis of randomised trials of antiplatelet therapy for prevention of death, myocardial infarction, and stroke in high-risk patients. *BMJ* 2002;324: 71–86. Erratum in *BMJ* 2002;324:141.

Bhatt DL, Fox KA, Hacke W, et al., for the CHARISMA Investigators. Clopidogrel and aspirin versus aspirin alone for the prevention of atherothrombotic events. *N Engl J Med* 2006;354:1706–1717.

CAPRIE Steering Committee. A randomized, blinded, trial of clopidogrel versus aspirin in patients at risk of ischemic events (CAPRIE). *Lancet* 1996;348:1329–1339.

Chi YW, Jaff MR. Optimal risk factor modification and medical management of the patient with peripheral arterial disease. *Catheterization Cardiovasc Intervent* 2008;71:475–489.

Chobanian AV, Bakris GL, Black HR, et al. The seventh report of the Joint National Committee on Prevention, Detection, Evaluation, and Treatment of High Blood Pressure. *JAMA* 2003;289:2560–2572.

Creager MA, White CJ, Hiatt WR, et al. Atherosclerotic peripheral vascular disease symposium II, executive summary. *Circulation* 2008; 118:2811–2825.

Dawson DL, Cutler BS, Hiatt WR, et al. A comparison of cilostazol and pentoxifylline for treating intermittent claudication. *Am J Med* 2000; 109:523–530.

Executive Summary of the Third Report of The National Cholesterol Education Program (NCEP) Expert Panel on Detection, Evaluation, and Treatment of High Blood Cholesterol in Adults (Adult Treatment Panel III). *JAMA* 2001;285:2486–2497.

Grundy SM, Cleeman JI, Bairey Merz CNB, et al. Implications of recent clinical trials for the National Cholesterol Education Program Adult Treatment Panel III guidelines. *Circulation* 2004;110:227–239.

Hirsch AT, Criqui MH, Treat-Jacobson D, et al. Peripheral arterial disease detection, awareness, and treatment in primary care. *JAMA* 2001;286: 1317–1324.

Hirsh AT, Haskal ZJ, Hertzer NR, et al. ACC/AHA 2005 Practice Guidelines for the management of patients with peripheral arterial disease (lower extremity, renal, mesenteric, and abdominal aortic): a collaborative report from the American Association for Vascular Surgery/Society for Vascular Surgery, Society for Cardiovascular Angiography and Interventions, Society for Vascular Medicine and Biology, Society of Interventional Radiology, and the ACC/AHA Task Force on Practice Guidelines (Writing Committee to Develop Guidelines for the Management of Patients With Peripheral Arterial Disease): endorsed by the American Association of Cardiovascular and Pulmonary Rehabilitation; National Heart, Lung, and Blood Institute; Society for Vascular Nursing; TransAtlantic Inter-Society Consensus; and Vascular Disease Foundation. *Circulation* 2006;113:e463–e654.

Norgren L, Hiatt WR, Dormandy JA, et al., for the TASC II Working Group. Inter-society Consensus for the Management of Peripheral Arterial Disease (TASC II). *Eur J Vasc Endovasc Surg* 2007;33:S1–S70.

Selvin E, Erlinger TP. Prevalence of and risk factors for peripheral arterial disease in the United States: results from the National Health and Nutrition Examination Survey, 1999–2000. *Circulation* 2004;110(6):738–743.

The Heart Outcomes Prevention Evaluation Study Investigators. Effects of an angiotensin-converting enzyme inhibitor, ramipril, on cardiovascular events in high-risk patients. *N Engl J Med* 2000;342:145–153.

Thompson PD, Zimet R, Forbes WP, Zhang P. Meta-analysis of results from eight randomized, placebo-controlled trials on the effect of cilostazol on patients with intermittent claudication. *Am J Cardiol* 2002;90:1314–1319.

Watson L, Ellis B, Leng GC. Exercise for intermittent claudication. *The Cochrane Library* 2008;4.

Chapter 17

Antithrombotic Trialists Collaboration. Collaborative meta analysis of randomized trials of antiplatelet therapy for prevention of death, myocardial infarction, and stroke in high risk patients. *BMJ* 2002;324:71–86.

Barnhorst DA, Barner HB. Prevalence of congenitally absent pedal pulses. *N Engl J Med* 1968;278:264–265.

Beebe HG, Dawson DL, Cutler BS, et al. A new pharmacological treatment for intermittent claudication: results of a randomized, multicenter trial. *Arch Intern Med* 1999;159:2041–2050.

Beks PJ, Mackaay AJ, de Neeling JN, et al. Peripheral arterial disease in relation to glycemic level in an elderly Caucasian population: the Hoorn Study. *Diabetologia* 1995;38:86–96.

Belch JJ, Bell PR, Creissen D, et al. Randomized, double blind, placebo controlled study evaluatiing the efficacy and safety of AS-013, a prostaglandin E1 prodrug, in patients with intermittent claudication. *Circulation* 1997;95:2298–2302.

Belch J, MacCuish A, Campbell I, et al. The prevention of progression of arterial disease and diabetes (POPADAD) trial: factorial randomized placebo controlled trial of aspirin and antioxidants in patients with diabetes and asymptomatic peripheral arterial disease. *BMJ* 2008; 337: a1840–a1850.

Boger RH, Bode-Boger SM, Thiele W, et al. Restoring vascular nitric oxide formation by L-arginine improves the symptoms of intermitten claudication in patients wit peripheral arterial occlusive disease. *J Am Coll Cardiol* 1998;32:1336–1344.

Bowers BL, Valentine RJ, Myers SI, et al. The natural history of patients with claudication with toe pressures of 40 mm Hg or less. *J Vasc Surg* 1993;18:506–511.

Brevetti G, Chiarello M, Ferulano G, et al. Increases in walking distance in patients with peripheral vascular disease treated with L-carnitine: a double blind, cross over study. *Circulation* 1988;77:767–773.

Brooks B, Dean R, Patel S, et al. TBI or not TBI: that is the question. Is it better to measure toe pressure than ankle pressure in diabetic patients? *Diabet Med* 2001;18:528–532.

Cacoub PP, Abola MTB, Baumgartner I, et al. on behalf of the REACH Registry Investigators. Cardiovascular risk factor control and outcomes in peripheral artery disease patients in the Reduction of Atherothrombosis for Continued Health (REACH) Registry. *Atherosclerosis* 2008, downloaded from www.elsevier.com.

CAPRIE Steering Committee, A randomized, blinded, trial of clopidogrel versus aspirin in patients at risk of ischemic events (CAPRIE). CAPRIE steering Committee. *Lancet* 1996;348:1329–1339.

Clifford PC, Davies PW, Hayne JA, et al. Intermittent claudication: is a supervised exercise class worth while? *Br Med J* 1980;280:1503–1505.

Coffman JD. Intermittent claudication: be conservative. *N Engl J Med* 1991;325:577–578.

Cohn JN, Goldstein SO, Greenberg BH, et al. A dose dependent increase in mortality with vesnarinone among patients with severe heart failure. Vesnarinone Trial Investigators. *N Engl J Med* 1998;339:1810–1816.

Collins TC, Petersen NJ, Suarez-Almazor M, et al. The prevalence of peripheral arterial disease in a racially diverse in a racially diverse population. *Arch Intern Med* 2003;163:1469–1474.

Collaborative overview of randomized trials of antiplatelet therapy I: prevention of death, myocardial infarction, and stroke by prolonged antiplatelet therapy in various categories of patients. Antiplatelet Trialists Collaborative. *BMJ* 1994;308:81–106.

Coordinating Committee of the National Cholesterol Education Program. Implications of recent clinical trials for the National Cholesterol Education Program Adult Treatment Panel III Guidelines. *Atherioscler Thromb Vasc Biol* 2004;24:e149–161.

Criqui MH, Fronek A, Klauber MR, Barrett-Connor E, Gabriel S. The sensitivity, specificity, and predictive value of traditional clinical evaluation of peripheral arterial disease: results from non-invasive testing in a defined population. *Circulation* 1985;71:516–522.

Criqui MH, Langer RD, Fronek A, et al. Mortality over a period of 10 yearrs in patients with peripheral arterial disease. *N Engl J Med* 1992; 326:381–386.

Criqui MH, Denenberg JO, Langer RD, et al. The epidemiology of peripheral arterial disease: importance of identifying the population at risk. *Vasc Med* 1997;2:221–226.

Criqui MH, Denenberg JO, Langer RD, et al. The epidemiology of peripheral arterial disease: Importance of identifying the population of risk. *Vasc Med* 1997;2:221–226.

Dawson DL, Cutler BS, Meissner MH, et al. Cilostazol has beneficial effects in treatment of intermittent cluaudication: results from a multicenter, randomized, prospective, double blind trial. *Circulation* 1998;98:678–686.

Dawson DL, Cutler BS, Hiatt WR, et al. A comparison of cilostazol and pentoxifylline for treating intermittent claudication. *Am J Med* 2000; 109:523–530.

Dawson DL, Zheng Q, Worthy SA, et al. Failure of pentoxifylline or cilostazol to improve blood and plasma viscosity, fibrinogern, and erythrocytes defrmability in claudication. *Angiology* 2002;53:509–520.

Degischer S, Labs KH, Hochstrasser J, et al. Physical training for intermittent claudication: a comparison of structured rehabilitation versus home-based training. *Vasc Med* 2002;7:109–115.

de Vries SO, Hunink MG, Polak JF. Summary receiver operating characteristic curves as a technique for meta analysis of the diagnostic performance of duplex ultrasonography in peripheral arterial disease. *Acad Radiol* 1996;3:361–369.

Donohoe ME, Fletton JA, Hook A, et al improving foot care for people with diabetes mellitus: a randomized controlled trial of an integrated care approach. *Diabet Med* 2000;17:581–587.

Dormandy JA, Murray GD. The fate of the claudicant: a prospective study of 1969 claudicants. *Eur J Vasc Surg* 1991;5:131–133.

Dormandy JA, Rutherford RB. For the TransAtlantic Inter-Society Consensus (TASC) Working Group. Management of peripheral arterial disease (PAD). *J Vasc Surg* 2000;31(Suppl 1, Pt 2): S1–S296.

Dormandy JA, Rutherford RB, for the TransAtlantic Inter-Society Consensus (TASC) Working Group. Management of peripheral arterial disease (PAD). *Int Angiol* 2000;19(Suppl 1):1–310.

Effect of intensive diabetes management on macrovascular events and risk factors in the Diabetes Control and Complications Trial. *Am J Cardiol* 1995;75:894–903.

Elhadd TA, Robb R, Jung RT, Stonebridge PA, Belch JJF. Pilot study of prevalence of asymptomatic peripheral arterial occlusive disease in patients with diabetes attending a hospital clinic. *Practical Diabetes Int* 1999;16:163–166.

Faulkner KW, House AK, Cstleden WM. The effect of cessation of smoking on the accumulative survival rates of patients with symptomatic peripheral vascular disease. *Med J Aust* 1983;1:217–219.

Franzini E, Sellak H, Babin-Chevaye C, et al. Effects of pentoxyifylline on the adherence of polymorphonuclear neurtophils to oxidant stimulated human endothelial cells: involvement of cyclic AMP. *J Cardiovasc Pharmacol* 1995;25 (Suppl 2):S92–S95.

Gardner AW, Katzel LI, Sorkin JD, et al. Exercise rehabilitation improves functional outcomes and peripheral circulation in patients with intermittent claudication: a randomized controlled trial. *J Am Geriatr Soc* 2001;49:755–762.

Gardner AW, Katzel LI, Sorkin JD, et al. Effects of long-term exercise rehabilitation on claudication distances in patients with peripheral arterial disease: a randomized controlled trial. *J Cardiopulm Rehabil* 2002;22:192–198.

Gardner AW, Poehlman ET. Exercise rehabilitation programs for the treatment of claudication pain: a meta-analysis. *JAMA* 1995;274:975–980.

Gardner AW, Katzel LI, Sorkin JD, et al. Exercise rehabilitation improves functional outcomes and peripheral circulation in patients with intermittent claudication: a randomized controlled trial. *J Am Geriatr Soc* 2001;49:755–762.

Gibellini R, Fanello M, Bardile AF, et al. Exercise training in intermittent claudication. *Int Angiol* 2000;19:8–13.

Girolami B, Bernardi E, Prins MH, et al. Treatment of intermittent claudication with physical training, smoking cessation, pentoxifylline, or nafronyl: a meta analysis. *Arch Intern Med* 1999;159:337–345.

Giswold ME, Landry GJ, Sexton GJ, et al. Modifiable patient factors are associated with reverse vein graft occlusion in the era of duplex scan surveillance. *J Vasc Surg* 2003;37:47–53.

Grundy SM, Cleeman JI, Bairey-Merz CN, et al. Implications of recent clinical trials for the National Cholesterol Education Program Adult Treatment Panel III Guidelines. *Circulation* 2004;110:227–239.

Guldager B, Jelnes R, Jorgensen SJ, et al. EDTA treatment of intermittent claudication: a double blind, placebo controlled study. *J Intern Med* 1992;231:261–267.

Heart Protection Study Collaborative Group. MRC/BHF Heart Protection Study of cholesterol lowering with simvastatin in 20,536 high-risk individuals: a randomized placebo-controlled trial. *Lancet* 2002; 360:7–22.

Hiatt WR, Hoag S, Hamman RF. Effect of diagnostic criteria on the prevalence of peripheral arterial disease. The San Luis Valley Diabetes Study. *Circulation* 1995;91:1472–1479.

Hiatt WR, Nawz D, Regensteiner JG, et al. The evaluation of exercise performance in patients with peripheral vascular disease. *J Cardiopulm Rehabil* 1988;8:525–532.

Hirsch AT, Criqui MH, Treat-Jacobson D, et al Peripheral arterial disease detection, awareness, and treatment in primary care. *JAMA* 2001;286: 1317–1324.

Hirsch AT, Ekers MA. A comprehensive vascular medical therapeutic approach to peripheral arterial disease: the foundation of effective vascular rehabilitation. In Fahey VA (ed). Vascular Nursing, 3rd ed. Philadelphia: WB Saunders;1999:188–211.

Hirsch AT, Halverson SL, Trat-Jacobson D, et al. The Minnesota Regional Peripheral Arterial Disease Screening Program: toward a definition of community standards of care. *Vasc Med* 2001;6:87–96.

Hirsch AT, Hiatt WR, PARTNERS Steering Committee. PAD awareness, risk, and treatment: new resources for survival-The USA PARTNERS Program. *Vas Med* 2001;6(3 Suppl):9–12.

Hirsch AT, Haskal ZJ, Hertzer NR, et al. ACC/AHA 2005 Practice Guidelines for the Management of Patients with Peripheral Arterial Disease (lower extremity, renal, mesenteric, and abdominal aorta). *Circulation* 2006;1131:1474–1547. Source: American Heart Associates, Inc.

Hood SC, Moher D, Barber GG. Mnagement of intermittent claudication with pentoxifylline: meta analysis of randomized controlled trials. *Can Med Assoc J* 1996;155:1053–1059.

Hooi JD, Stoffers HE, Kester AD, et al. Risk factors and cardiovascular diseases associated with asymptomatic peripheral arterial occlusive disease. The Limburg PAOD Study. Peripheral Arterial Occlusive Disease. *Scand J Prim Health Care* 1998;16:177–182.

Howell MA, Colgan MP, Seeger RW, et al. Relationship of severity of lower limb peripheral vascular disease to mortality and morbidity: a six year follow up study. *J Vasc Surg* 1989;9:691–696.

Igawa T, Tani T, Chijiwa T, et al. Potentiation of anti-platelet aggregating activity of cilostazol with vascular endothelial cells. *Thromb Res* 1990;57:617–623.

Ingolfsson IO, Sigurdsson G, Sigvaldason H, et al. A marked decline in the prevalence and incidence of intermittent claudication in Icelandic men 1968–1986: A strong relationship to smoking and serum cholesterol-The Reykjavik Study. *J Clin Epidemiol* 1994;47:1237–1243.

Joint National Committee on Prevention, Detection, Evaluation, and Treatment of High Blood Pressure. National Heart, Lung, and Blood Institute. Seventh report of the Joint National Committee on Prevention, Detection, Evaluation, and Treatment of High Blood Pressure. *Hypertension* 2003;42:1206–1252.

Jonason T, Bergstrom R. Cessation of smoking in patients with intermittent claudication: effects on the risk of peripheral vascular complications, myocardial infarction and mortality. *Acta Med Scand* 1987;221:253–260.

Kallio M, Forsblom C, Groop PH, et al. Development of new peripheral arterial occlusive disease in patients with type 2 diabetes during a mean follow-up of 11 years. *Diabetes Care* 2003;26:1241–1245.

Kannel WB, McGee DL. Update on some epidemiology features of intermittent claudication: the Framingham Study. *J Am Geriatr Soc* 1985; 33:13–18.

Katsilambros NL, Tsapogas PC, Arvanitis MP, et al. Risk factors for lower extremity arterial disease in non-insulin dependent diabetic persons. *Diabet Med* 1996;13:243–246.

Khilnani NM, Winchester PA, Prince MR, et al. Peripheral vascular disease: combined 3D bolus chase and dynamic 2D MR angiography compared with xray angiography for treatment planning. *Radiology* 2002;224:63–74.

Laine C, Goldman D. In the Clinic: Peripheral Arterial Disease. *Ann Intern Med* 2007;March;ITC3:2–14.

Lassila R, Lepantalo M. Cigarette smoking and the outcome after lower limb arterial surgery. *Acta Chir Scand* 1988;154:635–640.

Leng GC, Fowler B, Ernst E. Exercise for intermittent claudication. Cochrane Database Syst Rev 2000;CD000990.

Leng GC, Lee AJ, Fowkes FG, et al. Incidence, natural history and cardiovascular events in symptomatic and asymptomatic peripheral arterial disease in the general population. *Int J Epidemiol* 1996;25: 1172–1181.

Lowering blood homocysteine with folic acid based supplements: meta-analysis of randomized trials. Homocysteine Lowering Trialists Collaborative. *BMJ* 1998;316:894–898.

McPhail IR, Spitell PC, Weston SA, et al. Intermittent claudication: an objective office based assessment. *J Am Coll Cardiol* 2001;37: 1381–1384.

Mohler ER. Peripheral arterial disease: identification and implications. *Arch Intern Med* 2003;163:2306–2314.Money SR, Herd JA, Issacsohn JL, et al. Effect of cilostazol on walking distances in patients with intermittent claudication caused by peripheral vascular disease. *J Vas Surg* 1998;27:267–274.

Money SR, Herd JA, Issacsohn JL, et al. Effect of cilostazol on walking distances in patients with intermittent claudication caused by peripheral vascular disease. *J Vas Surg* 1998;27:267–274.

Most RS, Sinnock P. The epidemiology of lower extremity amputations in diabetic individuals. *Diabetes Care* 1983;6:87–91.

Muller-Buhl U, Wiesemann A, Oser B, Kirchberger I, Strecker EP. Correlation of hemodynamic and functional variables with the angiographic extend to peripheral occlusive disease. *Vasc Med* 1999;4:247–251.

Murabito JM, D'Agostino RB, Silbershatz H, et al. Intermittent claudication: a risk profile from the Framingham Heart Study. *Circulation* 1997;96:44–49.

Murabito JM, Evans JC, Nieto K, et al. Prevalence and clinical correlates of peripheral arterial disease in the Framingham Offspring Study. *Am Heart J* 2002;143:961–965.

Nelemans PJ, Leiner T, de Vet HC, et al. Peripheral arterial disease: meta-analysis of the diagnostic performance of MR agiography. *Radiology* 2000;217:105–114.

Newman AB, Siscovick DS, Manolio TA, et al. Ankle arm index as a marker of atherosclerosis in the Cardiovascular Health Study. Cardiovascular Heart Study (CHS) Collaborative Research Group. *Circulation* 1993; 88:837–845.

Novo S, Avellone G, DiGarbo V, et al. Prevalence of risk factors in patients with peripheral arterial disease: a clinical and epidemiological evaluation. *Int Angiol* 1992;11:218–229.

Otsuki M, Saito H, Xu X, et al. Cilostazol represses vascular cell adhesion molecule-1 gener transcription via inhibiting NF-kappaB binding to its recognition sequence. *Atherosclerosis* 2001;158:121–128.

Ouriel K, McDonnell AE, Metz CE, Zarins CK. Critical evaluation of stress testing in the diagnosis of peripheral vascular disease. *Surgery* 1982;91:686–693.

Packer M, Carver JR, Rodeheffer RJ, et al Effect of oral milrinone on mortality in severe chronic heart failure. The PROMISE Study Research Group. *N Engl J Med* 1991;325:1468–1475.

Patterson RB, Pinto B, Marcus B, et al. Value of a supervised exercise program for the therapy of arterial claudication. *J Vasc Surg* 1997;25: 312–318.

Pittler MH, Ernst E. Ginkgo biloba extract for the treatment of intermittent claudication: a meta analysis of randomized trials. *Am J Med* 2000;108:276–281.

Pradhan AD, Manson JE, Rossouw JE, et al. Inflammatory biomarkers, hormone replacement therapy, and incident coronary heart disease: prospective analysis from the Women's Health Initiative Observational Study. *JAMA* 2002;288:980–987.

Price JF, Mowbray PI, Lee AJ, et al. Relationship between smoking and cardiovascular risk factors in the development of peripheral arterial disease and coronary artery disease: Edinburgh Artery Study. *Eur Heart J* 1999;20:344–353.

Psaty BM, Smith NL, Siscovick DS, et al. Health outcomes associated with anti-hypertensive therapies used as first line agents: a systemic review and meta-analysis. *JAMA* 1997;277:739–745.

Radack K, Deck C. Beta-adrenergic blocker therapy does not worsen intermittent claudication in subjects with peripheral arterial disease: a meta-analysis of randomized controlled trials. *Arch Intern Med* 1991; 151:1769–1776.

Radack K, Wyderski RJ. Conservative management of intermittent claudication. *Ann Intern Med* 1990;113:135–146.

Ramsey DE, Manke DA, Sumner DS. Toe blood pressure: a valuable adjunct to ankle pressure measurement of assessing peripheral arterial disease. *J Cardiovasc Surg (Torino)* 1983;24:43–48.

Rao KM, Simel DL, Cohen HJ, et al. Effects of pentoxifylline administration on blood viscosity and leukocyte cytoskeletal function in patients with intermittent claudiction. *J Lab Clin Med* 1990;115:738–744.

Regensteiner JG. Exercise in the treatment of claudication: assessment and treatment of functional impairment. *Vasc Med* 1997;2:238–242.

Regensteiner JG, Meyer TJ, Krupski WC, et al. Hospital vs home based exercise rehabilitation for patients with peripheral arterial occlusive disease. *Angiology* 1997;48:291–300.

Regensteiner JG, Ware JE Jr, McCarthy WJ, et al. Effect of cilostazol on treadmill walking, community based walking ability, and health related quality of life in patients with intermittent claudication due to peripheral arterial disease: meta analysis of six randomized controlled trials. *J Am Geriatr Soc* 2002;50:1939–1946.

Ridker PM, Cushman M, Stampfer MJ, et al. Plasma concentration of C-reactive protein and risk of developing peripheral vascular disease. *Circulation* 1998;97:425–428.

Rieker O, Duber C, Schmiedt W, et al. Prospective comparison of CT angiography of the legs with intraarterial digital subtraction angiography. *Am J Roentgenol* 1996;166:269–276.

Roderick PJ, Wilkes HC, Meade TW. The gastrointestinal toxicity of aspirin: an overview of randomized controlled trials. *Br J Clin Pharmacol* 1993;35:219–226.

Rubin GD, Schmidt AJ, Logan LJ, et al. Multi-detector row CT angiography of lower extremity arterial inflow and runoff: initial experience. *Radiology* 2001;221:146–158.

Sanderson KJ, van Rij AM, Wade CR, et al. Lipid peroxidation of circulating low density lipoproteins with age, smoking in peripheral vascular disease. *Atherosclerosis* 1995;118:45–51.

Savage P, Ricci MA, Lynn M, et al. Effects of home versus supervised exercise for patients with intermittent claudication. *J Cardiopulm Rehabil* 2001;21:152–157.

Schratzberger P, Dunzendorfer S, Reinisch N, et al. Mediator dependent effects of pentoxyifilline on endothelium for transmigration of neutrophils. *Immunopharmacology* 1999;41:65–75.

Selvin E, Erlinger TP. Prevalence of and risk factors for peripheral arterial disease in the United States: results from the National Health and Nutruition Examination Survey 1999–2000. *Circulation* 2004;110: 738–743.

Steg PG, Bhatt DL, Wilson PW, et al. One year cardiovascular event rates in outpatients with atherothrombosis. *JAMA* 2007;297:1197–1206.

Strandness DE, Jr, Dalman RL, Panian S, et al. Effect of cilostazol in patiens with intermittent claudicatio: a randomized, double blind, placebo controlled study. *Vasc Endovascular Surg* 2002;36:83–91.

Strano A, Davi G, Avellone G, et al. Double blind crossover study of the clinical efficacy and the hemorheological effects of pentoxyifylline in patients with occlusive arterial disease of the lower limbs. *Angiology* 1984;35:459–466.

Strong JP, Malcom GT, McMahan CA, et al. Prevalence and extent of atherosclerosis in adolescents and young adults: implications for prevention from the pathobiological determinants of atherosclerosis in youth study. *JAMA* 1999;281:727–735.

Takahashi S, Oida K, Fujiwara R, et al. Effect of cilostazol, a cylic AMP phosphodiesterase inhibitor, on the proliferation of rat aortic smooth muscle cells in culture. *J Cardiovasc Pharmacol* 1992;20:900–906.

Takahashi S, Fukuhara A, Kobayashi T, et al. Impact of cilostazol on restenosis after percutaneous coronary balloon angioplasty. *Circulation* 1999;100:21–26.

UK Prospective Diabetes Study (UKPDS) Group. Intensive blood-glucose control with sulfonylureas or insulin compared with conventional treatment and risk of complications in patients with type 2 diabetes (UKPDS 33). *Lancet* 1998;352:837–853.

van der Heijden FH, Legemate DA, van Leeuwen MS, et al. Value of duplex scanning in the selection of patients for percutaneous transluminal angioplasty. *Eur J Vasc Surg* 1993;7:71–76.

van Rij AM, Solomon C, Packer SG, et al. Chelation therapy for intermittent claudication: a double blind, randomized, controlled trial. *Circulation* 1994;90:1194–1199.

Visser K, Hunink MG. Peripheral arterial disease: gadolinium enhanced MR angiography versus color-guided duplex US: a meta-analysis. *Radiology* 2000;216:67–77.

Weitz JI, Byrne J, Clagett GP, et al. Diagnosis and treatment of chronic arterial insufficiency of the lower extremities: a critical review. *Circulation* 1996;94:3026–3049.

White C. Intermittent claudication. *N Engl J Med* 2007;356:1241–1250.

Willigendael EM, Teijink JA, Bartelink ML, et al. Smoking and the patency of lower extremity bypass grafts: a meta analysis. *J Vasc Surg* 2005;42:67–74.

Woo SK, Kang WK, Kwon KI. Pharmacokinetic and pharmacodynamic modelingof the anitplatelet and cardiovascular effects of cilostazol in healthy humans. *Clin Pharmacol Ther* 2002;71:246–252.

Yusuf S, Sleight P, Pogue J, et al. Effects of an angiotensin converting enzyme inhibitor, ramipril, on cardiovascular events in high risk patients. The Heart Outcomes Prevention Evaluation Study Investigators. *N Engl J Med* 2000;342:748.

Chapter 18

Begg C, Cho M, Eastwood S, et al. Improving the quality of reporting of randomized trials: the CONSORT statement. *JAMA* 1996;276:637–639.

Harrington RA, Califf RM, Hodgson PK, et al. Careers in cardiovascular research. *Circulation* 2009;119:2945–2950.

Hopewell S, Clarke M, Moher D, et al., and the CONSORT Group. CONSORT for reporting randomized trials in journal and conference abstracts. Lancet online, at www.thelancet.com; 2008; vol. 371.

Kendall JM. Designing a research project: randomized controlled trials and their principles. *Emerg Med J* 2003;20:164–168.

Medpage Today Guide to Biostatistics. Retrieved June 23, 2009, from http://www.medpagetoday.com/Medpage-Guide-to-Biostatistics.pdf

Moher D, Schulz KF, Altman DG, for the CONSORT Group. The CONSORT Statement: Revised recommendations for improving the quality of reports of parallel-group randomized trials. *Ann Intern Med* 2001;134:657–662.

Sibbald B, Roland M. Understanding controlled trials: Why are randomized controlled trials important. *BMJ* 1998;316:201.

Index

Note: Italicized page locators indicate a figure/photo; tables are noted with a *t*.

B

C

E

G

H

I

J

K

L

M

Q

U

V

www.ingramcontent.com/pod-product-compliance
Ingram Content Group UK Ltd.
Pitfield, Milton Keynes, MK11 3LW, UK
UKHW020117290926
15471UKWH00003B/191